2/09

The Essential Guide to Psychiatric Drugs

REVISED AND UPDATED

Also by Jack M. Gorman, M.D.

The Essential Guide to Mental Health

The Essential Guide to
Psychiatric Drugs

· REVISED AND UPDATED FOURTH EDITION ·

JACK M. GORMAN, M.D.

ST. MARTIN'S GRIFFIN ☙ NEW YORK

Medical Caution

The information in this book is intended to guide potential patients and their families but not to substitute for the advice and directions of your personal physician. Do not take any medications or make changes in the way you take current medications without first consulting your doctor. Also, report all side effects or reactions you have to a medication to your doctor.

www.stmartins.com

Library of Congress Cataloging-in-Publication Data

Gorman, Jack M.
   The essential guide to psychiatric drugs / Jack M. Gorman.—Rev. and updated, 4th ed.
      p.   cm.
   Includes index.
   ISBN-13: 978-0-312-36879-1
   ISBN-10: 0-312-36879-8
   1. Psychotropic drugs—Popular works.   I. Title.

RM315.G67   2007
615'.788—dc22   2007032207

Fourth Edition: December 2007

10 9 8 7 6 5 4 3 2 1

Contents

Tables

Who Should Use This Book and How Should It Be Used?

Shelves in libraries and bookstores across the United States are loaded with psychological self-help books and home health care manuals. Daily newspapers regularly feature columns rendering advice on mental health interventions. Everybody seems to have access to information about health and medical treatment.

But over the years, as a practicing psychiatrist and scientist, I have been surprised by the number of patients with psychiatric problems and their families who have almost no idea what psychiatric drugs are supposed to do or why they are taking them. Many times I function as a consultant for patients who have already received psychiatric treatment, and I have found that most patients do not know if they are taking the right medication or even if they should be on medication at all. Nor do they recognize the side effects caused by the drugs.

I find that most patients and their families crave information about the reasons for taking psychiatric drugs, the benefits the drugs produce, and the risks the drugs entail. And they are quite able to grasp explanations that are neither condescending nor overly technical.

Despite popular myth, even very depressed or anxious patients can absorb great amounts of information about their illness and treatment options. I feel that all patients have a right and a responsibility to know why they are taking a drug, whether other options are available, and what the risks are. A fully informed patient is usually a doctor's ally, not an enemy.

This book is *not* intended to substitute for a personal psychiatrist, who will prescribe medication and monitor its effects. Because people are so different from each other and psychiatric drugs so complex, it is important that you ask your doctor about the information you read here, as not everything I have written could possibly fit every situation.

This guide will, however, help the person with a psychiatric problem. It will also help friends, relatives, and spouses of people who suffer from psychiatric illness to understand when drug therapy should be considered for their loved ones and which drug should be used, how long should treatment last, and what side effects should be expected.

It is important to stress that this book is not an attempt to "sell" psychiatric drugs. I hope I have clearly outlined the many situations in which drugs are *not* the best choice in treatment of a psychiatric problem and situations in which drugs may even be harmful.

Many books cover a specific psychiatric syndrome, like depression or panic disorder or obsessive-compulsive disorder, and describe the drugs useful in that particular condition. This guide is one of the few that include all psychiatric drugs. There are two ways to use the book:

First, it can be used as a reference book that provides information about individual psychiatric drugs. The middle section comprises separate descriptions of most available psychiatric drugs. You can simply look up the drug in which you are interested and read about its use, correct dose, special properties, and side effects. If you use the book in this way, it is not necessary to read all of the chapters to get the information you need about a particular drug.

Second, the book can be used to obtain a better general understanding of when and how to use psychiatric drugs. Part I tells you how to know if you should take medication for an emotional problem, how long to take the drug, how to stop use of psychiatric drugs, and how to choose the right doctor. Part III provides information on special topics concerning psychiatric drugs, for example, drugs given to the elderly, drugs used during pregnancy, and drugs that affect weight and sexual function.

The Essential Guide to Psychiatric Drugs is intended for three main groups: people who suffer from psychiatric problems, family members and friends of patients with psychiatric illnesses, and nonpsychiatric therapists and physicians who have clients and patients with emotional disorders. Although medical students, psychiatric residents, and even psychiatrists may find the book useful, it is deliberately written in a nontechnical manner. Essentially, I imagined that I was talking to a new patient and his or her relatives in my consulting room. This book should sound as if you had asked your doctor a question and he or she is taking the time to give you an answer you can understand.

A word about the cost of psychiatric drugs. In this, the fourth edition of

The Essential Guide to Psychiatric Drugs, I have eliminated estimated prices for each medication. Since the last edition, in 1977, this information has become widely available on the Internet and readers can go quickly to such sites as www.drugstore.com and look up prices for almost any medication in brand and generic forms, by strength of the tablets, and by quantity of pills. There are several important things to remember when doing this. First, the prices of drugs vary greatly from one region of the country to another, from one drugstore to the next, from one Internet source to the next, and especially by whether the medication is ordered in its generic or brand-name form. More will be said on this distinction in a later chapter, but generic forms of a drug, when available, usually cost a fraction of the cost of the brand-name form and with very rare exceptions are every bit as effective and safe. Nowadays, many people pay for their medications with health insurance and many health insurance plans have rules about which drugs they cover. Most of these plans insist on generic drugs unless there is a specific medical reason (which there usually isn't) that a brand-name drug is necessary. All of this so complicates giving prices for drugs that I offer the following advice instead: Consult the Internet to compare prices, shop around, try to use generic drugs whenever possible, and ask your physician to help you get the most value.

The case histories provided are of course fictional to protect the identities of my patients. They represent composites of actual cases and hence may be taken as accurate examples of common psychiatric problems.

Both generic and brand names are used throughout the book. Sometimes, brand names are so commonly used that it would be confusing to neglect them. The first letter of a brand name is always capitalized.

It is estimated that one out of every two Americans may at some point in his or her life suffer from a psychiatric problem, but only a very small number of these people will receive treatment. This book will help you decide if drug treatment might help you, or someone you care about, combat mental illness.

Acknowledgments

In my career as a doctor and scientist, many important and influential figures have shaped how I view my patients and my work. I have been fortunate to be guided by some truly outstanding mentors. Among these I especially acknowledge Dr. Donald F. Klein, the dean of American psychopharmacology; Dr. Roger MacKinnon, who teaches young psychiatrists the art of interviewing patients in the most elegant way possible; my father-in-law, Dr. Howard I. Kantor, one of the most caring physicians I have had the privilege to know; and Dr. Herbert Pardes, whose dedication to finding new treatments for psychiatric illness is an inspiration to all psychiatrists.

I also want to thank Drs. Stuart Yudofsky, Michael Sheehy, the late Fred Quitkin, Alexander Glassman, Robert Gould, Donald Kornfeld, Charles Nemeroff, Martin Keller, Steven Roose, Dwight Evans, Alan Schatzberg, Ned Kalin, David Dunner, Joseph LeDoux, Eric Kandel, Emanuel Landau, Stan Arkow, Cindy Aaronson, Robert Weil, Jerry Glicklich, David Leibow, Bruce and Polly McCall, and Jack Hirschfeld for all they taught me.

Physicians ultimately learn most from their patients, and I thank my own patients for their patience and courage.

Special gratitude is extended to my assistant, Diane Haimeck, and my agent, Vicki Bijur.

Many people in my personal life were extremely helpful to me in writing this book. They include my parents, Kate and Elliot Gorman; my mother- and father-in-law, Gloria and Howard Kantor, and our newest relatives Steve and Sylvia Berkowitz. My dear friends David and Susan Bressman deserve more gratitude than I can possibly give in a lifetime for all of their help and support. My younger daughter, Sara, is a star in the study of English literature at my alma mater, the University of Pennsylvania. I thank her for being a constant source of support and inspiration. My older daughter, Rachel, is a medical student at the College of Physicians and Surgeons of Columbia University, also my alma mater. I marvel at the fact that she has the time and energy to be so attentive to her father, always there to cheer me up and share bits of wisdom. Her husband, Avi Berkowitz, has so many talents it is impossible to enumerate them here, but without him this revision would never have been possible. The first edition of *The Essential Guide to Psychiatric Drugs* was written so long ago that no electronic copy of the original manuscript exists. Avi, a computer and electronics genius, solved the problem, and for this, along with so many other things, I am eternally grateful. Finally, and most of all, I thank my wife, Lauren Kantor Gorman. Sometimes I think I get involved in so many projects because otherwise I would be sitting around waiting for her to come home from work. She has a busy and very successful practice as a psychiatrist in New York City and is revered by her patients. That is how I feel, too.

Introduction to the Fourth Edition

It is now 2007, only five years after I predicted I would attempt a fourth edition of *The Essential Guide to Psychiatric Drugs.* One thing that has continuously gratified me is receiving letters and e-mails from patients and family members of patients with psychiatric illnesses telling me that the book helped them. That is why I wrote it, and to paraphrase a famous piece of advice, if I have helped even one person lighten the burden of mental illness, it has all been worth it.

I should explain why ten years have passed since I attempted a revision. Of course, I have been busy with other things, but that is a poor excuse because everyone is busy. The real reason is that in the last ten years so many new psychiatric medications have been introduced and so many controversies about psychiatric drugs have emerged that I found the task daunting. Nevertheless, I decided that I owe it to myself and all the interested consumers of psychiatric drugs at least to take one more crack at it. Hence, this new edition.

One major controversy that has plagued all of medicine is the issue of the relationship between the pharmaceutical industry and both scientists who study the effectiveness of medications and doctors who prescribe them. In the United States, with very few exceptions, all new medications are discovered and developed by corporations known as drug companies. Some of them are privately held, others have stockholders. Although the pharmaceutical industry is the most heavily regulated of any industry, mainly by the U.S. Food and Drug Administration (FDA) and its European Union counterpart, it is still a business that insists on making a profit. The pharmaceutical industry has brought us remarkable new medications that save lives and cure disease, and I believe that what motivates most of the people who work in it is the desire to benefit people with illness. Nevertheless, the pharmaceutical industry generates billions of dollars in profits, and competition among companies is strong. Each company must get its new drugs approved by the FDA, show the medical profession that its drugs are better than those of its competitors, and convince doctors to prescribe the drugs it makes if it is going to remain in business.

In recent years there have been many highly publicized cases of drug companies standing accused of manipulating or hiding results from research studies in order to make it seem that an ineffective drug really works or to cover up serious side effects. Drugs like Redux (fenfluramine) for weight loss and Vioxx have been pulled off the market when serious side effects that many believe the manufacturer knew about or should have known about before marketing emerged. In the case of psychiatric medications, I will discuss in detail in the appropriate chapter controversies like whether antidepressant drugs actually increase the risk for committing suicide and whether drugs used to treat agitation in elderly people with dementia increase the risk for stroke.

Compounding the criticism of the pharmaceutical industry has been increased scrutiny of its practices for "educating" physicians. Many see the millions of dollars spent each year by drug companies to support continuing medical education for physicians as thinly veiled marketing. Many prominent physicians, called "opinion leaders" by the companies, make considerable amounts of money either directly from the companies or via continuing medical education providers. Speakers at the educational events are supposed to be impartial. Nevertheless, there is no question that pharmaceutical companies are able to manipulate the material presented to prescribing physicians. Many new regulations have been put in place recently, often voluntarily by the companies, to create firewalls between industry and speakers, but skepticism abounds that this really makes the educators who are paid either directly or indirectly by the companies feel totally free to say what they think.

So what about this book and its author? It is critical, I believe, that I disclose my own involvement with the pharmaceutical industry. Until recently, I considered myself an equal opportunity offender—I regularly consulted to pharmaceutical companies and spoke at drug company–sponsored educational events. I believe that I never said anything that I didn't truly believe at any of these events, regardless of where the money was coming from, and I do not think, as many seem to, that the pharmaceutical industry is an "evil empire" bent on hurting people in order to make profits. Nevertheless, even

the appearance of conflict of interest is compromising, and I made the decision in 2003 to forgo accepting any money from the pharmaceutical industry. Although I have no specifics in mind, I do not guarantee that at some
point later on I might once again agree to accept compensation from a drug
company in return for professional services. I hope that this will reassure
readers that what I say here is what I truly believe, unencumbered by any
company influence.

Drug Directory

The following alphabetical list covers the drugs comprehensively described in this book and the page(s) where the drug is fully explained. Brand names are printed in capital letters and generic names in lowercase letters.

DRUG NAME	PAGE DESCRIBED
paliperidone (INVEGA)	272
PAMELOR (nortriptyline)	68
PARNATE (tranylcypromine)	83
paroxetine (PAXIL, PEVIA)	101
PAXIL (paroxetine)	101
PAXIPAM (halazepam)	163
pemoline (CYLERT)	129
PERMITIL (fluphenazine)	248
perphenazine (TRILAFON)	249
PERTOFRANE (desipramine)	61
PEXEVA (paroxetine)	101
phenelzine (NARDIL)	80
pimozide (ORAP)	256
pramipexole (MIRAPEX)	132
PROLIXIN (fluphenazine)	248
propranolol (INDERAL)	180
PROSOM (estazolam)	294
PROSTEP (nicotine patch)	322
protriptyline (VIVACTIL)	74
PROVIGIL (modafanil)	131
PROZAC (fluoxetine)	95
quetiapine (SEROQUEL)	267
ramelteon (ROZEREM)	302
REMERON (mirtazapine)	122
RESTORIL (temazepam)	291
REVIA (naltrexone)	318
RISPERDAL (risperidone)	260
risperidone (RISPERDAL)	260
RITALIN (methylphenidate)	127
ROZEREM (ramelteon)	302
selegiline patch (EMSAM)	89
SERAX (oxazepam)	165
SEROQUEL (quetiapine)	267
sertraline (ZOLOFT)	97
SERZONE (nefazodone)	115
SINEQUAN (doxepin)	70
SONATA (zalepon)	297
STELAZINE (trifluoperazine)	246

DRUG NAME	PAGE DESCRIBED
STRATTERA (atomoxetine)	129
SUBOXONE (buprenorphine)	320
SUBUTEX (buprenorphine)	320
SURMONTIL (trimipramine)	72
TEGRETOL (carbamazepine)	207
temazepam (RESTORIL)	291
thioridazine (MELLARIL)	244
thiothixene (NAVANE)	251
THORAZINE (chlorpromazine)	241
TOFRANIL (imipramine)	57
TRANXENE (clorazepate)	163
tranylcypromine (PARNATE)	83
trazodone (DESYREL)	116
triazolam (HALCION)	293
trifluoperazine (STELAZINE)	246
TRILAFON (perphenazine)	249
trimipramine (SURMONTIL)	72
VALIUM (diazepam)	161
valproic acid (DEPAKENE)	205
varenicline (CHANTIX)	323
venlafaxine (EFFEXOR)	110
VISTARIL (hydroxyzine)	300
VIVACTIL (protriptyline)	74
VIVITROL (naltrexone)	318
VYVANSE (amphetamine)	126
WELLBUTRIN (bupropion)	118, 324
XANAX (alprazolam)	166
zalepon (SONATA)	297
ziprasidone (GEODON)	269
ZOLOFT (sertraline)	97
zolpidem (AMBIEN)	295
ZYBAN (bupropion)	118, 324
ZYPREXA (olanzapine)	265

Part I

ESSENTIAL INFORMATION ABOUT PSYCHIATRIC DRUGS

Chapter 1

Be an Informed Consumer!

A psychiatrist practicing in a large northeastern city recently received a phone call from a surgeon. One of the surgeon's patients, who had had his gallbladder removed two days earlier, was found by a staff nurse in tears lying in his hospital bed. The patient reluctantly told the nurse he believed he was about to die and wanted to say good-bye to his wife and children. Without another word, the nurse called the surgeon, who immediately called the psychiatrist.

"Please get my patient on an antidepressant right away," the surgeon demanded.

"Are there any medical problems that might interfere with the safe use of antidepressants?" the psychiatrist asked.

"None," the surgeon quickly answered, and went on to state with clear anxiety in his voice, "but he is very depressed, maybe suicidal, and you better give him a drug right away."

The surgeon sounded nervous, but his assessment of the situation was probably correct. At least that was the psychiatrist's initial impression after the phone call. Within an hour, the psychiatrist was at the bedside of the tearful patient, who looked healthy and robust but thoroughly despondent. Already, the psychiatrist was running through his mind the many antidepressant medications currently available. Perhaps paroxetine. No, that might cause weight gain after a few months, and it takes four weeks to work. Venlafaxine? No, that takes some time to get to a dose high enough to be effective. And so on.

In the end, this patient was never placed on antidepressant medication. As the psychiatrist reviewed the patient's chart, he overheard a nurse discussing the case. Apparently, the patient had been admitted with severe jaundice, a yellowing of the skin caused by excess amounts of bilirubin in the blood. A tumor blocking the bile duct was suspected first, ruled out, and then suspected again. Because none of the tests were definitive, a decision was made to operate on the patient to see if a tumor was compressing any part of the system that connects the gallbladder to the liver. At the time of the operation, no tumor was found, but the surgeon had felt some stones in the gallbladder he thought might be causing the problem and therefore removed the gallbladder. Two days later, the patient's jaundice resolved.

"How did he react when he was told it wasn't cancer?" the psychiatrist wondered.

"I don't know," the nurse answered. "I'm not even sure who told him that no tumor was found."

In fact, no one had told the patient that only gallstones, no tumor, had been found. In one of those breakdowns in communication that occur all too often in large hospitals today, the surgeon thought the resident was going to explain things. The resident thought it was the intern's job, but the intern was barely awake enough to remember which patient was which. And the nurses expected that one of the doctors would certainly have set the patient straight.

Thirty minutes later, the patient was sitting up in bed, smiling and complaining that he wanted dinner. It took only that long—four weeks sooner than any antidepressant could have restored his good spirits—for the psychiatrist to find out that the patient had assumed that he had cancer, that no one wanted to break the news to him, and that he would never leave the hospital. He wanted to be brave, then found himself distraught and angry at himself for being so emotional. Mental images of his bereaved wife and children were torturing him and he wondered whether his life insurance company would find out he had told a small lie fifteen years earlier on his application.

Without administering a single drug, the psychiatrist "cured" this man's "suicidal depression." Most likely, the psychiatrist did not take much credit for the lifesaving intervention. This treatment was seemingly a matter of simple common sense. Yet, without this intervention, which took a good bit of detective work, we can imagine how horrible things might have gotten for the patient.

It may seem odd to begin a book about medications used to treat psychiatric disorders by telling a story in which drugs clearly were not the right treatment. I do this to drive home one of the central points behind this explanation of psychiatric drugs: Medicine is not the answer for many situations of depression, anxiety, and even psychosis. *Talking to patients with problems is absolutely essential and sometimes is curative.* If a patient feels that a doctor has decided to start a medication to treat a psychiatric problem very quickly, without taking a detailed personal history, he or she should get another opinion before taking a single pill.

Let me tell another story that gives the opposite perspective. A sixty-year-old woman was brought by relatives to the hospital emergency room. A month earlier, the woman's husband had died after a two-year battle with cancer. At first, she seemed stoic and perhaps even relieved that her husband's protracted suffering was at last over. But then she became increasingly depressed and withdrawn. She stopped eating and bathing, seemed confused and easily distracted, and refused to leave her apartment. The doctor in the emergency room recognized that the woman was depressed and reassured her family that this was a "natural" consequence of bereavement. "Just stay with her and be supportive," the doctor advised the family, "and she will soon pull out of it." The doctor seemed empathetic and wise; the family believed his advice and took the depressed widow home.

Two weeks later, the widow was brought by ambulance to the same emergency room, semicomatose, after an overdose of sleeping pills. Fortunately, she was revived and admitted to the hospital. She was immediately started on antidepressant medication and improved dramatically over the next two weeks. Although she remained very sad about her husband's death, she once again engaged her family, ate meals, took baths, and went shopping. She never again contemplated taking her own life.

The surgical patient and the widow had virtually the same symptoms of depression. To the casual observer, their complaints would have been indistinguishable. Yet in the first case, drugs would have been useless; without antidepressants, the second patient probably would have ultimately killed herself.

WHAT IS PSYCHOPHARMACOLOGY?

Psychopharmacology is the branch of medicine that specializes in the use of medication to correct psychiatric illness. A skilled psychiatrist must know a great deal about a wide variety of drugs. Because all of these drugs have different side effects, the psychiatrist must also understand a great deal of general clinical medicine. Much of this knowledge is highly technical and complex. There is a great deal of science underlying the drugs used to treat psychiatric patients.

Yet no amount of science could possibly help the doctor decide not to treat the surgical patient I have described with antidepressants but to immediately treat the widow. No X-ray, blood test, or finding on physical examination can be used to help make this decision. Nothing will show up in the urine, sputum, or blood of either patient that would tell which one will respond to medication and which one will not.

Psychiatrists make these decisions based largely on a combination of clinical lore, experience, and intuition. In only a few instances do we have scientifically indisputable facts on which to rely. Hence, the patient and his or her family must be involved in every step of the decision-making process. A correct decision can produce substantial, even dramatic, benefit; a mistake can lead to prolongation of suffering, adverse physical side effects, and sometimes even disaster. It is no wonder, then, that many patients and doctors alike avoid drug treatment of psychiatric disorders or even insist that drugs are universally bad and dangerous.

THE MANY CONTROVERSIES

In any human endeavor, and medicine is a cardinal example, whenever facts are sparse, strongly held theories proliferate. Because the pros and cons for the use of medicine in psychiatry are not absolutely clear or agreed upon, strong arguments have arisen on all sides. Radical biologists insist that all psychiatric illnesses result from abnormalities in the chemistry and physiology of the brain. Drugs are almost always seen as the answer and the adverse side effects as simply inconvenient. To these practitioners, "talking" therapies of whatever variety are a waste of time. Diametrically opposed to the radical biologists are the dogmatic psychologists, who insist that psychiatric problems are not medical problems but rather the products of unconscious conflict, bad life experiences, incorrect thinking, or adverse social circumstances. These theorists are fond of claiming that medications only "cover up" psychiatric symptoms, whereas psychological treatments—psychoanalysis, behavioral modification, cognitive restructuring, and so on—get to the true root of the problem. To the dogmatic psychologists, medications actually prevent patients from working on their problems and are almost always dangerous.

A more reasonable approach is increasingly being adopted by mental health professionals. Recent studies show that psychiatric illnesses are caused by complex interactions between what we inherit from our parents and the adverse experiences we confront during our lifetimes. Studies also show that sometimes psychotherapy is the most effective treatment for a particular problem, sometimes medication is, and sometimes a combination of the two is the best choice. Almost everyone agrees that whether the problem arises from abnormal genes or traumatic events and whether medication or psychotherapy is the answer, the problem resides in the brain, which is now recognized as the "organ of the mind." Although some iconoclasts still cling to old-fashioned dichotomies between "biology" and "psychology," this is fortunately on the way out.

Many different kinds of professionals are involved in mental health care, including psychiatrists, psychologists, social workers, and nurses. Only psychiatrists are medical doctors, however, and for the most part they are the only ones who can legally prescribe medication. Also permitted to prescribe medication are nurse practitioners, many of whom have had years of experience treating patients with psychiatric illness. A kind and experienced nurse practitioner is always better than a psychiatrist who lacks good interpersonal skills and doesn't know much psychopharmacology. In some jurisdictions, psychologists who take a special course in psychopharmacology are also permitted to prescribe medication. This has sparked a great deal of controversy, with organized psychiatry lobbying heavily against this practice. It was once the case that psychiatrists were the advocates for medication and other disciplines the advocates for psychotherapy, but even this is changing as more and more mental health professionals adopt the new, more scientific understanding that psychotherapy affects the brain just as medication does and that both kinds of treatment have their place.

There are a host of new and sometimes even more inflammatory controversies in psychopharmacology today. Most of them, as described in the introduction, relate to the influence of the pharmaceutical industry over what doctors prescribe. This issue has become so important I deal with it in Chapter 22, "Can We Trust Drug Companies?" In that chapter, the important phenomenon of the "Black Box Warning" also is discussed. Other controversies, such as whether antidepressants actually increase the risk for suicide, whether medications used to treat attention-deficit/hyperactivity disorder (ADHD)—called psychostimulants—increase the risk for heart problems, and whether medications used to treat agitation and other behavioral disturbances in elderly people with dementia such as Alzheimer's disease increase the risk for fatal illnesses, are discussed in the chapters dealing with these specific classes of medications.

DECIDING ON THE BEST TREATMENT

I feel sympathy for the patient suffering from depression, panic attacks, or bulimia who must decide what kind of treatment to get and from whom. Often, patients feel that if they go to a psychiatrist they will automatically be prescribed drugs, if they go to a psychoanalyst they will be prescribed psychoanalysis, and if they go to a behaviorist they will be prescribed behavioral treatment. Imagine if a person complaining of stomachache was offered digitalis by a cardiologist, cortisone cream by a dermatologist, and eyeglasses by an ophthalmologist!

Thus, the purpose behind this book. As I will describe, medications can be extremely helpful—even lifesaving—in treating mental health disorders. But the patient with a psychiatric problem must be an informed consumer and understand some guidelines before agreeing to take a drug. It is not my intention to justify psychiatric drugs or to argue in favor of medication for every psychiatric problem. Rather, I explain situations in which careful consideration should be given to the use of medication and situations in which drugs should be rejected as treatment. In addition, it is important to know something about how these drugs work, what side effects they produce, and what benefits can and cannot legitimately be expected. Finally, patients should have some way of judging whether they are getting proper care and consideration from their physician.

The advertising slogan of a large chemical corporation, "better living through chemistry," has been proposed sarcastically as the motto for psychiatrists who prescribe drugs. This book is intended as a primer in how to avoid the "better living through chemistry" approach in favor of application of sound clinical and scientific principles to the medical treatment of some very serious illnesses.

Chapter 2

How Do I Know If I Need
a Psychiatric Drug?

Let's say you haven't been feeling quite like yourself for the past few weeks. It's hard to get out of bed when the alarm clock goes off, even though you have been lying awake for a few hours. Nothing seems to interest you much, including sex and your favorite foods. Work suddenly seems impossible and you cannot concentrate. Recently, you have started to wonder whether you've made a mess of things. Maybe life isn't worthwhile. Maybe it would be better to be dead.

Or everything seems to be going just fine in your life when suddenly one day while you are driving the car, your heart starts to pound, you feel as if you can't catch your breath, you sweat, feel dizzy and faint, and are sure you must be having a heart attack. Maybe just a bad day, you think, until you get another of these attacks two days later while at work. A third attack wakes you up in the middle of the night, and another hits while you are playing with your children.

Or your twenty-year-old son has always been a model student, an athlete, and popular with other kids his age. Lately he seems to be acting strangely. He paces around the house at all hours of the night and sounds as if he is muttering to an imaginary person. He tells you he thinks the food you serve him is poisoned. Sometimes when he talks, he goes on and on without making any sense. Then, in the middle of a tranquil evening as the family is watching television, he suddenly screams and threatens to kill his father.

These are all examples of psychiatric conditions that may respond to drugs. The first is an obvious case of depression, the second is called panic disorder, and the third is the tragic but all too familiar early stage of schizophrenia. Many people feel unhappy from time to time, everybody experiences anxiety and a few palpitations when there are things to worry about, and what teenager or young adult does not go through a period of acting strangely as far as his or her parents are concerned? Obviously, we do not recommend drugs, or psychiatric intervention, for that matter, for the routine ups and downs of everyday life. How do you decide to see a psychiatrist and consider taking medicine?

WHAT TO CONSIDER BEFORE SEEING A PSYCHIATRIST

Here are some general guidelines to consider in trying to make that decision:

1. It is perfectly normal to feel sad or nervous sometimes, but usually there is an obvious reason. If you just received bad news, it is not abnormal to be unhappy; if you have a major presentation to make at work tomorrow, you may feel anxious and even have trouble falling asleep. But if you find yourself depressed, anxious, or panicky for no obvious reason, you may be suffering from a psychiatric disorder.

2. Even when people feel blue or worried with good cause, it usually does not completely ruin their ability to work, take care of their children, and function socially. When depression or anxiety has a big impact on the job or in the ability to perform your usual tasks at home, it's a good time to think about seeing a psychiatrist.

3. Normal worries and bad moods usually last only a day or two. If you can't shrug it off, especially when others tell you things aren't really as bad as you think they are, you might need help.

4. Take seriously the concern expressed by people close to you or whom you trust. Your spouse comments that you don't seem like yourself lately. Your boss or secretary mentions that you seem distracted and bothered. Your family doctor points out that you seem unduly worried about having a heart attack even though you are in perfectly good health. Many times, a person suffering from depression or anxiety disorder is the last to admit something is wrong. Especially difficut but important is to take seriously anyone's concern that you are drinking too much. Many people with alcohol abuse problems receive this caution and most, unfortunately, accuse the

bearer of the news of being wrong or puritanical. That may be true, but usually it isn't.

5. Watch out for "home remedies." If you start taking a drink every night because otherwise you'll never fall asleep, or if you borrow someone else's tranquilizers or think that aspirins or antihistamines are necessary for your "nerves," you are doing a poor job at self-medication. There are better medications for depression and insomnia than scotch and soda.

6. Anytime you seriously entertain the thought "I would be better off dead" or "My life is worthless and my family might be in better shape collecting my life insurance," you should pick up the phone and get help.

7. People are entitled to act strangely, entertain "unusual" ideas or opinions, or follow a "different drummer." You do no favor for a loved one, however, by allowing him or her to become lost in hallucinations, to be tortured by paranoid ideas, or to threaten harm to others. One out of every hundred people in the United States has schizophrenia; it is a devastating disease without a cure. But running away from schizophrenia only delays getting the help that is available. Instead of worrying about the stigma some people associate with seeing a psychiatrist, worry instead about what may happen if you do not follow your instinct that your child or spouse is acting in a bizarre manner and get help quickly.

To summarize these seven points, you (or someone close to you) may be a candidate to take a psychiatric drug if you have symptoms of anxiety or depression for no good reason; if your symptoms interfere with your ability to function at home or work; if your symptoms persist longer than a few days; if others tell you that you seem unusually moody, stressed, or anxious, or that you are drinking too much; if you have suicidal thoughts; if you use alcohol, street drugs, or unprescribed medications to ease tension, improve your mood, or help you sleep; or if you persistently exhibit odd, bizarre behavior, often to the point that others feel threatened (Table 1).

Remember, there is very little to be lost, and an awful lot to be gained, by consulting a psychiatrist in these circumstances. Don't succumb to the common myths about psychiatrists. We really are not interested in drumming up business by convincing people they are crazy; like most physicians, I like nothing better than to tell someone that nothing is seriously wrong and no treatment is necessary. Psychiatric illness is not a sign of personal weakness. Great scientists (S. E. Luria), heads of countries (Abraham Lincoln), sports figures (Terry Bradshaw), and famous artists (Vincent van Gogh) have suffered from psychiatric illnesses.

Table 1.

Warning Signs That a Psychiatric Drug May Be Needed

- You feel depressed, anxious, or panicky for no obvious reason.
- Depression or anxiety makes it difficult to do your usual work.
- Even though others tell you things are not that bad, you cannot stop worrying.
- Others tell you that you do not seem your usual self.
- You take other people's medication or over-the-counter drugs or drink more to "calm your nerves" or help you sleep.
- You have thoughts of suicide or feel that life isn't worth it.
- You are acting in a bizarre or frightening manner.

Finally, it is not true that everybody will know if you see a psychiatrist. Psychiatrists take the promise of confidentiality very seriously and are bound never to reveal to anyone that they saw you or what your problem is. One young woman suffering from depression burst into tears when I recommended she take medication for her illness. "If my boss ever finds out I am taking drugs for depression, he'll fire me in a minute!" she sobbed. As much as I wanted to relieve her unfounded fears, I of course could not tell her that her boss was, coincidentally, also a patient of mine and that he was taking antidepressants. No one has to know that you see a psychiatrist.

GETTING HELP

Once you have decided you may have a problem requiring professional help, the next step is to decide what kind of help to get. Here, you might become confused. Pick up any newspaper and you'll find advertisements from therapists promising cures for depression, anxiety, alcoholism, and cigarette smoking. Your best friend may recommend vitamins and exercise. Your family doctor may want to give you tranquilizers.

What you need is the advice of an expert in psychiatric illness who is familiar with the variety of treatments available and who can tailor a remedy to your personal situation. To get that, I advise first consulting a psychiatrist. The best way to find one is the same procedure you would use in choosing a dentist, pediatrician, or gynecologist. Ask your family doctor, call the local hospital or medical school, or rely on recommendations from family or friends.

In general, there are two kinds of treatment for psychiatric illness: medications and talking therapies. Sometimes a person needs one or the other, and sometimes both. In the next chapter, I consider how to decide which route is best for you.

Chapter 3

Psychotherapy, Drugs, or Both?

Surprisingly, some people are treated for emotional problems for many years without ever being told what is wrong with them. Some patients come to me after years of psychotherapy completely unable to explain how their treatment is affecting their symptoms.

The first task in deciding whether a psychiatric drug is appropriate is the diagnosis. This is no different from what happens when you go to the family doctor complaining of a stomachache or fever. The doctor asks many questions, sometimes performs a physical examination, and may obtain laboratory tests and X-rays. The only difference with psychiatric care is that psychiatrists rely more on answers to questions asked of the patient and family than on physical examinations or test results.

To diagnose, psychiatrists in the United States now use the American Psychiatric Association's *Diagnostic and Statistical Manual of Mental Disorders,* fourth edition, called the *DSM-IV* for short. It essentially gives very specific instructions on how to put together different kinds of emotional symptoms to make a psychiatric diagnosis. The *DSM-IV* forces the doctor to ask detailed questions about the nature of symptoms and how long they have lasted to figure out what is wrong.

The *DSM-IV* is admittedly imperfect. The system was conceived in its present form in 1980 with the publication of *DSM-III* (the third edition), and at the time it was a revolution for psychiatry. For the first time, a psychiatric diagnosis had some meaning because there were standardized criteria. The system has remained largely unchanged and has held up fairly well over two and a half decades, but cracks are increasingly noted. For one thing, as research has progressed, it is clear that not all of the diagnoses in *DSM-IV* match up that well with what appears in some cases to be the underlying brain abnormalities. For example, overactivity of a small structure in the brain called the amygdala seems to occur in patients with several different *DSM-IV* conditions, including depression, panic disorder, social anxiety disorder, and post-traumatic stress disorder (PTSD). Yet nothing in *DSM-IV* suggests a link among these conditions. Even more important is the finding that most patients with psychiatric illness suffer from more than one *DSM-IV* diagnosis. This is almost certainly because the *DSM-IV* categories are insufficiently precise. Finally, some of the definitions in *DSM-IV* do not make a whole lot of sense, even to experts in the field. The real difference between substance abuse and substance dependence, for example, is much debated, and whether undifferentiated schizophrenia really describes a distinct type of schizophrenia is far from clear. Committees are already working on *DSM-V*. For now, the DSM system is far better than what we had before 1980 and is extremely useful in making treatment decisions. A *DSM-IV* diagnosis is the start, although not necessarily the only factor, in deciding how to proceed with a psychiatric problem.

The diagnosis, made by *DSM-IV* criteria supplemented by the experience of the clinician and new insights from the psychiatric literature, then guides the psychiatrist in treatment recommentations. There are some psychiatric conditions that are almost always treated with medications, some for which medications are optional, and some for which medications are useless. Similarly, psychotherapy helps in some circumstances, is helpful but not required in others, and is a waste of time for still others. Let me give some examples.

THE IMPORTANCE OF DIAGNOSIS

Roger, a fifty-seven-year-old insurance salesman, is married, owns his own home, and enjoys playing golf on the weekends. He was doing very nicely at work until about six months ago, when he started feeling tired a lot of the time, then noticed he was waking up at three or four in the morning without being able to fall asleep again. Over the next few months he began to lose interest in playing golf, found he could not concentrate on what his coworkers or clients were saying to him, and began worrying that his business was nearly bankrupt, even though his partners assured him there was no danger of this. Four weeks before seeing a psychiatrist, his wife noticed that he had lost almost twenty pounds and asked him why he seemed so worried and tired all the time. Two weeks earlier he had had the first passing thought that he might be better off dead, and after that could not get the thought out of his head. By the time he saw the psychiatrist, he was too depressed to get out of bed in the morning to go to work, stopped shaving and taking showers, and gave only one-word answers after long pauses when asked questions. He admitted that given the opportunity, he would probably kill himself.

Roger is an obvious candidate for psychiatric drug treatment. Even though a detailed exploration might reveal the events in his life that triggered his severe depression, he is so withdrawn and uncommunicative that it is unlikely much psychotherapy could be conducted at this point. Furthermore, his condition is life threatening. If he doesn't actually kill himself, he might ultimately starve to death unless something is done to improve his appetite and make him start eating again. Roger should be put on antidepressant medication immediately. Incidentally, the official diagnosis we would give Roger is *major depression.* Some forms of psychotherapy, such as cognitive behavioral therapy and interpersonal psychotherapy, have also been proved by rigorous scientific studies to be effective in treating even severe depression. In Roger's case, however, the illness is so severe that medication is the best initial route.

Now let us turn to a less obvious case involving a different type of depression. Virginia is thirty-six and single but has lived with her boyfriend for three years. She is an architect, is well respected by her colleagues, and has many close friends. Still, Virginia has suspected more and more in recent years that she does not look at life the way other people do. She is successful but never happy. Most of the time she is convinced that her boyfriend is about to leave her or that she will lose her job. When these thoughts get very strong, she tends to eat everything in sight, often to the point of feeling sick to her stomach. Consequently, she is constantly battling her weight. Sometimes she gets horrible anxiety attacks and feels as if her heart is going to pop right out of her chest. On weekends she often spends most of her time in bed, complaining she is too tired to go out. If her friends convince her to go out, she usually has a good time and feels cheerful while she is with them. No one except her boyfriend and closest friends have any idea that she suffers from depression.

There is a very good chance that Virginia would get substantial benefit from medication for depression, but unlike the case of Roger, this is not an emergency. She is not suicidal, her life is not in jeopardy, and she is perfectly able to function at work. The "evidence-based" psychotherapies—that is, the types of psychotherapy that have been proved to work for depression by scientific studies—have a very good chance of helping Virginia. These include cognitive behavioral and interpersonal psychotherapy. These should be tried before medication, in my opinion, because psycotherapy obviously has fewer adverse side effects than medication. Also, studies suggest that patients with depression who respond to medication often relapse when the medication is discontinued. On the other hand, people who respond to a course of evidence-based psychotherapy, usually taking between three and six months, often stay well for long periods of time after the treatment is finished. Medication can be reserved for situations in which the evidence-based psycotherapies are insufficiently effective. Longer-term psychotherapies that follow psychoanalytic principles might also be helpful if the therapist can identify the underlying causes of the depression. However, there is no scientific evidence at the present time that psychoanalytic-based treatments are effective for depression. In the case of Virginia, before making a definite decision on treatment, a psychiatrist might recommend a few more meetings to determine whether psychotherapy has potential benefit and might ultimately recommend a combination of talking therapy and drug therapy. Virginia, by the way, suffers from *atypical depression.* I have more to say about this in the chapter on depression.

At the opposite end of the spectrum from Roger is Donna. She is an English professor at a university and is about to find out whether she will get a promotion. She is anxious and moody just thinking about the meeting she must have with her department chairman in two weeks when she will be told her professional fate. But there is more than this simple anxiety and moodiness. As the big meeting approaches, Donna realizes that she really hasn't done everything she could to improve her chances. She knows she is bright and qualified, but she always avoids making the right political moves. Consequently, she seems to be passed up for less qualified professors on many occasions. Donna wonders why she can't push ahead those last few inches and put herself over the top. What holds her back from expending the extra effort to ensure professional success?

Donna does not suffer from depression or anxiety disorder. She has a *conflict* about success. Drugs will not help. Of course, a tranquilizer might help her sleep better the night before the big meeting with the chairman, but that is not her real problem. Donna will benefit most from one of a variety of psychotherapies aimed at improving her self-confidence, making her assertive, and removing her conflicts about success.

I have deliberately made these examples somewhat extreme to illustrate the main point: Diagnosis is as essential when dealing with psychiatric disorders as it is in dealing with any medical problem. The question of what treatment—psychotherapy, drugs, or both—is best can be answered only when the symptoms are clear and the diagnosis made.

Psychiatrists are obviously not the only specialists in emotional problems who know how to make diagnoses and provide useful treatment. A few features of psychiatrists should be kept in mind, however.

First, psychiatrists are medical doctors who must graduate from medical school just like internists, surgeons, and pediatricians. Medical illnesses can sometimes cause psychiatric illnesses, and psychiatrists are specially trained to recognize the situations in which physical disease is the cause of emotional problems. Many people therefore feel most comfortable seeing a psychiatrist at least once to be sure they are not suffering from a neurological or medical problem.

Second, only psychiatrists among the many mental health practitioners are legally qualified to prescribe drugs. (Exceptions to this are nurse practitioners, but they are in very short supply, and psychologists in a very few jurisdictions.) Remember, prescribing drugs means much more than simply writing a prescription. Only a physician can appreciate the side effects, dose requirements, and drug interactions involved in administering psychiatric drugs.

Third, in deciding whether a drug might help a psychiatric problem, one of the best guidelines is how well similar patients have done with drugs in the past. Although that information can be obtained from textbooks, the truth is that most doctors and therapists find experience to be the best teacher. By observing how patients with different emotional problems react to the various psychiatric drugs, the psychiatrist learns which patient is the best candidate for a specific treatment. As only psychiatrists have this training and experience, they are often in the best position to recognize who might benefit from drug treatment.

If drug therapy is not required, a referral should be made to a qualified psychotherapist. Psychiatrists are often very skilled in psychotherapy; indeed, some psychiatrists are much more comfortable treating patients with psychotherapy than with drugs. Many psychologists and social workers are also excellent psychotherapists.

Psychologists do graduate work in clinical psychology after college. This usually includes at least a one-year internship in which they evaluate and treat patients. Many also do dissertations and receive a Ph.D. They are often highly qualified to make diagnoses and conduct psychotherapy. Social workers receive a graduate master of social work degree (M.S.W.), usually requiring two years of course work and patient contact. Many do extra training in psychotherapy after getting the M.S.W. degree and some do dissertations and receive a doctorate of social work.

In most states, there is no legal definition of psychotherapist. Anyone who thinks he or she has an understanding ear and good advice to give can call himself or herself a psychotherapist. Studies have shown that the best predictor of how well a psychotherapy will work is the "fit" or relationship between patient and therapist at the start of the therapy. I recommend getting a referral from a physician or someone who has been in therapy before, selecting only therapists with a degree in a mental health field (a psychiatrist with an

M.D., a psychologist with a Ph.D., or a social worker with an M.S.W.), and then interviewing two, three, or more therapists until you find one with whom you feel comfortable.

If drug therapy is recommended, there are many things you will need to know before putting the first pill in your mouth. In the next chapter, I offer some guidelines to help you ensure that you are receiving the best possible drug treatment.

Chapter 4

How Do I Get Psychiatric Drugs?

The task of finding a competent practitioner to prescribe and manage psychiatric medication may seem perilous. You may reasonably wonder how to avoid falling into the hands of a doctor who "drugs" everybody who walks into the office.

In many respects, choosing a psychiatrist is not very different from choosing a physician. A doctor with good credentials who listens carefully, explains things, weighs all of the options out loud, and promises easy access during the treatment period is obviously required. This is probably what you would look for if you needed a doctor to prescribe eyeglasses, remove a gallbladder, or treat the flu.

There is, of course, an important aspect of psychiatric illness that makes choosing a proper physician more difficult. By its very nature, mental illness affects a person's judgment and motivation to get help. Psychiatric patients often suffer from excessive guilt; thus, they are prone to avoid challenging a doctor's advice or asking for a second opinion. Some psychiatrists unfortunately promote this attitude, acting as if they have all the answers and reacting angrily if a patient questions the treatment or requests a consultation. Patients with high levels of anxiety may grab at the first suggestion of a cure without thinking things over; they may feel that a strong-willed physician is just what they need to relieve their worries, even if the treatment plan doesn't sound right. Psychotic patients usually have serious distortions of reality and use little logic to make many of their decisions, including their choice of doctor or commitment to adhere to a treatment plan.

TEN POINTS TO REMEMBER

So in choosing a doctor to prescribe psychiatric drugs, keep these ten guidelines in mind:

1. Doctors with an M.D. or D.O. degree, that is, medical doctors, are licensed to prescribe psychoactive medication. Psychiatrists are mental health experts who went to medical school; many now specialize in prescribing drugs, and in general they are the most knowledgeable and experienced in prescribing psychiatric medications. At present, there are no specific requirements that a psychiatrist must meet to specialize in drug treatment. Almost all medical school departments of psychiatry can refer you to a psychiatrist with special experience in medication treatment, and this is often a good place to start. Psychopharmacology is the use of medication to treat psychiatric illness, and physicians who place special emphasis on this in their work call themselves psychopharmacologists. However, there is no official designation or subspeciality of psychopharmacology as there is for cardiology as a subspeciality of internal medicine. At present, psychopharmacologist is what a psychiatrist with a special interest in medication calls himself or herself.

In any event, it is perfectly reasonable to ask psychiatrists if they have special interest and experience in prescribing psychiatric drugs, what proportion of their patients actually receive drugs, where they learned to do this, and if they treat specific types of patients. In answering these questions, the psychiatrist should be direct and clear. A psychiatrist who becomes defensive or tries to "interpret" the questions as hostile or representing an unconscious conflict is probably trying to cover up a lack of expertise in psychopharmacology.

2. Do not take drugs from a non-M.D. practitioner who gets the prescription for you from a doctor. A patient may be in therapy with a social worker, nurse, or psychologist who thinks that medication is required. Many such therapists are extremely knowledgeable about psychiatric drugs and are in fact very qualified to recognize a need for medication. The proper procedure in this case is for the patient to consult a psychiatrist to decide whether medication is needed and for the psychiatrist then to manage the medication side of treatment.

Unfortunately, some therapists are afraid to refer a patient to another practitioner for fear of losing the patient and therefore merely describe the case to a psychiatrist who writes a prescription without ever seeing the patient. When side effects or questions arise, the therapist asks the doctor and relays the answer to the patient. This is like having your dentist take out your appendix under the direction of a surgeon in the next room.

Incidentally, the failure to refer patients is not limited to non-M.D. therapists. Very often, a psychiatrist will feel that a patient treated with drugs isn't getting better or has additional problems that drugs won't solve. Instead of getting a consultation from a skilled professional in psychotherapy, the psychiatrist may blame the patient for not trying hard enough or change the medications.

This brings up a very important principle of all health care: There is nothing wrong with a doctor asking a patient to consult another doctor for another opinion. The best doctors do this regularly. No one doctor can know everything. Furthermore, it is entirely possible for the best, smartest, most conscientious doctor to miss some aspect of a case. I am not talking here about doctors who miss heart attacks, strokes, cancer, or mania. Many more subtle problems can arise in treatment that can be misinterpreted or missed entirely. Physicians should always know when to ask for help and patients should always respect a doctor who has the sense to request advice.

3. Know how to work with primary care physicians when you think you have a psychiatric problem. It is no longer realistic to tell people who may be suffering from a psychiatric problem to go directly to see a psychiatrist. More and more people are enrolled in managed health care programs that require the permission of a "gatekeeper," usually a family physician or general practitioner, before a specialist can be consulted. Many such primary care doctors are very interested in psychiatry and are knowledgeable, but they are up against a difficult set of practical problems in trying to address their patients' psychiatric problems themselves. The usual HMO allows a primary care doctor less than twenty minutes to evaluate a new patient and discourages him or her from frequent follow-up visits. This is hardly enough time to make a psychiatric evaluation. Because of this, primary care physicians are sometimes reluctant to get into psychiatric discussions with patients, fearing it will take too long. They also may restrict themselves to prescribing the simplest psychiatric drugs, ones, for example, that do not require any changes in dose, so that they do not have to see the patient too many times (if at all) after the initial visit.

Here is what I advise: If you think you have a psychiatric problem and are required by your health plan to see the primary care physician first, ask if he or she is comfortable dealing with psychiatric issues. If the answer is yes, give him or her a chance to help you. Use all of the information in this book to become informed about psychiatric drugs and to know what questions you must ask the doctor. Follow your doctor's instructions and see if you improve over the next four to six weeks. Do not hesitate to call him or her if you experience any problems with the medication. If, however, the primary care doctor seems uncomfortable with psychiatric problems or if you are not getting better after one or at most two months, then insist on being referred to a psychiatrist.

4. When consulting a psychiatrist, make sure the initial appointment lasts at least an hour and that you have an opportunity to explain your situation in depth. There is no way to take an adequate medical and psychiatric history in a short period. Without such a history, a doctor cannot possibly determine the psychiatric diagnosis and the need for medication.

Remember, except in rare instances, psychiatrists do not yet have the luxury of laboratory tests and X-rays to help them make a diagnosis or design a treatment strategy. Sometimes, very subtle differences in symptom patterns make a large difference. For example, two very depressed people may see a psychiatrist to inquire about the possible benefit of antidepressants. The psychiatrist may quickly determine that medication is indicated but then face the difficult problem of deciding which of the many available medications should be tried first. In one case, further history reveals that the patient has a specific abnormality on the electrocardiogram that makes the use of one class of antidepressants risky. In the second case, the patient reveals after close questioning that the depressed mood is occasionally alleviated when good things happen to him. This suggests the use of different kinds of antidepressants. It takes time to tease apart the various life situations and emotional symptoms to determine the right treatment; a patient is entitled to that time.

5. It is very important that you feel that the doctor has tailored his or her treatment recommendations to your specific needs. I have seen patients in consultation who believe that the psychiatrist they previously saw gave everybody lithium regardless of the specifics, or that the doctor didn't listen carefully to a specific request that medication likely to cause weight gain be avoided. You must feel that the doctor has taken your situation into account and is willing to be as flexible as possible in designing treatment. Sometimes, of course, flexibility is not possible. Patients often wish for medication with absolutely no side effects. No such drugs exist for the treatment of any medical condition and definitely not for the treatment of psychiatric disorders. However, it is often possible to design a treatment plan that comes close to meeting a particular person's specific needs, and this should always be attempted.

6. The psychiatrist should always be willing to justify the choice of treatment. As much as possible, the patient should be made to feel like an informed consumer. Brain science is indeed a complicated field, but a good psychiatrist knows how to simplify things sufficiently—without being condescending—so that a patient can understand how the various drugs recommended work. More important, the doctor should be able to detail all of the possible alternatives to drug treatment and why they were not chosen.

For every psychiatric condition there is a nondrug treatment that someone, somewhere will recommend. With more than one hundred different psychotherapies, there are obviously many alternatives to drugs. And many times, the psychiatrist, after taking a careful history, decides that psychotherapy is a superior choice to drugs. The patient should feel free to ask about alternatives to drug treatment and should be completely satisfied that the doctor has considered them and is not dogmatically opposed to them.

7. Unless there is an emergency, consider getting a second opinion before starting medication. This does not mean that the first doctor should not be trusted. Two doctors are very likely to have slightly different opinions of a person's psychiatric problems and to recommend slightly different treatments. In such a case, it is probably wise to stick with the original physician. For example, if both consultants agree that the diagnosis of depression is correct and that antidepressants are warranted, it probably does not make a great deal of difference if one doctor recommends fluoxetine (Prozac) and the other recommends sertraline (Zoloft), as both belong to the same class of drugs. Such differences usually have more to do with which drug the psychiatrist is used to prescribing than with diagnosis or recommended treatment.

On the other hand, if one consultant feels a patient is depressed and should seek psychotherapy, and the other feels the diagnosis is depression as part of manic-depressive illness and long-term treatment with lithium is indicated, obviously there is a serious difference. In later chapters, I explain how to decide what to do in these situations, but for now it is important to stress that to a limit, obtaining more information and opinions is usually a good idea. No one should avoid getting additional facts.

8. Psychiatric drug treatment is not a "take two aspirins and call me in the morning" situation. If medication is prescribed after the initial consultation, there should be an arrangement for regular follow-up. Often, patients think they can simply take medication for a few weeks and that will be the end of it. Unfortunately, health insurance coverage for psychiatric care is shockingly inadequate, so patients avoid making further visits to see the doctor. But psychiatric drug treatment is complex and patients must be followed on a regular basis.

For example, antidepressants of the monoamine oxidase inhibitor (MAOI) class are extremely useful and powerful drugs for relief of depression. Sometimes, however, patients actually become "high" from the drug after several weeks, a condition technically called hypomania. Unfortunately, this high is often missed by patients and their families, who are so glad the patient is no longer depressed that they fail to recognize that something new is wrong. The signs of hypomania include rapid speech, excess energy, inappropriate optimism, and decreased sleep requirement. It can often be treated simply by reducing the dose of medication, but it must first be recognized. For that reason, doctors are correct in insisting that the patient on monoamine oxidase inhibitors be seen in the office about once a month, even after the depression has resolved.

It is often the case that one drug, whether prescribed or bought over the counter, causes problems when another drug is taken. Doctors call this problem "drug-drug interaction." The list of such drug-drug interactions is so long that it would be impossible to give all the details here. In general, however, antidepressants of the monoamine oxidase class should never be coprescribed with another antidepressant or with a number of other drugs, such as the painkiller meperidine (Demerol), the antianxiety drug buspirone (Buspar), or over-the-counter cold remedies, such as drugs containing pseudoephedrine (including Sudafed) and many antihistamines (including Benadryl). Similarly, some of the antidepressants called tricyclic antidepressants, like imipramine (Tofranil) and amitriptyline (Elavel), should not be coprescribed with several of the antidepressants in the class called selective serotonin reuptake inhibitors (SSRIs), such as paroxetine (Paxil), fluoxetine (Prozac), or sertraline (Zoloft). In these cases, coprescription of two drugs will cause the levels in the blood of one or both of them to be much higher than expected, which can cause dangerous adverse side effects and even be lethal. In other cases, adding one drug to another can lower the blood level of one of them. Combining either carbamazeine (Tegretol) or modafinil (Provigil) with birth control pills will lower the blood level of the birth control pills and can cause an unexpected pregnancy.

How can a patient be sure this doesn't happen? Of course you should inform each doctor you see of all the other prescribed and over-the-counter drugs you are taking. Unfortunately, sometimes a patient will forget one of them. The best thing to do is to take all your medications off your night table and out of your medicine cabinet, put them in a bag, take them to your doctor, and go through them one at a time.

In addition to regular office visits, patients need to know that they can contact the doctor or an associate twenty-four hours a day, seven days a week, twelve months a year (even in August, when many psychiatrists seem to take their vacation). Psychiatrists must have the same kind of around-the-clock availability as internists, obstetricians, and cardiologists because psychiatric illness severe enough to require drug treatment may produce complications at any time and psychiatric drugs can produce side effects that need immediate attention. If your doctor is hard to get hold of, switch to a different doctor.

9. Make sure important side effects are described before you start taking a drug. This guideline applies to any medical treatment, but special problems

arise with psychiatric illness. First, psychiatric patients worry so much in general that the last thing they need is to worry about the rare side effects of drugs. Second, some psychiatric patients suffer from temporary impairment of judgment and may therefore overestimate the risk of a side effect and make an incorrect decision to refuse drug treatment. Third, some psychiatric patients cannot understand the implications of various side effects and make an informed decision.

All of this has led some psychiatrists to adopt a paternalistic approach and edit what they tell patients about the "downside" of a particular drug. Although understandable, this attitude is rarely correct. We all have a right to know the adverse consequences of a treatment. We also have the right to refuse treatment. Hence, it is hard to think of instances in which the doctor should not explain the common and most important side effects. A patient should never feel that a doctor is withholding information about the adverse effects of drugs.

10. It is appropriate, and often desirable, for family members and significant others to be involved in drug treatment of psychiatric disorders. There are many reasons for this. First, by their very nature psychiatric illnesses often make it difficult for patients to give a complete and accurate history of the problem and symptoms. Manic patients usually talk so fast and give so many extraneous details that the doctor has a hard time figuring out what happened at what time without a family member to help. Depressed patients have trouble concentrating and often omit important facts. It is also very hard for psychiatric patients to remember ever feeling well, so that the doctor may not get a true picture of when the trouble began.

Second, having a regular observer available to help chart the progress of a patient taking medication is very useful. Many antidepressants, for example, improve sleep and appetite before improving mood. The patient may feel nothing is happening because he or she still feels depressed, but the family member may notice that the patient has started sleeping through the night and eating regular meals. Without hearing from this family member, the patient and the doctor might miss the early evidence of a positive drug effect and prematurely discontinue the medication. Finally, it is important to review side effects with family members so that they also know what to watch for. Psychiatric patients may feel so terrible in general that they will not bother to call the doctor if a rash develops or nausea occurs, symptoms the doctor must be aware of.

Of course, maintaining confidentiality is always crucial in treating patients with mental illness. The psychiatrist, like all mental health practitioners, is absolutely bound never to divulge information about a patient to anyone without permission. Sometimes, family members make intrusive and inappropriate demands for information about a patient's progress. There exist situations in which family members have a vested interest in seeing that the patient does not recover. For example, I have seen many husbands who are threatened by the idea of having their depressed or phobic wives suddenly become happier and therefore more assertive and independent. Thus, it is best that the patient select family members who can be part of the treatment effort and decide with the doctor exactly what role these members will have and what information they should be given access to. Always be wary of a doctor who flatly refuses to discuss anything with a patient's family, even at the patient's request.

Table 2 summarizes the ten guidelines for choosing a psychiatrist and starting drug treatment. In general, the first person to ask is a trusted

Table 2.

Guidelines for Getting Psychiatric Drugs

1. Only medical doctors (with an M.D. or a D.O. degree) can prescribe medication (exceptions are nurse practitioners and, in a very few jurisdictions, psychologists).
2. See the psychiatrist yourself; don't get the medication from a non-M.D. therapist who speaks to the psychiatrist and gets the prescription for you.
3. If you are getting psychiatric drugs from a physician who is not a psychiatrist but things are either not getting better after a few weeks or getting steadily worse, ask to see a psychiatrist.
4. The first consultation with the psychiatrist should be long enough (usually at least an hour) for you to completely explain all your symptoms.
5. Treatment should feel as if it is designed for your particular situation and needs.
6. The psychiatrist should be able to explain and justify the particular choice of drug recommended for you.
7. Feel free to get a second opinion from another psychiatrist before you swallow the first pill.
8. Follow-up visits are necessary. You cannot see the doctor once, get a prescription, and do the rest on your own.
9. Get a description of important side effects before you start the medication.
10. Don't hesitate to have your family or significant others be with you when you see the psychiatrist and be involved with your treatment.

family doctor, who often will know a good psychiatrist. A non-M.D. practitioner with whom a patient is already in psychotherapy will often have the names of psychiatrists who can prescribe medication and who have done a good job in the past. A phone call to the nearest medical school department of psychiatry is often fruitful. Psychiatrists who specialize in drug treatment tend to be on university medical school faculties. Finally, to the extent possible, be open with family members and friends when contemplating seeing a psychiatrist. Unfortunately, in some circles there remains a stigma attached to psychiatric illness that dissuades people from discussing their problems. Studies have shown that 50 percent of the American population suffers from psychiatric illness; in other words, an awful lot of people have psychiatric problems and many have sought treatment. Often, it is the successfully treated patients who keep their experience with psychiatry a secret, and only the relatively few disgruntled patients who openly describe their experience. Many people have had a good experience with psychiatric medication treatment and this is probably the best recommendation one could receive in selecting a doctor.

After your first appointment, review the ten guidelines to determine whether you have chosen the right doctor. Above all, never be afraid to ask questions and expect serious, well-thought-out answers.

Chapter 5

What Are Side Effects?

Every drug, psychiatric or otherwise, has side effects. Some side effects are serious; some may seem worse than the illness for which the drug was prescribed; others are merely inconvenient. Side effects may occur early in drug treatment or may not start until many months into treatment. Most side effects are alleviated when the patient stops taking the drug, but in a few instances side effects persist.

Chapters 7 to 12 list the side effects for each drug. Here, I make some general comments about side effects.

Side effects are unwanted physical and emotional changes caused by drugs that usually have nothing to do with the drugs' ability to cure illnesses. No drug is specific enough to affect only the sick part of the body; all drugs do at least one thing more than what we want them to do.

It is important to find out what side effects may be expected before putting the first pill in your mouth. There are basically two ways to obtain this information.

USING DRUG GUIDES SELECTIVELY

The first way is to look up the side effects in a reference book. I usually encourage patients to read whatever they want to about drug treatment.

Sometimes, patients unnecessarily worry themselves by referring to such books as the *Physicians' Desk Reference (PDR)*. For example, one patient who had been taking a drug for about a month told me the medication was giving her headaches. "I've never heard or observed that to be a side effect of this particular drug," I told her.

Now, she thought she had me. "Oh yes, it says right in the *PDR* that headaches are a side effect of this drug you have me on."

That was news to me so I got out my copy of the *PDR* (actually, nowadays I usually use the even more convenient Palm Pilot program called Epocrates to keep up-to-date on medications and their adverse side effects) and looked it up. What we found was a table listing about twenty different side effects. There were two columns in the table: One column showed the number of patients who took the drug and experienced each side effect, and the other column showed the number of patients who took a placebo pill—an identical sugar pill used in drug studies—and manifested the side effects. For the side effect *headache,* the number of patients in the placebo column was higher than the number of patients in the active drug column. This means that the drug is not any more responsible than a sugar pill for causing headaches.

This is one of the pitfalls of reading a book like the *PDR*. Much of the language is technical and often refers to findings from scientific tests of drugs rather than actual clinical experience.

Another problem with these reference books is that they often list every side effect ever reported for a drug, even if it occurred in only one of a thousand cases. Doctors who treat a large number of patients need to know that information; they might run into that one patient who develops a very rare side effect. An individual patient, however, has a very small chance of experiencing that side effect.

Also consider what can be found with respect to very common drugs in the *PDR* or similar books. Although penicillin is a highly effective antibiotic that rarely hurts anyone, there are a few patients who have a severe allergic reaction that can be fatal. The risk is so small, however, that few people refuse to take such an effective drug as penicillin. Even aspirin has some pretty serious side effects in some people. A listing for aspirin in the *PDR* or similar books would include such side effects as ulcers and uncontrolled bleeding. Aspirin overdose can even be fatal! So merely reading through a list of side effects could deter a person from taking an aspirin for a headache.

ASK THE DOCTOR

The second way to get information is to ask the doctor prescribing the medication to explain all of the side effects and to give you an idea of how likely they are to occur in a given individual. This varies from person to person. Some antidepressants can make it difficult for a person to urinate. For a twenty-year-old woman who is otherwise perfectly healthy, this effect is usually very mild and hardly noticeable; however, a sixty-year-old man with an enlarged prostate gland might end up in the emergency room and have a catheter inserted.

The best advice is to read books like the *PDR* and also to ask the psychiatrist prescribing the medication to give you a list of the more common side effects. The doctor should alert you to the serious effects that need immediate attention and also reassure you about those side effects for which there is no need to worry. In other cases, the doctor may know of side effects to a drug that do not even appear in the *PDR*. For example, at a recent meeting attended by several hundred psychiatrists, mostly in private practice, a speaker asked the audience to "raise your hand if you think Paxil [an antidepressant] causes weight gain more often than the other antidepressants in its class [the class being the SSRI or selective serotonin reuptake inhibitor antidepressants]." Virtually all of the doctors in the audience raised their hands. Yet, for a variety of reasons to be discussed later, this side effect does not appear in the *PDR*. Above all, don't hesitate to call the doctor if you are not sure whether a new symptom is serious. A good doctor would rather be called than find out that something bad has happened to his or her patient but the patient was too embarrassed to call. Naturally, we all like to sleep through the night, but it is always worth my while to get out of bed at four in the morning to decide if some possible drug side effect is serious rather than have one of my patients become sick unnecessarily.

Chapter 6

How Long Should I Take a Psychiatric Drug?

You should continue to take a drug as long as it helps and you should keep taking it until the illness is gone.

For each psychiatric drug described in Chapters 7 to 12, you will find information on how long to stay on the drug and the best way to discontinue use of the drug. Some general principles are useful.

We usually start out with very small doses of psychiatric medication and build up to the full therapeutic dose over a few days or even weeks. This gradual buildup minimizes the side effects and gives the body a chance to adjust. Also, some drugs take weeks before they start to work, especially antidepressants, lithium, and the antianxiety drug BuSpar. You should definitely give the drug a fair chance to know if it is going to help.

Many people are concerned that the effects of a psychiatric drug will wear off. Technically, this is called tolerance. A patient becomes tolerant to a drug when a dose that has worked for a while stops working. In such situations it is necessary to increase the dose or switch to a different drug.

Fortunately, tolerance is almost never a factor with psychiatric drugs. Once a dose of antidepressant, lithium, or antianxiety drug is found that works, it usually remains effective as long as drug treatment is required. The exceptions are sleeping pills, which sometimes lose their effectiveness after two to three weeks, and amphetamines, which are only rarely used as antidepressants.

Now, let's say the drug works and you are feeling much better. You might want to stop taking the medication, and, in certain situations, that is exactly the right thing to do (Table 3).

Table 3.

How Long to Stay on Psychiatric Drugs

DRUG	RECOMMENDED TREATMENT LENGTH
Antidepressants	Six months after remission, longer if depression is recurrent
Lithium, Depakote	Indefinitely for bipolar (manic-depressive) patients
Antipsychotics	One year after first episode; indefinitely after second episode
Antianxiety drugs	Shortest possible period (except when treating panic disorder)
Antipanic drugs	Six months after remission, longer if panic disorder is recurrent
Sleeping pills	Shortest possible period

SHORT-TERM TREATMENT

A thirty-four-year-old man who had always been a bit on the nervous side learned one morning that the company at which he had worked for five years had just lost a great deal of money. Rumors around the office convinced him that the company was about to go out of business and he would soon lose his job. Over the next few weeks, despite the lack of official confirmation of these rumors from his boss, he found himself paralyzed with worry, fear, and anxiety. Unable to sleep, he could not concentrate on looking for a new job. A psychiatrist prescribed an antianxiety medication at a low dose and recommended counseling. The man took the medication every morning for a week and met with the psychiatrist two more times. He focused on the need to formulate a plan of action to find out if his job was secure and, if not, to find a new one. At the end of the week he felt more relaxed and was determined to take control of the situation. The psychiatrist recommended that he stop the medication but continue the counseling sessions a few more weeks. Within a month he was working at a new and better job.

In this case, a medication that took action very quickly was prescribed, and combined drug therapy and relatively simple counseling allowed the patient to calm down quickly and get his life under control. Long-term drug therapy was not necessary.

Table 4.

Are Psychiatric Drugs Habit-Forming?

DRUG CLASS	EXAMPLES	HABIT-FORMING	NOT HABIT-FORMING
Antidepressants[a]	Celexa		✓
	Zoloft		✓
	Effexor		✓
	Cymbalta		✓
Ampthetamines	Adderall	✓	
	Methylphenidate	✓	
Mood stabilizers	Lithium		✓
	Depakote		✓
	Lamictal		✓
Antianxiety drugs	Valium	✓	
	Librium	✓	
	Ativan	✓	
	BuSpar		✓
Sleeping pills	Ambien[b]		✓
	Sonata[b]		✓
	Lunesta[b]		✓
	Trazodone		✓

[a]If stopped abruptly, however, there can be an uncomfortable set of withdrawal symptoms.
[b]Some experts believe that there is evidence that these drugs can be habit-forming.

MEDIUM-LENGTH TREATMENT

After the death of her mother, a forty-six-year-old woman developed a deep depression that continued for several months. It quickly became apparent to her family and friends that the depression went beyond normal bereavement. The woman lost twenty pounds, slept only two or three hours a night, complained constantly of muscle pain and headache, and burst into tears almost daily at work. One day she explained to her husband that she was sure she was responsible for her mother's death, even though she fully recognized that her mother had died of an inoperable tumor. A psychiatrist placed the woman on an antidepressant. The medication caused side effects for the first two weeks, then the woman's husband noticed she was sleeping through the night and eating again. After four weeks she became noticeably less depressed, stopped complaining of physical ailments, and no longer cried at work. She asked the psychiatrist if she could stop taking the medication. The doctor advised her that the risk of relapse is relatively high during the six months after a depression has resolved. The patient remained on the antidepressant for six months and then discontinued use; she has remained free of depression.

Even though a patient may feel better after a few weeks on a medication, there is good evidence that for many psychiatric illnesses, at least six months of treatment is required to avoid relapse.

At the other extreme are situations in which medication should be taken indefinitely. Many such situations exist in other areas of medicine as well. We would not criticize the diabetic for taking insulin for the rest of her life; without it, she would die. Some people with high blood pressure or thyroid conditions take medications for years because the underlying illness can only be controlled, never cured, by the continuous use of drugs.

For some reason, however, many people are horrified by the idea of taking a psychiatric drug for many years. Nevertheless, the next description is of a patient for whom this was clearly necessary.

LONG-TERM TREATMENT

A well-known movie actor in his early thirties was brought to the emergency room in a coma after having ingested about one hundred of a friend's sleeping pills. Fortunately, his friend found him lying on the living room floor only a few minutes after he passed out and called an ambulance. His stomach was pumped and he was transferred to the intensive care unit. After more than twenty-four hours he woke up, angry that he had survived his suicide attempt. Friends told the hospital psychiatrist that the actor had been increasingly despondent during the last six months, but that before that he had exhibited the completely opposite behavior. In fact, prior to becoming depressed the actor had gone through six months of nonstop activity. He had been to five or six auditions a week, stayed up very late almost every night writing screenplays and letters, spent enormous amounts of money on clothes and gifts, and told everybody he was a sure shot for an Academy Award. He irritated even close friends with his nonstop talking and bragging, his drinking, and his quick temper.

The hospital psychiatrist called the actor's parents and learned that he had repeatedly exhibited such highs and lows since he was nineteen years old and that he had one previous serious suicide attempt. The parents revealed that the actor's older brother and one paternal uncle had similar problems. The psychiatrist easily diagnosed manic depression—now known officially as bipolar disorder—and recommended treatment with the mood-stabilizing drug lithium. Once it was established that lithium was helpful, the doctor recommended that the patient continue treatment at least five years, because the risk of a relapse, which might lead to a successful suicide attempt, far outweighed the inconvenience of taking the pills every day.

WHEN TO STOP DRUGS QUICKLY

There are three main reasons to stop a medication as soon as possible.

• If a drug does no good, it should be stopped. Patients and doctors should constantly ask themselves and each other what good the medicine is doing. It is wrong to keep taking pills when the symptoms persist.

• If a drug causes intolerable side effects, it should be stopped. For example, an antidepressant that cures a patient's depression but makes him so sleepy he cannot work or makes it impossible for him to have sex is simply substituting one set of problems for another. Usually it is possible to find a drug that alleviates a psychiatric problem without producing side effects worse than the illness.

• Some drugs are habit-forming (Table 4) and those drugs become harder to stop the longer they are used. This is especially true of some medications of the benzodiazepine class used to treat anxiety, for example, diazepam (Valium) and clorazepate (Tranxene), and most sleeping pills. Although these drugs are usually very safe and useful, it is best to discontinue use as soon as possible. Antidepressants (except amphetamines), lithium, and antipsychotic drugs are generally not habit-forming.

Prematurely stopping a psychiatric drug often leads to the return of symptoms. Patients with depression or panic attacks, for example, usually need to take the medication for at least six months to avoid relapse. Patients with schizophrenia or bipolar mood disorder may need to stay on the drugs the rest of their lives or risk very serious symptoms that necessitate hospitalization. Thus, you should ask your doctor if you can stop the medication. Do not give in to pressure from others who think that taking drugs reflects a "weakness" or "only covers up the problem" and stop taking the drugs too soon. The goal is to take the drug long enough to control the illness.

GETTING OFF PSYCHIATRIC DRUGS

After you and your doctor decide that you should stop taking a psychiatric drug, one word can usually sum up how to do it: slowly.

With few exceptions, it is always best to reduce the dose of a psychiatric drug over several days or even weeks, rather than stop abruptly. Stopping a drug too quickly may produce withdrawal or rebound symptoms.

Many changes occur in the brain and the rest of the body after medications have been taken for a long time. In a sense, the body gets used to the drug and makes changes to accommodate it. If you then withdraw a drug too quickly, your body may not have enough time to prepare for the change and may, therefore, react in what seems a chaotic way. For example, some drugs produce anticholinergic side effects. These drugs actively inhibit a part of the nervous system called the cholinergic nervous system. If the drug is stopped suddenly, the cholinergic nervous system loses its brakes and may overreact for several days. You'll feel as if you have the flu; there is discomfort but not danger.

The anticholinergic drugs with which this can be a problem include imipramine (Tofranil), amitriptyline (Elavil), doxepin (Sinequan), nortriptyline (Aventyl), protriptyline (Vivactil), desipramine (Norpramin), maprotiline (Ludiomil), clomipramine (Anafranil), phenelzine (Nardil), chlorpromazine (Thorazine), thioridazine (Mellaril), loxapine (Loxitane), and perphenazine (Trilafon).

Abruptly stopping the newer antidepressants—fluoxetine (Prozac), sertraline (Zoloft), paroxetine (Paxil), fluvoxamine (Luvox), venlafaxine (Effexor XR), and nefazodone (Serzone)—can produce dizziness, nausea, and "shocklike" sensations in the body. These are harmless but uncomfortable. The problem is especially noticeable with rapid discontinuation of Paxil, Luvox, and Effexor XR. Slow tapering is obviously recommended. Although some people who seem negative about psychiatric drugs in general have used this information to claim that these antidepressants are addictive, that is really a mischaracterization of the facts. Patients do not crave antidepressants the way a cocaine addict craves cocaine. Rather, there is an uncomfortable but not medically dangerous set of withdrawal symptoms that may motivate the patient to want to go back on the medication. With gradual tapering, most of these problems can be significantly reduced if not avoided altogether.

More uncomfortable is what happens if an antianxiety drug like Valium, Ativan, Xanax, Serax, or Librium is suddenly stopped. The whole nervous system may suddenly become very active. You develop a withdrawal syndrome with shakiness, anxiety, difficulty sleeping, ringing in the ears, and, very rarely, convulsions. (This is described in more detail in Chapter 8.)

The only psychiatric drugs that routinely cause serious withdrawal effects are the stimulant drugs very occasionally prescribed to treat depression that has not responded to other treatment and often prescribed to treat the adult version of attention-deficit/hyperactivity disorder. These drugs include amphetamines (for example, Dexedrine and Adderall) and the psychostimulants Ritalin, Concerta, Metadate, and Cylert. Abrupt cessation of stimulant drugs can cause severe, often suicidal, depression in adult patients. (The special factors to consider in deciding when to stop antipsychotic medications are discussed in Chapter 10.)

In this respect, psychiatric drugs are really no different from other medications. If you have been taking medication for high blood pressure for many years and stop taking it too quickly, your blood pressure can shoot way up, even higher than it was before you started taking the drug. After taking thyroid hormone medication for a few weeks, your own thyroid gland may completely shut down and stop producing hormone. Again, if you stop the thyroid medication abruptly, your thyroid gland may not have time to start working again, leaving you with no thyroid hormone at all.

Except in the case of emergencies or surgery with general anesthesia, there is usually no reason to discontinue a psychiatric drug suddenly. In general, the longer you have been on medication and the higher the dose, the longer it will take to safely stop it. The doctor usually outlines a schedule for gradual reduction of the dose of the drug, called a tapering schedule, until zero medication is reached. When this is done, there may be slight discomfort but rarely danger. Withdrawal syndromes usually disappear entirely within two weeks of the last dose.

This is why psychiatrists want you to tell them every time you change their dose of medication. I always warn patients not to stop a drug suddenly and to call me if they think they want or need to lower the dose.

Many patients taking psychiatric drugs worry about what will happen if they require emergency surgery. Suppose your appendix needs to be removed or a broken bone must be repaired in an operation. There would be no time to stop the psychiatric drug.

There is, fortunately, little need to worry. In these emergency situations, operations can almost always proceed safely. The anesthesiologist will have to work a bit harder to take into account the effects of the psychiatric drug on blood pressure, heart rate, and breathing during the surgery. Sometimes, the anesthesiologist stops the psychiatric drug and administers other medications to prevent drug withdrawal symptoms; at other times, the anesthesiologist continues the psychiatric drug and makes the necessary compensations during the operation. There is now convincing literature that in emergency situations, even patients taking monoamine oxidase inhibitor antidepressants—which have very important effects on blood pressure—can safely undergo general anesthesia and surgery.

Hospitalization to stop use of psychiatric drugs is rarely needed. However, a very small percentage of psychiatric patients abuse their medication, usually the benzodiazepine antianxiety drugs (for example, Valium and Librium) or the psychostimulants (Adderall abuse is becoming, in my observation, an increasingly severe problem among teenagers and college-age people), and take much higher doses than prescribed. These patients often see several different doctors at the same time. Each doctor writes a prescription, thinking he or she is the patient's only doctor. Patients who abuse benzodiazepines usually have alcohol and other drug abuse problems as well. Patients who take extremely high doses of benzodiazepines, such as 40 or 50 mg a day of Valium or 10 mg a day of Ativan, can still often be tapered off the drug as long as it is done very slowly. Some, however, cannot comply with the tapering regimen and are best hospitalized. This situation is rare and involves less than 1 percent of patients who are prescribed antianxiety drugs.

Part II

PSYCHIATRIC DRUG REFERENCE GUIDE

Chapter 7

Drugs Used to Treat Depression

No one should ever accept living with depression. In fact, it is now comparatively rare—although unfortunately not rare enough—for a depressed patient to be unable to realize substantial improvement through psychiatric treatment. One of the saddest things a doctor sees is a patient who has suffered from depression for years, believing the situation was "all my fault," "something I just needed to get over," or "the way things are in life—nothing is perfect."

Depression as an illness is extremely common. Good scientific studies indicate that a person has about a one in five chance of developing a depression serious enough to warrant treatment sometime in his or her lifetime. It is possible, although not certain, that having a parent or a first-degree relative with a history of depression may increase the lifetime risk of suffering a severe depression. Like red hair or blue eyes, various forms of depression, such as bipolar depression (formerly known as the depressed phase of manic-depressive illness), seem to run in families, and children show a higher risk of inheriting the gene from a parent with strong depressive tendencies. Some, but not all, research studies have indicated that the same may be true of a family history of alcoholism. Depression is about twice as common in women as in men, although the reason for this is still not clear. Finally, recent studies have identified some of the specific genes that seem to increase the risk for depression but also show that traumatic life experiences explain more of the reason why people become depressed than genes do.

Depression is very serious. This may sound simple, but I once saw an otherwise rather good article titled "Depression: The Common Cold of Psychiatry" in the magazine section of a Sunday newspaper. Although depression may be analogous to the common cold in terms of frequency of occurrence, the two are hardly similar in terms of severity and the headline seriously trivialized the illness. People get over colds with no lasting problems. Depression, on the other hand, can be fatal. The ominous complication of depression is, of course, suicide. Most suicides are committed by people who had a depression that should and could have been diagnosed. In this country, suicide remains a leading cause of death—third among all causes of death for people twenty-five to thirty-four years of age and tenth for adults overall. The highest risk group is elderly men, especially those with other medical problems. Teenage suicide is an increasing problem; even children commit suicide. Thus, depression must be taken seriously as a potential killer by patients, their families, and their doctors.

Even when it doesn't result in death, depression is an awful illness. The depressed person feels consistently down, blue, and sad. There is no glimmer of hope and everything that happens seems to be wrong. The patient with depression usually wishes he or she were dead and may voice these feelings, for example, "I wouldn't mind if a truck hit me." Appetite, concentration, sleep, and energy are usually grossly altered. In short, to be depressed is often to experience a living hell.

The decision to use drugs to treat depression depends largely on the answers to two questions: Does the patient have a form of depression that is likely to respond to medication? How quickly must the depression be relieved? Remember that there is now very good scientific evidence that certain forms of psychotherapy, particulary cognitive behavioral therapy (CBT) and interpersonal psychotherapy (IPT), are effective for depression. Some studies have shown that these forms of psychotherapy are just as effective as antidepressant medication, have fewer adverse side effects than medication, and have longer-lasting effects. Some studies have also suggested that the combination of medication and a scientifically proven psychotherapy is more effective than either intervention alone. Studies also suggest, although this is controversial, that medication is superior to psychotherapy for severe forms of depression. While this is not a book about psychotherapy, it is important to know these facts and to ask anyone recommending medication for you whether psychotherapy would be a reasonable alternative or should be combined with medication to get the best result.

DIFFERENT KINDS OF DEPRESSION

There are innumerable systems for classification of depression. Despite popular belief, depression comes in many varieties, with great variation in the associated symptoms. Unfortunately, many of the classification systems used by doctors are not especially helpful in deciding the best treatment for a particular patient. A number of terms used in the classification of depression are given in Table 5 so that you can gain some familiarity with these different systems; however, most of these terms have only limited usefulness. Furthermore, a person can suffer from several forms of depression at the same time.

The main distinction among different kinds of depression to remember is between major depression and dysthymia. Major depression refers to a classically defined syndrome in which a person becomes ill over a relatively short period of time, usually months, and gradually becomes incapacitated. Major depression tends to be episodic and recurrent. In its most serious form, major depression becomes psychotic depression when the patient has psychotic symptoms (such as hearing voices or delusions) along with depressed mood. When major depression occurs in someone who also has periods of mania, it is called bipolar depression. Dysthymia, on the other hand, refers to a chronic, low-grade depression that may be a lifelong problem. Patients with dysthymia are rarely incapacitated.

One more category to remember is atypical depression. Most people with major depression or dysthymia have characteristic changes in a number of areas. That is, they tend to have trouble sleeping and eating, and feel worse in the morning. It is also difficult to cheer them up. When a depressed person has these changes in the opposite direction—eats and sleeps too much, feels worse in the evening, and is able to be cheered up—we say he or she has depression with atypical features, or atypical depression.

In major depression, there is almost a complete loss of ability to derive pleasure from anything. Mood is no longer reactive; that is, no one or no event can cheer the patient up, even briefly. Assessing a patient as having a reactive or a nonreactive mood does not imply anything about the cause of the depression. By reactive mood is meant the capacity of the patient to be cheered up.

FEATURES OF MAJOR DEPRESSION

If you compliment someone with major depression, you'll find that your kind words fall on deaf ears. The person with major depression who suddenly gets good news will somehow attach a negative interpretation to it and never crack a smile. Everything that happens seems only to make these people feel more guilty, more worried, and sadder.

Along with this loss of mood reactivity and interest in life, someone with major depression usually exhibits a characteristic group of symptoms. First,

Table 5.

Some Terms Used to Classify Depression

TERM	DESCRIPTION
Unipolar	Depression that occurs in a person who never experiences manic highs
Bipolar[a]	Depression that occurs in a person who sometimes also experiences manic highs
Reactive	Depression that is supposedly caused by an obvious traumatic life event, like death of a family member or dismissal from a job
Endogenous	Depression that supposedly comes out of the blue, with no obvious cause
Primary	Depression that is unaccompanied by other psychiatric illness
Secondary	Depression that occurs after the onset of another illness, like alcoholism, drug dependency, or medical illness
Seasonal	Depression that regularly begins in the late fall when the length of day shortens and resolves in the spring
Postpartum	Depression that occurs in a woman who has recently had a baby; generally the same as major depression
Involutional	Depression that occurs in an elderly person; generally the same as major depression
Atypical[a]	Depression characterized by an ability to be cheered up by some things
Major[a]	Depression characterized by an inability to be cheered up
Dysthymia[a]	Low-grade, chronic depression
Psychotic[a]	Depression accompanied by hallucinations and/or delusions

[a]Clinically useful terms; see Table 6.

the person tends to have a sleep disturbance called early morning awakening: although often able to fall asleep without trouble, the person wakes up very early in the morning and finds himself or herself totally unable to fall asleep. There is loss of appetite, usually leading to some degree of weight loss, and difficulty concentrating. In trying to read a newspaper article, for

Table 6.

Features of Different Forms of Depression

	MAJOR	ATYPICAL	BIPOLAR	PSYCHOTIC	DYSTHYMIA
Reactive mood	No	Yes	No	No	Yes
Course	Episodic	Chronic	Episodic	Episodic	Chronic
Worst time of day	Morning	Evening	Morning	Morning	Evening
Appetite	Decreased	Increased	Increased or decreased	Decreased	Increased or decreased
Sleep	Disturbed (early morning awakening)	Increased	Increased or decreased	Decreased	Increased or decreased
Energy	Decreased	Very decreased	Extremely decreased	Decreased but agitated	Decreased
Psychotic signs	No	Very rarely	Sometimes	Always	No
Anxiety symptoms	Common	Common, especially panic attacks	Common	Common	Common
Hospitalization required	Sometimes	Occasionally	Often	Usually	No
Effective treatments	SRIs,[a] SNRIs,[b] cyclic antidepressants, electroconvulsive therapy	Monoamine oxidase inhibitors, SRIs,[a] psychotherapy	Lithium, Depakote, Lamictal, thyroid hormone, antidepressants	Antidepressants plus antipsychotic or electronvulsive therapy	SRIs,[a] SNRIs,[b] psychotherapy

[a]SRIs = Prozac, Zoloft, Paxil, Luvox, Serzone, Celexa, Lexapro
[b]SNRIs = Effexor XR, Cymbalta

example, the person with major depression may find that he or she reads and rereads the same paragraph five times and still can't follow the story. This problem can get so bad that the person appears to have dementia. The lack of concentration and difficulty remembering are sometimes called *pseudodementia*.

Major depression tends to occur in discrete episodes. The person is usually well and then slowly begins to show signs of depressed mood, loss of interest in life, and the other symptoms already described. Suicide is always a risk. An example of a person suffering from major depression follows:

Thomas is a very successful fifty-five-year-old businessman, who built his small investment company into a multimillion-dollar business. He has been happily married for almost thirty years and has three children who are happy and love him. About two months after his last birthday, Thomas began complaining of insomnia; he would wake up at three or four in the morning and then toss and turn without falling back asleep until the alarm clock went off. He began to lose weight and suffered from various aches and pains including headaches and stomachaches. His family doctor performed a thorough physical examination and blood tests; Thomas was the picture of physical health. Then he started to make mistakes at work, looked dreary and distracted to his coworkers, and lacked energy. His wife noticed that his usually robust sex drive had dwindled to complete lack of interest and that nothing, including visits from his children, favorable financial news, and his favorite hobbies, seemed to cheer him up.

One day, Thomas let slip to his wife, "I wonder how much longer I'll be able to go on?" He explained to her that he knew he was a "fraud" as a businessman, an inadequate husband and father, and a boring person. After much persuasion and pleading, Thomas was convinced to see a psychiatrist, who diagnosed major depressive disorder and recommended an antidepressant. Four weeks later, Thomas was again sleeping through the night, his appetite returned to normal, and he was noticeably more interested in life and more energetic.

FEATURES OF PSYCHOTIC DEPRESSION

Sometimes, major depression can become so severe that a person begins to show signs of psychosis. That is, he or she exhibits symptoms otherwise associated with diseases such as schizophrenia in which there is a major break with reality. So-called psychotic depression involves hallucinations—hearing or seeing things that are not really there—or delusions—false ideas that a person believes despite all reasonable attempts to convince him or her otherwise. A psychotically depressed person may hear a voice telling him that he is a bad person, has committed terrible crimes, or should die. These voices sound real, and he is sometimes surprised that no one else can hear them.

In typical delusions, a psychotically depressed person may believe that she has an incurable disease even though all medical tests are normal, that she has caused a terrible event like an automobile crash or a war, or that someone close to her has died even though the person is alive. It is important to emphasize that these hallucinations and delusions are all depressing in nature and quality; psychotically depressed people do not hear friendly or encouraging voices talking to them and they do not believe they are kings or presidents or millionaires.

Studies and clinical practice have indicated that major depression responds best to antidepressants of the serotonin reuptake inhibitor (SSRI), the serotonin norepinephrine reuptake inhibitor (SNRI), and the cyclic classes (described later in this chapter), and to electroconvulsive therapy (ECT) (discussed at the end of this chapter). When psychotic features coexist with major depression, an antipsychotic medication (for example, Risperdal or Zyprexa) is added to the antidepressant, or electroconvulsive therapy is given. Unless there is an urgent need to resolve the depression immediately, such as an extreme suicide threat or life-threatening weight loss, most psychiatrists treat the patient with major depression with an antidepressant first. If this treatment fails, a deicision is usually made either to switch to a different antidepressant or to add an "augmenting" agent, also discussed later. For so-called treatment refractory depression, that is, depression that does not respond to any medications or psychotherapies, electroconvulsive therapy is generally the next step. Recently, alternatives to ECT have emerged, including repetitive transcranial magnetic stimulation (rTMS) and vagal nerve stimulation (VNS). Antidepressants of the monoamine oxidase inhibitor (MAOI) class, including a new version that comes as a patch instead of a pill (Emsam, the selegiline patch), are prescribed by some experienced psychopharmacologists to patients whose depression does not respond to more traditional drugs. Finally, there is some evidence that the so-called morning after pill, RU-486 or mifepristone, may be an effective drug for psychotic depression, although much more testing is necessary before this can be used outside of experimental studies.

FEATURES OF BIPOLAR DEPRESSION

An episode of what seems to be major depression may actually be part of the illness now called bipolar disorder. People with bipolar disorder suffer from recurrent cycles of depression and mania. When they are depressed, they have most of the features of major depression, although sometimes they overeat and oversleep instead of experiencing insomnia and loss of appetite. The suicide rate during bipolar depression is extremely high. In addition to treatment with an antidepressant, people with bipolar depression should usually receive lithium, Depakote, or Lamictal (lamotrigine). Such treatment will help resolve the current depression and, more important, will greatly reduce the risk of future depressions and manic episodes.

It is important to distinguish bipolar or psychotic depression from major depression. Bipolar depression usually requires lithium or Depakote therapy or sometimes therapy with Lamictal (lamotrigine) or one of the atypical antipsychotic medications (such as Zyprexa or Abilify); psychotic depression requires antipsychotic medication along with the antidepressant. (Bipolar disorder and its treatment are described in more detail in Chapter 9.)

FEATURES OF DYSTHYMIA

Dysthymia is such a chronic condition that some people are not even aware that they have it. They have been depressed since childhood and, for them, depression has almost become a way of life. People with dysthymia are usually able to function at jobs and have social lives. They don't generally want to kill themselves, although they often entertain the thought that dying might not be such a bad thing. The main problem is that they are never happy or satisfied. They have difficulty finding meaning or interest in things and do not anticipate with pleasure or relish future events. Life for a person with dysthymia is generally filled with worry and fear. When people with dysthymia develop major depression, the situation is sometimes referred to as double depression. When the major depression is resolved, they return to their chronic, low-grade depressed mood. This is not a normal state of being and responds quite well to medication (and sometimes to psychotherapy also).

FEATURES OF ATYPICAL DEPRESSION

People with atypical depression maintain a reactive mood throughout their depression. Again, this has nothing to do with how deeply depressed they feel; their suffering is real. Rather, from time to time something good happens that temporarily cheers the person up to the point that he or she actually experiences pleasure. Unless this illness is treated, however, the depression usually returns all too quickly.

Many of the vegetative signs observed in major depression and dysthymia are reversed in atypical depression. People with atypical depression tend to overeat and oversleep. Some develop a particular craving for sweet food; others eat more because it seems to calm them down. Weight gain is not uncommon. People with atypical depression often have no trouble falling asleep or staying asleep; in fact, they sleep whenever they can, sometimes twelve to fourteen hours a day, including multiple naps. They may explain the sleeping as the only escape from feeling depressed.

Along with this oversleeping come a very pronounced decrease in energy and constant complaints of fatigue and lack of motivation. People with major depression usually feel worst in the morning; those with atypical depression find the end of the day hardest.

As already described, people with major depression seem oblivious to what is going on in the world. Nobody or nothing can make any difference in the relentlessly depressed mood. Atypical depression is often the complete opposite. These people feel as if they are entirely under the influence of external events. Everything that even hints of criticism or rejection immediately makes them feel horribly depressed and creates a desire to go to bed or even die. Praise and attention can temporarily lift their mood, which is why I think this illness is particularly common in performers who have the unique opportunity to get on stage, receive applause, and temporarily get better.

In his groundbreaking work on classifying depression, Donald F. Klein, M.D., likened the life of someone with atypical depression to being on a roller coaster. Getting attention is like taking a stimulant drug such as amphetamine or cocaine; there is a temporary high almost like euphoria, followed by a deep crash when the effect of the applause wears off. In fact, I have noted that many patients with atypical depression have used amphetamines or cocaine in the past and seem to get particular mood benefit from its use.

Again, unlike the discrete episodic nature of major depression, atypical depression seems to last for years and sometimes, if untreated, for a lifetime. Atypically depressed people may say they cannot remember a time in their life, going back to adolescence, when they did not feel depressed. Here is an example of a patient with atypical depression:

Marjorie is a thirty-four-year-old dermatologist with a successful practice and many hobbies and interests. She is highly regarded by her colleagues and patients. For as long as she can remember, however, she has been plagued by feeling "blue," lonely, and abandoned for periods lasting a few days to a few months. Many times she has contemplated talking to a therapist about this, but usually something has occurred to cheer her up. Most recently, for example, she became very depressed when a man she had been dating for three months ended their relationship. After hearing the news she stayed in bed an entire weekend, getting up only to binge on chocolate ice cream and peanut butter sandwiches. She alternated between crying and feeling murderously angry. Although she was able to go to work on Monday morning, she felt tired and listless. All of this changed, however, when a man she had met a few months before at a party called and asked her to dinner. A few hours later her mood was much better and she felt very energetic again.

The reason for spending so much time in making this distinction between major and atypical depression was more important before the widespread use of the SSRI and SNRI antidepressants. Cyclic antidepressant drugs, like Tofranil, Elavil, and Norpamin, were once the first-line treatments for major depression. They sometimes produced an improvement in patients with atypical depression, but clinical experience and some very good studies done in the 1970s and 1980s, especially by my late colleague Frederick Quitkin, M.D., showed that atypical depression responded better to monoamine oxidase inhibitor (MAOI) antidpressants like Nardil and Parnate than to the cylic antidepressants. Nowadays, cyclic antidepressants are rarely used as first-line agents, and drugs of the SSRI and SNRI classes seem to work equally well for both major and atypical depression. Hence, regardless of whether it is major or atypical, most psychiatrists will start the patient with depression with drugs like Celexa (citalopram), Zoloft (sertraline), Effexor XR (venlafaxine) or Cymbalta (duloxetine). Emsam, the new MAOI patch, may also catch on for some patients as an initial choice. For patients with atypical depression who do not respond to one of these first-line agents, however, consideration should be given to an MAOI.

Of course, no single individual's illness in any branch of clinical medicine is ever entirely pure. A patient with major depression may eat too much or may not have trouble sleeping, or a patient with atypical depression may feel worse in the morning than in the evening or actually lose his or her appetite. It is not uncommon for a person with a long history of atypical depression to develop major depression at some point. This is sometimes called "double depression." Hence, the differential diagnosis between the two, and consequently the decision about drug choice, is not always straightforward. A very careful history and description of symptoms and course of illness are clearly required.

SEASONAL DEPRESSION

Some people note that their depressions always seem to start in the late fall as the temperature drops and the length of daylight (technically known as the photoperiod) shortens. Often, but not always, their depressions take the form of atypical depression. With late spring and warmer temperatures and longer days, the depression goes away on its own. Some of these people actually find themselves getting on the high side during the summer and turn out to have bipolar disorder. Many people who think there is a seasonal pattern to their mood problems turn out to be wrong; a careful history shows that their depressions actually begin at different times of the year. But for those people who do really have seasonal depression, one very good treatment is daily exposure to a light box. (Light boxes can either be rented or bought from several companies.) The effective dose of light appears to be 10,000 lux, actually much less than a very sunny day, and the person is instructed to have the light box on, but not to gaze directly at it, for about thirty minutes every morning. People with seasonal depression usually begin this automatically around Thanksgiving and stop around Memorial Day.

DEPRESSION AFFECTING WOMEN ONLY

As mentioned earlier, major depression and dysthymia occur in women about twice as often as men. There are many theories for why this might be but no definitive explanations. Neverthess, these types of depression have the same features regardless of sex. On the other hand, there are at least three kinds of depression that are unique to women: depression related to the menstrual cycle, postpartum depression, and perimenopausal depression. Some women describe episodes of depression that routinely begin in the week or so before onset of menstruation, technically called the late-luteal phase of the menstrual cycle, and resolve once menstruation begins. Again, careful history is necessary because often a woman is under the impression that her depressive episodes are linked to the menstrual cycle but in fact occur at various times during the month. For patients who do have depressive episodes that are synchronized with the premenstrual period, a surprising finding is that they often respond to antidepressants like Zoloft (sertraline) or Celexa (citalopram) after just a few days of administration. For most patients with depression, it takes weeks for any antidepressant to work and the reason for this rapid response of premenstrual depression is unknown. Many women with this problem begin to take the antidepressant automatically about ten days before their periods to prevent depression altogether.

Postpartum depression occurs in three varieties. The most common is known as postpartum blues—a woman feels moody, let down, and irritable after delivering a baby. This usually responds to support and reassurance. True postpartum depression can occur anywhere from immediately after delivery to several months after childbirth. It resembles major depression in almost every way and, in addition to being a terrible ordeal for the new mother, can compromise her ability to bond with and care for her new baby. Antidepressant medication is usually highly effective for these women. Finally, psychotic postpartum depression is rare but a medical emergency. Women who develop psychotic postpartum depression often hear voices and have delusions that tell them that the new baby is defective or dangerous. The horrible stories in newspapers of women killing their newborn babies and themselves usually occur in women with psychotic postpartum depression. Most women who develop psychotic postpartum depression turn out to have bipolar disorder. Immediate intervention is necessary to protect the mother and baby from harm, often by hospitalizing the mother and administering antidepressant and antipsychotic medication. Later, mood stabilizers are often started if the woman indeed turns out to have bipolar disorder.

There has been great controversy about whether women who are about to enter or who have recently entered menopause have an elevated risk for depression. Studies vary on this, but it is probably sensible to be particularly on the alert for mood problems during the perimenopausal time. This does not mean that all or even most menopausal women have depression, but simply that it is possible that this is a time when the risk for developing depression is higher than other times in a woman's life. Depression during the perimenopausal period often responds to hormone replacement therapy, but this is controversial given recent studies suggesting that HRT increases the risk for serious health consequences. Consequently, when depression occurs during the perimenopausal period, it should be evaluated and treated like any other case of depression.

SEVERITY OF DEPRESSION

The second issue in deciding whether drug treatment is necessary for depression—how quickly must the depression be resolved—is really one of severity. Someone who has been depressed for more than two weeks, does not eat, cannot sleep beyond three in the morning, and constantly thinks of committing suicide should be treated with medication immediately. Remember that antidepressant medications usually work after four weeks, sometimes sooner, whereas psychotherapies may take months or longer, so it is important not to delay the start of treatment too long. On the other hand, someone who has an occasional bad day and once in a while gets into a bad mood probably won't respond to antidepressants and doesn't need them anyway. Patients who have tried various forms of psychotherapy and still feel depressed should seek consultation with a psychiatrist.

There are two basic rules of thumb. First, if a depression lasts longer than two weeks, interferes with the ability to function in school or at work, and disturbs vegetative functions like sleeping and eating, then drug treatment should be considered. Second, even when depression is clearly the product of some adverse life event, like loss of a job, death of a family member, or divorce, if mood does not improve with reassurance and support and persists over time, drug treatment should be considered. Studies have shown over and over again that these so-called reactive depressions actually do respond to antidepressants. Finally, whenever someone feels suicidal, there should be a psychopharmacologic consultation.

STEPS INVOLVED IN GETTING TREATMENT

Now let us suppose you and your doctor have decided that drug treatment of depression is a good idea. Here is what needs to be done.

1. Your psychiatrist should establish the type(s) of depression you are suffering from (major, dysthymia, bipolar, psychotic, atypical).

2. All possible medical causes of depression should be ruled out. Many medical conditions can masquerade as depression, including thyroid problems, certain types of cancer, neurological problems like small strokes that otherwise go unrecognized, HIV infection, and diseases of the immune system such as lupus. Some medications used to treat medical problems are also known to cause depression, including many drugs used to treat high blood pressure and steroid drugs like prednisone. Medical illness is more likely to be the cause of depression in elderly patients. A careful medical history is always needed, and sometimes a physical examination and laboratory tests are advisable. Some psychiatrists do these themselves; others request a consultation with an internist or a family practitioner. Remember, however, that most depressed patients do not have underlying medical problems. It is wrong to spend months undergoing complex medical tests to find the cause of depression. This only delays effective treatment.

3. Blood tests, X-rays, or other medical tests may be necessary either to help confirm that an underlying medical problem is causing your depression or that antidepressants are safe for you to take. However, none of these will

make a diagnosis of depression. Some people ask if they can have brain-imaging studies like PET, SPECT, or functional magnetic imaging scans to make or confirm a psychiatric diagnosis. While these are marvelous research tools for us to learn more about brain function in psychiatric illness, they cannot be used yet as diagnostic tests for an individual who may be suffering from any psychiatric illness. I believe that within the next decade that will begin to change and psychiatrists will indeed be able to order brain-imaging tests to help make a diagnosis, but not yet.

4. You and your doctor should discuss the exact drug recommended—the dose, the side effects, and when you should expect to start feeling better.

5. You should discuss with the psychiatrist whether medication alone is sufficient or if some form of psychotherapy along with the drugs will be beneficial. Make sure you are satisfied the doctor has thought about this carefully and given you a recommendation that makes sense for your own personal situation.

6. Make another appointment to see the doctor in about a week so your progress can be checked. Some suggested treatment plans for five different forms of depression are shown in Tables 7 to 11. Please remember that these are only blueprints: The treatment you need can be decided on only by you and your doctor.

REVIEW OF ANTIDEPRESSANTS

We are now ready to review all of the drugs used in the treatment of depression. These are divided into five classes: cyclic antidepressants; monoamine oxidase inhibitors; stimulants; the newer antidepressants (these are the drugs we actually prescribe most often for depression); and a category I will call psychostimulants which, among other uses, includes drugs used to boost the response to other antidepressants (Table 12).

CYCLIC ANTIDEPRESSANTS

Cyclic antidepressants were an important part of the "psychopharmacological revolution" in the late 1950s and 1960s when psychiatric drugs first became a major component of the treatment of mental illnesses. Nowadays, they have largely been replaced as first-line treatments for most types of depression. The newer medications, introduced in the late 1980s and early 1990s, beginning with Prozac, are safer than the cyclic antidepressants. However, none of the new drugs is more effective than cyclic antidepressants, and some studies suggest that for severe depression the cyclic antidepressants are more effective than the newer drugs. Hence, they still have a place but are usually reserved for patients who do not respond to a serotonin reuptake inhibitor (like Zoloft or Celexa) or to a serotonin norepinephrine reuptake inhibitor (like Effexor XR or Cymbalta).

IMIPRAMINE

Brand Names: Tofranil, Tofranil-PM.

Used For: Mostly major depression, also some of the anxiety disorders (see Chapter 8). In children, imipramine is used to treat bed-wetting (enuresis).

Do Not Use If: You have narrow-angle glaucoma, you have certain abnormal heart rhythms (your doctor will tell you if you have these), your prostate gland is very enlarged, or if you are given an antidepressant of the monoamine oxidase inhibitor class or some of the antidepressants of the serotonin reuptake inhibitor (SSRIs) class.

Tests to Take First: You may need an electrocardiogram first, especially if you are over age fifty.

Tests to Take While You Are on It: A blood test can tell how much of the drug is actually getting into your body. Called an imipramine level, this

---

Table 7.

Suggested Treatment Plan for Major Depression

1. Rule out underlying medical illness that may be causing depression.
2. Begin a serotonin reuptake inhibitor (SRI) such as Prozac, Celexa, Paxil, or Zoloft, or a serotonin norepinephrine reuptake inhibitor (SNRI) such as Effexor XR or Cymbalta.
3. Start at a low dose and gradually increase the dose to the therapeutic level.
4. Wait four to six weeks for a response. If there is no response, consider adding an augmenting agent like Wellbutrin (bupropion) or thyroid hormone, or switching to a different antidepressant.

test is necessary only if you are not responding to the usual dose of the drug and your doctor is considering an increase in dose.

Usual Dose: You will probably start between 25 and 75 mg a day and build up to 100–200 mg. Sometimes, psychiatrists prescribe 300 mg or more daily as long as side effects are not a problem. You should probably have an electrocardiogram before taking more than 300 mg. The entire day's medication can be taken in a single dose at bedtime.

How Long Until It Works: Usually after about four weeks of taking the drug daily. Sometimes, an effect is seen as early as two weeks; other

---

Table 8.

Suggested Treatment Plan for Bipolar Depression

1. Rule out underlying medical illnesses that may be causing depression.
2. Carefully evaluate for suicide potential; hospitalize if necessary.
3. Begin lithium, Depakote, or Lamictal and an antidepressant (an SRI or Wellbutrin).
4. Watch for development of signs of mania.
5. Stop the antidepressant as soon as the depression resolves, but remain on lithium, Lamictal, or Depakote indefinitely to prevent future depressions and manic episodes.

Table 9.

Suggested Treatment Plan for Psychotic Depression

1. Rule out underlying medical illnesses that may be causing depression.
2. Carefully evaluate for suicide potential; hospitalization often is advised.
3. Begin an antidepressant (Effexor XR or a cyclic antidepressant are good choices) and an antipsychotic drug (such as Trilafon or Risperdal).
4. Wait four to six weeks for a response. Stop the antipsychotic drug when the hallucinations and delusions are completely resolved.
5. If there is no response, consider electroconvulsive therapy.

Table 10.

Suggested Treatment Plan for Atypical Depression

1. Rule out underlying medical illnesses that may be causing depression.
2. Begin an SRI, SNRI, or Wellbutrin.
3. Start at a low dose and gradually increase the dose to the therapeutic level.
4. If the first medication does not work, even with augmenting agents, consider a monoamine oxidase inhibitor (Emsam, Nardil, Parnate, Marplan).

Table 11.

Suggested Treatment for Dysthymia

1. Consider psychotherapy *and* begin an SRI antidepressant (Prozac, Celexa, Zoloft) or SNRI (Effexor XR, Cymbalta) or Wellbutrin.
2. If no. 1 works, consider tapering off antidepressant after six months to a year and completing psychotherapy.
3. If no. 1 does not work, reevaluate psychotherapy and switch medications.
4. If dysthymia is still a problem, consider an MAOI.

times, it takes as long as six weeks. Usually, sleep and appetite return to normal before the actual depressed mood is alleviated.

Common Side Effects: The following effects occur in 10 percent or more of patients who take Tofranil: dry mouth, constipation, blurry vision, difficulty urinating, increased sensitivity to the sun, dizziness after standing up quickly, weight gain, increased sweating, drowsiness.

Less Common Side Effects: Confusion, agitation, memory impairment, nausea, changes in heart rhythm.

What to Do About Side Effects: Dry mouth—don't suck on hard candies containing sugar as you will ruin your teeth; try sugarless hard candies or mouthwash. Constipation—drink at least six glasses of water or juice daily. Laxatives may be prescribed. Blurry vision—normal vision usually returns in a couple of weeks, but a change in eyeglass prescription can help. Difficulty urinating—this problem is more frequent in men than women and can become a serious problem in older men; usually it is only annoying. The drug bethanechol (Urecholine) can be prescribed to counteract this effect. Increased sensitivity to the sun—use a very good sunblock with an SPF of at least 30 when out in the sun. You should do this even if you aren't taking imipramine. Dizziness after standing up quickly—this is caused by a brief drop in blood pressure. The best remedy is to sit down and get up slowly. In elderly people this side effect can be more serious and for that reason imipramine is not always the best antidepressant for people over age sixty-five. Weight gain—this can range from just a few pounds to twenty or more pounds. No one knows why imipramine does this and not a lot can be done except to diet. Severe weight gain is sometimes a reason to switch to a different antidepressant. Drowsiness—taking the whole dose at night, right before bedtime, minimizes daytime sleepiness. Less common side effects—these are generally a problem only in elderly people, in whom confusion, agitation, and memory impairment may necessitate switching to another drug. For younger patients these side effects are rarely of concern. (See Table 13 for a summary of the common side effects of cyclic antidepressants and remedies.) Most patients do not experience heart problems with imipramine, but the drug should almost never be given to a patient with a history of heart disease, including angina, heart attack, or arrhythmia.

If It Doesn't Work: After four to six weeks at a good dose (at least 200 mg), the doctor may first add another drug to try to increase imipramine's effectiveness. These are called augmenting agents and include thyroid hormone, lithium, Wellbutrin, psychostimulants (like Ritalin, Concerta, Adderall, and Mirapex), and atypical antipsychotic drugs (like Risperdal, Abilify, and Geodon). If this doesn't work, the doctor will probably recommend switching to another antidepressant.

If It Does Work: Once the depression is lifted, the patient is usually advised to keep taking the medication for six months, at which time the dose is reduced and then stopped over about two weeks. For patients with a history of three or more episodes of major depression, longer-term treatment is recommended. You should see your doctor about once a month for medication management, more often if there are other complications. Tofranil should be tapered rather than abruptly stopped to avoid withdrawal symptoms (similar to those of flu); however, Tofranil is not addictive and is easy to stop.

Cost: Generic imipramine is as effective and safe as the brand-name drug and costs a fraction of the brand name.

Special Comments: Imipramine was the first tricyclic (meaning "three-ringed") antidepressant introduced in the United States. It is a tried-and-true drug that is very effective in relieving major depression. It has relatively more side effects than some of the other drugs discussed here but is still sometimes used by psychopharmacology experts for patients with severe depression who do not respond to other medications.

DESIPRAMINE

Brand Names: Norpramin, Pertofrane.

Used For: Major depression.

Do Not Use If: You have narrow-angle glaucoma, you have certain abnormal heart rhythms (your doctor will tell you if you have these), your prostate gland is very enlarged, or if you are given an antidepressant of the monoamine oxidase inhibitor class or some of the antidepressants of the serotonin reuptake inhibitor (SSRIs) class.

Tests to Take First: You may need an electrocardiogram first, especially if you are over age fifty.

Tests to Take While You Are on It: A blood test can tell how much of the drug is actually getting into your body. Called a desipramine level, this test is necessary only if you are not responding to the usual dose of the drug and your doctor is considering an increase in dose.

Usual Dose: Usually starts at 25–75 mg a day and is increased over one to two weeks to about 200 mg. Doses up to 300 mg are often administered and occasionally doctors prescribe more than 300 mg. The entire day's medication can be taken in one dose at night.

How Long Until It Works: Usually after about four weeks of taking the drug daily. Sometimes an effect may be seen as early as two weeks and other times it takes as long as six weeks. Usually, sleep and appetite return to normal before the actual depressed mood is alleviated.

Common Side Effects: Dry mouth, constipation, difficulty urinating, blurry vision, increased sensitivity to the sun, weight gain, increased sweating, dizziness after standing up quickly. Side effects occur less frequently with desipramine than with imipramine.

Less Common Side Effects: Confusion, agitation, memory impairment, nausea. These side effects are the same as those for imipramine although less likely to occur. Changes in heart rhythm can be serious but usually occur only in people with a history of heart disease. Most patients do not experience heart problems with desipramine, but the drug should almost never be given to a patient with a history of heart disease, including angina, heart attack, or arrhythmia.

What to Do About Side Effects: Dry mouth—don't suck on hard candies containing sugar as you will ruin your teeth; try sugarless hard candies or mouthwash. Constipation—drink at least six glasses of water or juice

Table 12.

Checklist for Antidepressants

DRUG	USE	ANTICHOLINERGIC[a]	SEDATIVE	INSOMNIA	WEIGHT GAIN	DIZZINESS[b]	SEXUAL PROBLEMS	WITHDRAWAL PROBLEMS
Cyclic Antidepressants								
Tofranil	MD, PD, BD[c]	✓✓[d]	✓	✓	✓	✓✓	✓	✓
Norpramin	MD, PD, BD	✓		✓	✓	✓✓	✓	✓
Elavil	MD, PD, BD	✓✓✓	✓✓		✓✓	✓✓	✓	✓
Pamelor, Sinequan	MD, PD, BD	✓✓✓	✓✓	✓	✓✓	✓✓✓	✓	✓
Surmontil	MD	✓✓✓	✓✓	✓✓	✓	✓	✓	✓
Vivactil	MD, AD	✓✓✓				✓✓	✓	✓
Ludiomil	MD	✓	✓		✓	✓✓	✓	
Monoamine Oxidase Inhibitors								
Nardil	AD	✓	✓	✓	✓✓	✓✓✓	✓✓	✓
Parnate	AD			✓✓	✓✓✓	✓✓✓	✓✓	✓
Marplan	AD	✓	✓	✓✓	✓✓✓	✓✓✓	✓✓	✓
Emsam	AD			✓	✓		✓	✓
SRIs and SNRIs								
Prozac	MD, AD			✓✓	✓✓		✓✓	
Desyrel	MD		✓✓		✓	✓✓		

Wellbutrin	MD, BD			✓✓✓		✓✓✓	✓✓✓
Paxil	MD, AD			✓✓		✓✓	✓✓
Zoloft	MD, AD		✓	✓✓✓			✓
Serzone	MD, AD			✓		✓	✓✓
Effexor XR	MD, AD		✓	✓✓✓		✓✓	✓✓
Remeron	MD	✓✓	✓✓		✓	✓✓✓	✓✓
Celexa	MD, AD		✓				✓✓
Lexapro	MD, AD		✓✓				✓✓✓
Cymbalta	MD, AD		✓✓✓				✓✓
Stimulants							
Dexedrine	AD		✓✓	✓✓✓			✓✓✓
Ritalin	AD		✓✓✓				✓✓✓
Adderall	AD		✓✓				✓✓✓
Mirapex	AD		✓	✓	✓		✓

[a] Anticholinergic side effects are mainly dry mouth, constipation, blurry vision, and difficulty urinating.
[b] Refers to the drug's capacity to cause dizziness by lowering blood pressure.
[c] MD: major depression; PD: psychotic depression; BD: bipolar depression; AD: atypical depression and dysthymia.
[d] ✓: mild; ✓✓: moderate; ✓✓✓: a great deal.

Table 13.

Common Side Effects of Cyclic Antidepressants

SIDE EFFECT	SPECIAL PRECAUTIONS	POSSIBLE REMEDIES
Dry mouth[a]	Can cause tooth decay	Suck on sugarless hard candies, use mouthwash
Constipation[a]	Rarely causes complete inability to move bowels	Increase fluid intake, eat raw bran, take laxatives
Difficulty urinating[a]	Dangerous for men with enlarged prostate	Physician may add the drug bethanechol (Urecholine)
Blurry vision[a]	Not dangerous, but those drugs should never be given to patients with narrow-angle glaucoma	Usually transient, may require eyeglasses
Increased sensitivity to sun	Can lead to severe sunburn	Use sunblock when outside
Increased sweating	Mild dehydration in very hot weather	Increase fluid intake
Increased heart rate	Usually not a problem	Physician may want to check electrocardiogram
Weight gain	Usually only a few pounds, but can be more	Restrict calories

[a]These are called anticholinergic side effects.

daily. Laxatives may be prescribed. Blurry vision—normal vision usually returns in a couple of weeks, but a change in eyeglass prescription can help. Difficulty urinating—this problem is more frequent in men than women and can become a serious problem in older men. Usually it is only annoying. The drug bethanechol (Urecholine) can be prescribed to counteract this effect. Increased sensitivity to the sun—use a very good sunblock with an SPF of at least 30 when out in the sun. You should do this even if you aren't taking desipramine. Dizziness after standing up quickly—this is caused by a brief drop in blood pressure. The best remedy is to sit down and get up slowly. In elderly people this side effect can be more serious, and for that reason desipramine is not always the best antidepressant for people over age sixty-five. Weight gain—this can range from just a few pounds to twenty or more pounds. No one knows why desipramine does this and not a lot can be done except to diet. Severe weight gain is sometimes a reason to switch to a different antidepressant. Less common side effects—these are generally a problem only in elderly people, in whom confusion, agitation, and memory impairment may necessitate switching to another drug. For younger patients these side effects are rarely of concern.

If It Doesn't Work: After four to six weeks at a good dose (at least 200 mg), the doctor may first try adding another drug to try to increase desipramine's effectiveness. These are called augmenting agents and include thyroid hormone, lithium, Wellbutrin, psychostimulants (like Ritalin, Concerta, Adderall, and Mirapex), and atypical antipsychotic drugs (like Risperdal, Abilify, and Geodon). If this doesn't work, the doctor will probably recommend switching to another antidepressant.

If It Does Work: Once the depression is lifted, the patient is usually advised to keep taking the medication for six months, at which time it is reduced and then stopped over about two weeks. For people with a history of three or more episodes of major depression, longer-term treatment is recommended. You should see your doctor about once a month for medication management, more often if there are other complications. It is best to taper desipramine instead of abruptly stopping, but withdrawal symptoms are usually not a problem and it is easy to get off the drug.

Cost: Generic desipramine is every bit as safe and effective as brand name and is a fraction of the cost,

Special Comments: Desipramine is a derivative of imipramine. In fact, the body naturally turns imipramine into desipramine. Desipramine generally has milder side effects than imipramine, especially with respect to dry mouth, constipation, difficulty urinating, and blurry vision. For that reason, many clinicians and patients prefer it to imipramine. Desipramine has different chemical effects on the brain than imipramine and for that reason some psychiatrists believe it is less effective in some circumstances. The choice between imipramine and desipramine is often a toss-up. Like imipramine, desipramine is usually prescribed now only by psychopharmacology experts and only to patients with severe depression who have not responded to SSRI or SNRI medications.

AMITRIPTYLINE

Brand Names: Elavil, Endep.

Used For: Major depression, control of certain kinds of chronic pain.

Do Not Use If: You have narrow-angle glaucoma, you have certain abnormal heart rhythms (your doctor will tell you if you have these), your prostate gland is very enlarged, or if you are given an antidepressant of the monoamine oxidase inhibitor class or some of the antidepressants of the serotonin reuptake inhibitor (SSRIs) class.

Tests to Take First: You may need an electrocardiogram first, especially if you are over age fifty.

Tests to Take While You Are on It: None.

Usual Dose: Starts at 25–75 mg daily and is raised over one to two weeks to about 200 mg. Doses of 300 mg are often given and occasionally doctors prescribe higher doses. The entire day's medication can be taken in one dose at bedtime.

How Long Until It Works: Elavil is very sedating so a depressed patient with insomnia will experience an improvement in sleep after a day or two. The antidepressant effect takes two to six weeks, with appetite improving before alleviation of the depressed mood.

Common Side Effects: The following effects occur in at least 10 percent of patients who take Elavil: dry mouth, constipation, blurry vision, difficulty urinating, increased sensitivity to the sun, dizziness after standing up quickly, weight gain, sleepiness, increased sweating.

Less Common Side Effects: Confusion, agitation, memory impairment, and nausea are generally a problem only in elderly people who take Elavil. In older people these side effects may necessitate switching to another drug. For younger patients these side effects are rarely of concern. Changes in heart rhythm can be serious but usually occur only in people with a history of heart disease. Most patients do not experience heart problems with Elavil, but the drug should almost never be given to a patient with a history of heart disease, including angina, heart attack, or arrhythmia.

What to Do About Side Effects: Dry mouth—don't suck on hard candies containing sugar as you will ruin your teeth; try sugarless hard candies or mouthwash. Constipation—drink at least six glasses of water or juice daily.

Laxatives may be prescribed. Blurry vision—normal vision usually returns in a couple of weeks, but a change in eyeglass prescription can help. Difficulty urinating—this problem is more frequent in men than women and can become a serious problem in older men. Usually it is only annoying. The drug bethanechol (Urecholine) can be prescribed to counteract this effect. Increased sensitivity to the sun—use a very good sunblock with an SPF of at least 30 when out in the sun. You should do this even if you aren't taking Elavil. Dizziness after standing up quickly—this is caused by a brief drop in blood pressure. The best remedy is to sit down and get up slowly. In elderly people this side effect can be more serious and for that reason amitriptyline is not always the best antidepressant for people over age sixty-five. Weight gain—this can range from just a few pounds to twenty or more pounds. No one knows why Elavil does this and not a lot can be done except to diet. Severe weight gain is sometimes a reason to switch to a different antidepressant. Sleepiness or sedation—the best approach is to take the medication as close to bedtime as possible; however, many patients still complain of feeling drowsy during the day and this sometimes limits the drug's usefulness.

If It Doesn't Work: After four to six weeks at a good dose (at least 200 mg), the doctor may first try adding another drug to try to increase Elavil's effectiveness. These are called augmenting agents and include thyroid hormone, lithium, Wellbutrin, psychostimulants (like Ritalin, Concerta, Adderall, and Mirapex), and atypical antipsychotic drugs (like Risperdal, Abilify, and Geodon). If this doesn't work, the doctor will probably recommend switching to another antidepressant.

If It Does Work: Once the depression is lifted, it is usually recommended to keep taking the medication for six months, at which time it is reduced and stopped over about two weeks. For patients with a history of three or more episodes of depression, longer-term treatment is recommended. You should see your doctor about once a month for medication management, more often if there are other complications. Elavil should be tapered rather than abruptly stopped to avoid withdrawal symptoms (flulike symptoms); however, it is relatively easy to withdraw from this drug.

Cost: Generic amitriptyline is every bit as effective and as safe as brand-name Elavil and is a fraction of the cost.

Special Comments: The main difference between imipramine and Elavil is that Elavil has more side effects. It causes more dry mouth, constipation, blurry vision, and difficulty urinating than either imipramine or desipramine, and, unlike those two drugs, it makes patients feel sleepy. For patients with extreme agitation, the sedating property of Elavil is sometimes desirable. Older psychiatrists have a fondness for Elavil because it is very effective; in fact, it is unlikely that if antidepressants were systematically tested head to head any would prove more effective than

Elavil. Because of its many side effects and potential cardiac risks, however, it is now mostly prescribed only by experienced psychopharmacologists to patients with severe depression who have not responded to SSRI or SNRI antidepressants.

NORTRIPTYLINE

Brand Names: Aventyl, Pamelor.

Used For: Major depression.

Do Not Use If: You have narrow-angle glaucoma, certain heart rhythm irregularities that can be easily detected with a standard electrocardiogram (ECG), or a very enlarged prostate gland, or if you are given an antidepressant of the monoamine oxidase inhibitor class or some of the antidepressants of the serotonin reuptake inhibitor (SSRIs) class.

Tests to Take First: Your doctor may want you to have an ECG before starting the medication, especially if you are over fifty years old.

Tests to Take While You Are on It: In contrast to imipramine, desipramine, Elavil, and almost every other antidepressant, a blood test to determine the amount or level of nortriptyline in your body is almost always required. The reason is that nortriptyline is effective only when the amount of drug in the blood is maintained within a narrow range. If there is too little or too much, the drug will simply not work against depression. So the doctor usually requests a blood level a few weeks after you start taking nortriptyline to make sure that the dose is right. This has nothing to do with side effect control.

Usual Dose: Doses of nortriptyline are lower than those of imipramine, desipramine, and Elavil. The starting dose is between 10 and 25 mg and the usual therapeutic dose ranges from as low as 50–75 mg to as high as 150 mg. The blood level of the drug determines the dose the patient should take. The entire day's medication can be taken in a single dose at bedtime.

How Long Until It Works: On average, four weeks but sometimes as quickly as two weeks. Don't give up if it takes a little longer. Six weeks is long enough to know whether it will help.

Common Side Effects: Dry mouth occurs in about 20 percent of people who take nortriptyline. Unlike imipramine, desipramine, and Elavil, nortriptyline does not seem to lower blood pressure much when a person stands up quickly. Although this effect usually poses no problem for younger people, blood pressure drops can sometimes cause the elderly to pass out and fall. A few elderly people have sustained hip fractures while on cyclic antidepressants. Because this side effect occurs less often with nortriptyline, it is often recommended as the best cyclic antidepressant for elderly patients. Difficulty urinating, constipation, and blurry vision occur in 10 percent or less of patients who take nortriptyline. Weight gain and increased sensitivity to the sun can also occur.

Less Common Side Effects: Confusion, agitation, memory impairment, nausea. These side effects are the same as those for imipramine although less likely to occur. Changes in heart rhythm can be serious but usually occur only in patients with a history of heart disease. Most patients do not experience heart problems with nortripyline, but the drug should almost never be given to a patient with a history of heart disease, including angina, heart attack, or arrhythmia.

What to Do About Side Effects: Dry mouth—don't suck on hard candies containing sugar as you will ruin your teeth; try sugarless hard candies or mouthwash. Constipation—drink at least six glasses of water or juice daily. Laxatives may be prescribed. Blurry vision—normal vision usually returns in a couple of weeks, but a change in eyeglass prescription can help. Difficulty urinating—this problem is more frequent in men than women and can become a serious problem in older men. Usually it is only annoying. The drug bethanechol (Urecholine) can be prescribed to counteract this effect. Increased sensitivity to the sun—use a very good sunblock with an SPF of at least 30 when out in the sun. You should do this even if you aren't taking nortriptyline. Dizziness after standing up quickly—this is caused by a brief drop in blood pressure. The best remedy is to sit down and get up slowly. Weight gain—this ranges from just a few pounds to twenty or more pounds. No one knows why nortriptyline does this and not a lot can be done except to diet. Severe weight gain is sometimes a reason to switch to a different antidepressant. Less common side effects—these are generally a problem only in elderly people, in whom confusion, agitation, and memory impairment may necessitate switching to another drug. For younger patients these side effects are rarely of concern.

If It Doesn't Work: After four to six weeks at a therapeutic blood level, the doctor may first add another drug to try to increase nortriptyline's effectiveness. These are called augmenting agents and include thyroid hormone, lithium, Wellbutrin, psychostimulants (like Ritalin, Concerta, Adderall, and Mirapex), and atypical antipsychotic drugs (like Risperdal, Abilify, and Geodon). If this doesn't work, the doctor will probably recommend switching to another antidepressant.

If It Does Work: Once the depression is lifted, the patient is usually advised to keep taking the medication for six months, at which time it is reduced and then stopped over about two weeks. For people with a history of three or more episodes of depression, longer-term treatment is recommended. You should see your doctor about once a month for medication management, more often if there are other complications. Nortriptyline should be tapered instead of abruptly stopped to avoid withdrawal symptoms (flulike symptoms); however, nortriptyline causes very mild withdrawal and it is very easy to stop use.

Cost: Generic nortriptyline is every bit as safe and effective as the brand-name drug at a fraction of the cost.

Special Comments: Nortriptyline is the best of the cyclic drugs for elderly people with major depression who do not have certain specific heart problems, although it has generally been replaced by SSRIs and other newer drugs such as Remeron as the first-line antidepressant for older patients. The need to get blood levels a few times during treatment is only a minor inconvenience. Because the effective dose is lower for nortriptyline than for some of the other cyclic antidepressants, even younger people sometimes find it has fewer side effects.

DOXEPIN

Brand Names: Adapin, Sinequan.

Used For: Major depression.

Do Not Use If: You have narrow-angle glaucoma, a very enlarged prostate, certain heart rhythm abnormalities (your doctor will determine if this is an important consideration for you), or if you are given an antidepressant of the monoamine oxidase inhibitor class or some of the antidepressants of the serotonin reuptake inhibitor (SSRIs) class.

Tests to Take First: You may need an electrocardiogram first, especially if you are over age fifty.

Tests to Take While You Are on It: None at present.

Usual Dose: Starts at 25–75 mg daily and is raised over one to two weeks to about 200 mg. Doses of 300 mg are often given and occasionally doctors will prescribe even higher doses. The entire day's medication can be given as a single dose at bedtime.

How Long Until It Works: Sinequan is very sedating, so a depressed patient with insomnia will experience improved sleep after a day or two. The antidepressant effect takes two to six weeks, with appetite improving before alleviation of the depressed mood.

Common Side Effects: Dry mouth, constipation, blurry vision, difficulty urinating, increased sensitivity to the sun, dizziness after standing up quickly, weight gain, sleepiness, increased sweating.

Less Common Side Effects: Confusion, agitation, memory impairment, nausea. Generally a problem only in elderly people, in whom these side effects may necessitate switching to another drug. For younger patients these side effects are rarely of concern. Changes in heart rhythm can be serious but usually occur only in patients with a history of heart disease. Most patients do not experience heart problems with Sinequan, but the drug should almost never be given to a patient with a history of heart disease, including angina, heart attack, or arrhythmia.

What to Do About Side Effects: Dry mouth—don't suck on hard candies containing sugar as you will ruin your teeth; try sugarless hard candies or mouthwash. Constipation—drink at least six glasses of water or juice daily. Laxatives may be prescribed. Blurry vision—normal vision usually returns in a couple of weeks, but a change in eyeglass prescription can help. Difficulty urinating—this problem is more frequent in men than women and can become a serious problem in older men. Usually it is only annoying. The drug bethanechol (Urecholine) can be prescribed to counteract this effect. Increased sensitivity to the sun—use a very good sunblock with an SPF of at least 30 when out in the sun. You should do this even if you aren't taking doxepin. Dizziness after standing up quickly—this is caused by a brief drop in blood pressure. The best remedy is to sit down and get up slowly. In elderly people this side effect can be more serious and for that reason doxepin is not always the best antidepressant for people over age sixty-five. Weight gain—this ranges from just a few pounds to twenty or more pounds. No one knows why doxepin does this and not a lot can be done except to diet. Severe weight gain is sometimes a reason to switch to a different antidepressant. Sleepiness or sedation—the best approach is to take the medication as close to bedtime as possible; however, many patients still complain of feeling drowsy during the day and this sometimes limits the drug's usefulness.

If It Doesn't Work: An initial step if Sinequan doesn't work is to add one of the augmenting agents such as thyroid hormone, lithium, Wellbutrin, psychostimulants (like Ritalin, Concerta, Adderall, and Mirapex), and atypical antipsychotic agents (like Risperdal, Abilify, and Geodon). If this fails, a next strategy is usually to switch to a different antidepressant.

If It Does Work: Once the depression is lifted, the patient is usually advised to keep taking the medication for six months, at which time it is reduced and then stopped over about two weeks. For people with a history of three or more episodes of major depression, longer-term treatment is recommended. You should see your doctor about once a month for medication management, more often if there are other complications.

Cost: Generic doxepine is every bit as safe and effective as the brand-name drugs at a fraction of the cost.

Special Comments: Doxepin has an interesting history. It was originally advertised as having fewer important side effects than other cyclic antidepressants and was supposed to be especially gentle on the heart. This made it very popular. It turns out that doxepin really has no fewer heart-related side effects than the other cyclic antidepressants, but it does cause sedation, dizziness after standing quickly, and dry mouth. Many psychiatrists also insist it doesn't work all that well against depression. Consequently, it has fallen out of favor a great deal in recent years. Imipramine, desipramine, amitriptyline, and nortriptyline are better choices among the cyclic drugs.

TRIMIPRAMINE

Brand Name: Surmontil.

Used For: Major depression.

Do Not Use If: You have narrow-angle glaucoma, certain abnormal heart rhythms (your doctor will be able to tell you if you have these), a very enlarged prostate gland, or a history of seizures (epilepsy), or if you are given an antidepressant of the monoamine oxidase inhibitor class or some of the antidepressants of the serotonin reuptake inhibitor (SSRIs) class.

Tests to Take First: You may need an electrocardiogram first, especially if you are over age fifty.

Tests to Take While You Are on It: None required.

Usual Dose: Probably starts between 25 and 75 mg daily and builds up to 100–200 mg. Sometimes psychiatrists prescribe 300 mg or more daily as long as side effects are not a problem. You should probably have an electrocardiogram before taking doses greater than 300 mg.

How Long Until It Works: Usually after about four weeks of taking the drug daily. Sometimes an effect may be seen as early as two weeks; at other times, it takes as long as six weeks. Usually, sleep and appetite return to normal before alleviation of the depressed mood.

Common Side Effects: Dry mouth, constipation, blurry vision, difficulty urinating, increased sensitivity to the sun, dizziness after standing up quickly, weight gain, increased sweating, drowsiness.

Less Common Side Effects: Confusion, agitation, memory impairment, nausea. Changes in heart rhythm can be serious but usually occur only in people with a history of heart disease. Most patients do not experience heart problems with Surmontil, but the drug should almost never be given to a patient with a history of heart disease, including angina, heart attack, or arrhythmia.

What to Do About Side Effects: Dry mouth—don't suck on hard candies containing sugar as you will ruin your teeth; try sugarless hard candies or mouthwash. Constipation—drink at least six glasses of water or juice daily. Laxatives may be prescribed. Blurry vision—normal vision usually returns in a couple of weeks, but a change in eyeglass prescription can help. Difficulty urinating—this problem is more common in men than women and can become a serious problem in older men. Usually it is only annoying. The drug bethanechol (Urecholine) can be prescribed to counteract this effect. Increased sensitivity to the sun—use a very good sunblock with an SPF of at least 30 when out in the sun. You should do this even if you aren't taking trimipramine. Dizziness after standing up quickly—this is caused by a brief drop in blood pressure. The best remedy is to sit down and get up slowly. In elderly people this side effect can be more serious and for that reason trimipramine is not always the best antidepressant for people over age sixty-five. Weight gain—this ranges from just a few pounds to twenty or more pounds. No one knows why trimipramine does this and not a lot can be done except to diet. Severe weight gain is sometimes a reason to switch to a different antidepressant. Drowsiness—taking the whole dose at bedtime reduces the amount of daytime sleepiness, but some patients still feel drowsy during the day and prefer a different antidepressant. Less common side effects—these are generally a problem only in elderly people, in whom confusion, agitation, and memory impairment may necessitate switching to another drug. For younger patients these side effects are rarely of concern.

If It Doesn't Work: After four to six weeks at a good dose (at least 200 mg), the doctor may first add another drug to try to increase trimipramine's effectiveness. These are called augmenting agents and include thyroid hormone, lithium, Wellbutrin, psychostimulants (like Ritalin, Concerta, Adderall, and Mirapex), and atypical antipsychotic agents (like Risperdal, Abilify, and Geodon). If this doesn't work, the doctor will probably recommend switching to another antidepressant.

If It Does Work: Once the depression is lifted, the patient is usually advised to keep taking the medication for six months, at which time it is reduced and then stopped over about two weeks. For people with a history of three or more episodes of depression, longer-term treatment is recommended. You should see your doctor about once a month for medication management, more often if there are other complications.

Cost: After Surmontil went off patent, a generic form of the drug, known as trimipramine, was briefly made available. Then, for several years, no form of Surmontil was manufacturered. Recently, a small company began producing Surmontil, but there is no generic form available. Hence, this is a fairly expensive drug.

Special Comments: Obviously, trimipramine is pretty much the same as imipramine—a perfectly good antidepressant with no special features. Consequently, it never caught on much and is infrequently prescribed.

PROTRIPTYLINE

Brand Name: Vivactil.

Used For: Major depression.

Do Not Use If: You have narrow-angle glaucoma, certain heart rhythm abnormalities, very bad insomnia, an enlarged prostate, or if you are given an antidepressant of the monoamine oxidase inhibitor class or some of the antidepressants of the serotonin reuptake inhibitor (SSRIs) class.

Tests to Take First: If you are over fifty, and in certain other situations, your doctor will probably want an electrocardiogram first.

Tests to Take While You Are on It: None required.

Usual Dose: Starts at 5–10 mg daily and is increased to as high as 60 mg. It is best to take the medication in divided doses, one in the morning and one in the afternoon. Vivactil lasts a long time in the body, so even after stopping use, it will remain in the body for about a week.

How Long Until It Works: The antidepressant effect takes the usual four weeks that is common to all drugs in this class; however, this is a very "activating" drug and patients may feel a burst of energy from Vivactil after being on it only a few days.

Common Side Effects: Dry mouth, constipation, blurry vision, and difficulty urinating are especially common with Vivactil; increased sensitivity to the sun and dizziness after getting up quickly may occur. Vivactil also causes insomnia and may temporarily make a patient feel jittery or even anxious. It does not produce weight gain and may even induce a modest weight loss.

Less Common Side Effects: Confusion, agitation, memory impairment. Changes in heart rhythm can be serious but usually occur only in people with a history of heart disease. Most patients do not experience heart problems with Vivactil, but the drug should almost never be given to a patient with a history of heart disease, including angina, heart attack, or arrhythmia.

What to Do About Side Effects: Dry mouth—don't suck on hard candies containing sugar as you will ruin your teeth; try sugarless hard candies or mouthwash. Constipation—drink at least six glasses of water or juice daily. Laxatives may be prescribed. Blurry vision—normal vision usually returns in a couple of weeks, but a change in eyeglass prescription can help. Difficulty urinating—this problem is more common in men than women and can become a serious problem in older men. Usually it is only annoying. The drug bethanechol (Urecholine) can be prescribed to counteract this effect. Increased sensitivity to the sun—use a very good sunblock with an SPF of at least 30 when out in the sun. You should do this even if you aren't taking Vivactil. Dizziness after standing up quickly—this is caused by a brief drop in blood pressure. The best remedy is to sit down and get up slowly. In elderly people this side effect can be more serious. Less common side effects—these are generally a problem only in elderly people, in whom confusion, agitation, and memory impairment may necessitate switching to another drug. For younger patients these side effects are rarely of concern.

As mentioned earlier, Vivactil has unique side effects. The modest amount of weight loss is usually not regarded as a problem by most patients and nothing needs to be done about this. The occasional jitteriness and anxiety are temporary; tranquilizers can be prescribed, although this should be only for a week or less and in low doses. Insomnia can be a problem; patients complain it takes more than an hour to fall asleep and they wake up in the middle of the night. Taking the medication in the morning may help. Sleeping pills also help, but this is to be avoided whenever possible.

If It Doesn't Work: If Vivactil is not sufficiently effective after four weeks, many doctors will try to add a second drug to boost the response. These are called augmenting agents and include thyroid hormone, lithium, Wellbutrin, psychostimulants (like Ritalin, Concerta, Adderall, and Mirapex), and atypical antipsychotic agents (like Risperdal, Abilify, and Geodon). If this doesn't work, it is usually best to switch to a different medication.

If It Does Work: Once the depression is lifted, the patient is usually advised to keep taking the medication for six months, at which time it is reduced and then stopped over about two weeks. For people with a history of three or more episodes of depression, longer-term treatment is recommended. You should see your doctor about once a month for medication management, more often if there are other complications. It is best to taper off Vivactil rather than stop abruptly to minimize withdrawal symptoms (flulike symptoms); however, Vivactil is relatively easy to stop taking.

Cost: After several years of being totally unavailable in brand-name or generic forms, a small company has recently begun to manufacture Vivactil again. For a brand-name drug it is relatively inexpensive but still more expensive than generic antidepressants.

Special Comments: Vivactil isn't prescribed very much anymore because the side effects of dry mouth, constipation, urinary difficulties, and so on, are about the worst among the cyclic drugs and because some patients complain of anxiety. The one advantage it has over the other cyclic drugs is its "activating" property, which makes the patient feel more energetic and thus is not bad for someone with depression. It also doesn't produce weight gain. It has been suggested that Vivactil is similar to monoamine oxidase inhibitor antidepressants in having a particular effect in cases of atypical depression. Overall, Vivactil's advantages are usually outweighed by its disadvantages.

MAPROTILINE

Brand Name: None available. It used to be called Ludiomil but is no longer produced in brand-name form.

Used For: Major depression.

Do Not Use If: You have narrow-angle glaucoma, certain abnormal heart rhythms (your doctor will be able to tell you if you have these), a very enlarged prostate gland, or a history of seizures (epilepsy), or if you are given an antidepressant of the monoamine oxidase inhibitor class or some of the antidepressants of the serotonin reuptake inhibitor (SSRIs) class.

Tests to Take First: You may need an electrocardiogram first, especially if you are over age fifty.

Tests to Take While You Are on It: None required.

Usual Dose: Starts at about 50 mg daily and goes as high as 225 mg daily. Dose should not exceed 225 mg because this increases the risk of a seizure.

How Long Until It Works: Usually after about four weeks of taking the drug daily. Sometimes an effect may be seen as early as two weeks; at other times, it takes as long as six weeks. Usually, sleep and appetite return to normal before alleviation of depressed mood.

Common Side Effects: Dry mouth, constipation, increased sensitivity to the sun, dizziness after standing up quickly, weight gain, drowsiness. These side effects are pretty much the same as those for imipramine, although they may be slightly milder.

Less Common Side Effects: Confusion, agitation, memory impairment, nausea, difficulty urinating, blurry vision. These side effects are pretty much the same as those for imipramine, although they may be slightly milder. Although not common, convulsions may occur in about one in a thousand people. This risk is higher than that with other cyclic drugs. The risk is probably greater for patients with a history of seizures. Risk is reduced by keeping the dose below 225 mg. Changes in heart rhythm can be serious but usually occur only in people with a history of heart disease. Most patients do not experience heart problems with maprotiline, but the drug should almost never be given to a patient with a history of heart disease, including angina, heart attack, or arrhythmia.

What to Do About Side Effects: Dry mouth—don't suck on hard candies containing sugar as you will ruin your teeth; try sugarless hard candies or mouthwash. Constipation—drink at least six glasses of water or juice daily. Laxatives may be prescribed. Blurry vision—normal vision usually returns in a couple of weeks, but a change in eyeglass prescription can help. Increased sensitivity to the sun—use sunscreen with SPF of at least 30 when out in the sun. You should do this even if you aren't taking maprotiline.

Dizziness after standing up quickly—this is caused by a brief drop in blood pressure. The best remedy is to sit down and get up slowly. In elderly people this side effect can be more serious and for that reason maprotiline is not always the best antidepressant for people over age sixty-five. Drowsiness—taking the whole dose at bedtime should reduce daytime sleepiness. Weight gain—this ranges from just a few pounds to twenty or more pounds. No one knows why maprotiline does this and not a lot can be done except to diet. Less common side effects—these are generally a problem only in elderly people, in whom confusion, agitation, and memory impairment may necessitate switching to another drug. For younger patients these side effects are rarely of concern.

If It Doesn't Work: After four to six weeks at a good dose (not above 225 mg), the doctor may first try adding another drug to try to increase maprotiline's effectiveness. These are called augmenting agents and include thyroid hormone, lithium, Wellbutrin, psychostimulants (like Ritalin, Concerta, Adderall, and Mirapex), and atypical antipsychotic agents (like Risperdal, Abilify, and Geodon). If this doesn't work, the doctor will probably recommend switching to another antidepressant.

If It Does Work: Once the depression is lifted, the patient is usually advised to keep taking the medication for six months, at which time it is reduced and then stopped over about two weeks. For people with a history of three or more episodes of depression, longer-term treatment is recommended. During this maintenance period the dose should be kept below 200 mg/day. You should see your doctor about once a month for medication management, more often if there are other complications. Maprotiline should be tapered, not stopped abruptly, but it is not hard to stop.

Cost: Because only a generic form of maprotline is available, it is relatively inexpensive.

Special Comments: The chemical structure of all the cyclic drugs described so far has three rings, hence they are called tricylics. Maprotiline has four rings and so is called a tetracylic. The company that originally made maprotiline in its brand-name form, Ludiomil, emphasized its chemical composition in its advertising when it first released the drug onto the American market. As it turns out, this change in chemical structure does not make maprotiline act much differently in people than imipramine or the other tricylic drugs. Hence, it has nothing that distinguishes it from imipramine.

Summary of Cyclic Antidepressant Drugs

Imipramine (Tofranil), desipramine (Norpramin), amitriptyline (Elavil), and nortriptyline (Aventyl, Pamelor) are the standard drugs in this class. Of these four, amitriptyline has the most side effects and is probably the poorest choice for outpatients who want to keep on working and functioning without feeling sedated. Thus, when a cyclic antidepressant is called for, most psychiatrists will probably prescribe imipramine, desipramine, or nortriptyline, with a preference for nortriptyline in the elderly. Keep in mind, however, that the cyclic drugs have fallen to second place after the newer antidepressants listed later in this chapter. Because they are very effective, particularly for patients with severe depression, they are mainly used by specialists in psychopharmacology after a newer drug has failed to work.

MONOAMINE OXIDASE INHIBITORS

Every year when I was teaching residents in psychiatry, I would ask those at the beginning of their final year of training whether they had ever prescribed a monoamine oxidase inhibitor. In the last five or so years, the answer has been a unanimous no. This is unfortunate because there are instances, although fortunately not many these days, in which nothing else works. MAOIs are powerful antidepressants that produce dramatic improvement in some cases of depression. They also have many side effects and require a special diet. Therefore, these drugs should be prescribed only by a psychiatrist who is experienced in giving them to patients. My fear is that when my generation dies off, there won't be very many such doctors. I should add here that a newly available MAOI obtainable in a patch form, Emsam (selegiline patch), does not require the special diet at lower doses. More on this below.

Before describing the drugs in this class, it is important to explain the need for the special diet. MAOIs block or inhibit the work of an important brain chemical. (Readers interested in understanding more about this should read Chapter 21.) One of the consequences of the way these drugs work is that a person taking an MAOI will not be able to handle a substance called tyramine found in specific foods. After eating a tyramine-containing food, a person taking an MAOI can develop a very high level of tyramine, which can cause the blood pressure to soar out of control. This is called a "hypertensive crisis" and can cause severe headache, stiff neck, nausea, stroke, or even death.

To prevent a hypertensive crisis, certain foods and medications should be eliminated from the diet. The list of foods and drugs to avoid that I use is shown in Table 14, but you should ask your doctor for a complete explanation before taking an MAOI.

There are two main reasons for prescribing an MAOI:

Table 14.

Food and Drugs to Avoid While Taking Monoamine Oxidase Inhibitors[a]

Foods to Avoid
Cheese, except cottage cheese, cream cheese, and farmer cheese
Homemade yogurt (commercial yogurt is okay)
Aged meats and fish (e.g., aged corned beef, salami, fermented sausage, pepperoni, summer sausage, pickled herring, smoked lox)
Liver and liverwurst
Broad beans (Italian green beans, Chinese pea pods, English pea pods)
Bovril or Marmite yeast extract (baked products like bread and cake made with yeast are perfectly safe)
Meat tenderizers
Overripe bananas and banana skins
Red wine, Chianti, vermouth, liquors, beer, ale, sherry, cognac

Foods to Eat in Moderation
White wine and distilled alcoholic beverages (e.g., gin, vodka, whiskey)
Caffeinated drinks (coffee, tea, soda)
Avocados
Chocolate
Figs, raisins, dates
Soy sauce

Drugs to Avoid
Cocaine
Demerol (meperidine)
Cold medications (aspirin, ibuprofen, and acetaminophen are okay)
Other antidepressants
Buspirone (BuSpar)
Nasal decongestants (cromolyn sodium, Nasalcrom, Flovent, and Intal are okay, but check with your doctor before taking any allergy or asthma medications)
Sinus, allergy, hay fever, and asthma medications (check with your doctor, because some may be permitted)
Amphetamines
Diet pills
Local anesthetics containing epinephrine (your dentist can give you Novocain without epinephrine)

[a]Please review this with your doctor and make additions that he or she recommends.

1. Although some patients with atypical depression may improve on an SSRI, SNRI, or similar newer antidepressant, MAOI antidepressants probably work best for this kind of depression. Most psychiatrists will try an SSRI like Celexa or Zoloft, an SNRI like Effexor XR or Cymbalta, or Wellbutrin before an MAOI.

2. Many patients who do not respond to a six-week trial of an antidepressant will go on to have a good response to an MAOI.

The typical person placed on an MAOI has a long-standing depression, often dating to childhood or adolescence. These patients tend to function more or less adequately on a daily basis and are not generally candidates for emergency hospitalization. They are often unusually sensitive to criticism and rejection, complain of chronic fatigue and lethargy, overeat when they feel depressed, and sleep whenever possible. They also commonly are anxious and may experience panic attacks.

Nardil, Parnate, and Marplan are the MAOIs used for these people. Emsam, the selegiline patch, is too new to know if it will have the same effectiveness. Nardil causes more weight gain than Parnate, but Parnate disturbs sleep more than Nardil. Marplan seems to me to have the best side effect profile and to work about as well as Nardil and Parnate, but it is sometimes difficult to get and I am always nervous that a patient who is taking it will suddenly be unable to find a drugstore that carries it. In other respects, the medications are very similar, so the decision about which to take depends mainly on what side effects are more acceptable to the individual patient and with which drug the physician is more familiar. An interesting variant on the MAOIs is a drug called moclobemide, which is available only in Canada and Europe. It does not require a special diet but is also not as potent as Nardil and Parnate. MAOIs are also used to treat some anxiety disorders, as discussed in the next chapter. Now for the specific drugs in this class.

PHENELZINE

Brand Name: Nardil.

Used For: Atypical depression, major depression that has not responded to a cyclic antidepressant or newer antidepressant.

Do Not Use If: You do not think you can stick to the diet and medication restrictions (see Table 14), use cocaine (which may precipitate a hypertensive crisis), or ever have to take the painkilling drug meperidine (Demerol).

Tests to Take First: It is probably a good idea for the doctor to record your blood pressure before you start taking the drug to know how the drug affects it.

Tests to Take While You Are on It: There is a blood test that shows how effectively the drug is blocking the work of the brain chemical monoamine oxidase, which Nardil is supposed to inhibit. This is sometimes done if a person doesn't seem to be responding and the doctor wants to know if increasing the dose would be helpful. Usually, however, the simplest thing is to increase the dose and see what happens.

Usual Dose: Nardil is available in 15-mg tablets. The starting dose is usually one or two pills, taken either together or divided. The therapeutic dose can be 45 or 60 mg, but some patients need 90 mg or even higher doses to get a good response. After the first week or two, the whole day's dose can be taken at bedtime.

How Long Until It Works: At least two weeks, usually four weeks, and sometimes as long as six weeks.

Common Side Effects: Low blood pressure and dizziness after standing up fast (in at least 10 percent of patients); weight gain, sometimes as much as twenty pounds (in at least 10 percent of patients and probably more); swelling around the ankles from fluid retention; sleep disturbance, which can be insomnia for some people or sleepiness for others; trouble having an orgasm, for both men and women (in about 20 percent of patients). Tingling or shocklike sensations in the fingers and toes, nausea or diarrhea, and muscle twitching are also common side effects.

Less Common Side Effects: Hypertensive crisis is quite rare as long as the patient sticks to the dietary and medication restrictions. It is really not very hard to do this and very rarely does a patient object to these restrictions. Some of the side effects caused by the cyclic antidepressants—dry mouth, constipation, blurry vision, difficulty urinating—can also occur with Nardil but to a much smaller degree. Patients may experience a hypomanic (opposite of depression) high; they feel happy all the time, without a care in the world, and are very self-confident. They experience little need for sleep and have tremendous energy and a high sex drive. Some patients actually enjoy this effect, but those around them complain that they are irritable, intrusive, grandiose, and talk too much. Because patients may not identify hypomania as a problem, it is important to enlist the aid of a spouse, parent, sibling, close friend, or adult child to monitor the progress of the patient on phenelzine.

What to Do About Side Effects: Low blood pressure and dizziness—even younger people find these effects troublesome. The best remedies are to rise slowly from a lying or sitting position; avoid saunas and dehydration, which lower blood pressure further; and drink fluids throughout the day. Some doctors prescribe salt tablets or recommend extra salt intake during meals to keep blood pressure up. Special surgical stockings that compress the legs may also help, but most people hate to wear them. Finally, a pill called Florinef can be prescribed for a few weeks to keep blood pressure up. Occasionally, this side effect is bad enough to warrant stopping the drug. Weight gain—like low pressure, this side effect sometimes limits the ability of people to use Nardil. Calorie restrictions and exercise help. Most people lose the weight once they stop the drug. Swelling—fingers and ankles sometimes swell as a result of water retention. The swelling usually goes down; a water pill (called a diuretic) may help, but it may lower blood pressure further and should therefore be prescribed cautiously. Sleep disturbances—these usually level out in time. One strategy in battling insomnia is to take the medication in the morning. If sleepiness is the problem, the drug can be taken at bedtime. The daytime sleepiness sometimes caused by Nardil is difficult to eliminate but usually lasts only an hour or two in the afternoon. It is best to be cautious about prescribing sleeping pills to counteract insomnia, but this is sometimes the only solution. Avoid drinking a lot of coffee to counteract sedation. Trouble with orgasm—both men and women frequently complain that the length of time to orgasm is longer. As this effect usually goes away with time, patience is important. If it persists, lowering the dose may help. Hypertensive crisis—this can be avoided by following the prescribed diet. If dietary restrictions are violated and the blood pressure suddenly increases, the first symptom is usually a severe, throbbing headache. In this medical emergency, the patient should go to an emergency room immediately because rapid treatment can bring the blood pressure back down before anything serious happens. Some psychiatrists give patients a medication called nifedipine (Procardia, Adalat) to carry with them at all times. The patient is instructed to place a capsule under the tongue at the first sign of a headache. This can bring the blood pressure down again very quickly (see Table 15 to learn what to do if you get a headache) but also has resulted in some serious medical complications. Therefore, I do not recommend it but rather make sure that patients understand fully the seriousness of strict adherence to the dietary restrictions. Hypomania—the dose of the drug should be lowered or the drug stopped. Sometimes, counteracting medications are prescribed. Tingling and shocklike feelings—as a decrease in vitamin B_6 causes this effect, vitamin B_6 pills are usually administered.

If It Doesn't Work: There are several strategies available to the person who does not respond to Nardil after six weeks. Thyroid pills and lithium are sometimes added to boost the response. Some of the atypical antipsychotic drugs, like Risperdal, Zyprexa, Seroquel, and Geodon, may also work, but unlike with other classes of medications, it is not safe to add Wellbutrin or a psychostimulant (like Ritalin, Cogentin, Adderall, or Mirapex) to an MAOI. Very experienced psychiatrists may try to combine Nardil with

---

Table 15.

What to Do If You Have a Headache While on Monoamine Oxidase Inhibitors

1. Don't panic.
2. Call your doctor immediately.
3. Proceed to the nearest emergency room, preferably accompanied by another person.
4. Tell the staff in the emergency room you are on a monoamine oxidase inhibitor (Nardil, Parnate, Emsam [selegiline patch], or Marplan). They should check your blood pressure immediately, begin treatment if it is too high, and call your doctor.

---

other antidepressants, but this must be done with great caution. Patients should *never* do this on their own. Often, a failure to respond to Nardil means that more intense efforts at psychotherapy will be required.

If It Does Work: Nardil almost always works, so the major issue is usually coping with the side effects. Most patients find that the benefits of freedom from depression far outweigh the side effects. Patients on Nardil should be seen about once a month by the doctor and will usually need to raise and lower the dose many times to maintain as much freedom from side effects as possible without sacrificing the antidepressant effect. The usual rule of remaining on the drug at least six symptom-free months applies. Atypical depression, however, is often a chronic condition and some patients slump right back into depression when they try to stop the medicine. For that reason, many patients elect to stay on Nardil for years. There are no known long-term health risks.

Cost: Only the brand-name drug is available, making it fairly expensive.

Special Comments: From the list of side effects, patients may wonder who would be bold enough to try Nardil. But for people who get relief after years of chronic depression, the side effects are usually tolerable. MAOIs should be prescribed cautiously but not avoided when necessary.

TRANYLCYPROMINE

Brand Name: Parnate.

Used For: Atypical depression; major depression that has not responded to SSRI, SNRI, or other antidepressants.

Do Not Use If: You don't think you can stick to the diet and medication restrictions, suffer from severe insomnia, use cocaine, or need the painkilling drug meperidine (Demerol). (See table 14.)

Tests to Take First: It is probably a good idea for the doctor to record your blood pressure before you start taking the drug to know how the drug affects it.

Tests to Take While You Are on It: There is a blood test that shows how effectively the drug is blocking the work of the brain chemical monoamine oxidase, which Parnate is supposed to inhibit. This is sometimes done if a person doesn't seem to be responding and the doctor wants to know if increasing the dose would be helpful. Usually, however, the simplest thing is just to increase the dose and see what happens.

Usual Dose: Parnate comes in 10-mg tablets. The usual starting dose is one or two tablets. It may take from 30 mg to as much as 60 mg to get a good response. The dose should be raised slowly by about one pill every three to four days. It is usually taken as one or two doses in the morning or early afternoon.

How Long Until It Works: May be faster than Nardil, often about two weeks, but may take up to six weeks. Some people experience a "speeded-up," amphetaminelike effect first, but this passes in about a week.

Common Side Effects: Low blood pressure and dizziness after standing up quickly (more common than with Nardil); weight gain, but less than that with Nardil; swelling around the ankles from fluid retention; sleep disturbance (usually insomnia) that is often troublesome; trouble having an orgasm, for both men and women, but less than with Nardil. Tingling or shocklike sensations in the fingers and toes and muscle twitching are also side effects.

Less Common Side Effects: Hypertensive crisis is quite rare as long as the patient sticks to the dietary and medication restrictions. It is really not very hard to do this and very rarely does a patient object to these restrictions. Occasionally, hypertensive crisis has been reported with Parnate even when the dietary and medication restrictions were followed. Some of the side effects caused by the cyclic antidepressants—dry mouth, constipation, blurry vision, difficulty urinating—can also occur with Parnate but to a much smaller degree. Patients may experience a hypomanic (opposite of depression) high; they feel happy all the time, without a care in the world, and are very self-confident. They experience little need for sleep and have tremendous energy and a high sex drive. Some patients may actually enjoy this effect, but others around them complain that they are irritable, intrusive, and grandiose, and talk too much. Because patients may not identify hypomania as a problem, it is important to enlist the aid of a spouse, parent, sibling, close friend, or adult child to monitor the progress of someone on Parnate.

What to Do About Side Effects: Low blood pressure and dizziness—even younger people find these effects troublesome. The best remedies are to rise slowly from a lying or sitting position; avoid saunas and dehydration, which lower blood pressure further; and drink fluids throughout the day. Some doctors prescribe salt tablets or recommend extra salt intake during meals to keep blood pressure up. Special surgical stockings that compress the legs may also help, but most people hate to wear them. Finally, a pill called Florinef can be prescribed for a few weeks to keep the blood pressure up. Occasionally, this side effect is bad enough to warrant stopping the drug. Weight gain—like low blood pressure, this side effect sometimes limits the ability of people to use Parnate. It occurs less often with Parnate than with Nardil. Calorie restriction and exercise help. Most people lose the weight once they stop the drug. Swelling—fingers and ankles swell from water retention. The swelling usually goes down; a water pill (called a diuretic) may help, but it may lower blood pressure further and should therefore be prescribed cautiously. Sleep disturbances—these usually level out in time. Parnate often produces insomnia. The antidepressant Desyrel (trazodone), which is very sedating, is sometimes prescribed for the insomnia (50 mg at night). Some doctors prescribe sleeping pills (usually Ambien or Lunesta). Parnate should be taken early in the day, so taking one dose when you wake up and one in the afternoon or early evening at the latest is best. Trouble with orgasm—both men and women frequently complain that the length of time to orgasm is longer than usual, but this is less of a problem than with Nardil. As this effect usually goes away in time, patience is important. If it persists, lowering the dose can help. Hypertensive crisis—this can be avoided by following the prescribed diet. If dietary restrictions are violated and blood pressure suddenly increases, the first symptom is usually a severe, throbbing headache. Rarely, a patient on Parnate can have a hypertensive crisis even without violating the dietary restrictions. In this medical emergency, the patient should go to an emergency room immediately because rapid treatment can bring the blood pressure back down before anything serious occurs. Some psychiatrists give patients a medication called nifedipine (Procardia, Adalat) to carry with them at all times, but this also has resulted in some serious medical complications. Therefore, I do not recommend it but rather make sure that patients understand fully the seriousness of strict adherence to the dietary restrictions and agree to go right to the emergency room after calling me if they experience one of the symptoms of a hypertensive crisis (see Table 15 to learn more about what to do if you get a headache while on Parnate). Hypomania—the dose should be lowered or the drug stopped. Sometimes, counteracting medications are prescribed. Tingling or shocklike feelings—as a decrease in vitamin B_6 causes this effect, vitamin B_6 pills are usually administered.

If It Doesn't Work: Several strategies are available to the person who does not respond to Parnate after six weeks. Thyroid hormone or lithium is sometimes added to boost the response. Some of the atypical antipsychotic drugs, like Risperdal, Zyprexa, Seroquel, and Geodon, may also work, but unlike with other classes of medications it is not safe to add Wellbutrin or a psychostimulant (like Ritalin, Cogentin, Adderall, or Mirapex) to an MAOI. Very experienced psychiatrists may try to combine phenelzine with other antidepressants, but this must be done with great caution. Patients should *never* do this on their own. Often, a failure to respond to Parnate means that more intense efforts at psychotherapy are required.

If It Does Work: Parnate almost always works, so the major issue is usually coping with the side effects. Most patients find that the benefits of freedom from depression far outweigh the side effects. Patients on Parnate should be seen about once a month by the doctor; the dose usually needs to be raised and lowered many times to maintain as much freedom from side effects as possible without sacrificing the antidepressant effect. The usual rule of remaining on the drug at least six symptom-free months applies. Atypical depression, however, is often a chronic condition and some patients slump right back into depression when they try to stop the medicine. For that reason, many patients elect to stay on Parnate for years. There are no known long-term health risks.

Cost: No generic version is available, making Parnate relatively expensive.

Special Comments: Parnate is very similar to Nardil but tends to be more activating. Some people experience fewer side effects on it than with Nardil and some people experience more. A very thin person not too worried about weight gain might prefer Nardil; patients who feel sleepy and lethargic because of their depression may prefer Parnate. The MAOI special diet (see Table 14) is again of crucial importance.

ISOCARBOXAZID

Brand Name: Marplan.

Used For: Atypical depression, major depression that has not responded to a cyclic antidepressant or newer antidepressant.

Do Not Use If: You do not think you can stick to the diet and medication restrictions, use cocaine (which may precipitate a hypertensive crisis), or ever have to take the painkilling drug meperidine (Demerol; see Table 14).

Tests to Take First: It is probably a good idea for the doctor to record your blood pressure before you start taking the drug to know how the drug affects it.

Tests to Take While You Are on It: There is a blood test that shows how effectively the drug is blocking the work of the brain chemical monoamine oxidase, which Marplan is supposed to inhibit. This is sometimes done if a person doesn't seem to be responding and the doctor wants to know if increasing the dose would be helpful. Usually, however, the simplest thing is to increase the dose and see what happens.

Usual Dose: Marplan is available in 10-mg tablets. The starting dose is usually one or two pills, taken either together or divided. The therapeutic dose can be 30 or 60 mg. After the first week or two, the whole day's dose can be taken at bedtime.

How Long Until It Works: At least two weeks, usually four weeks, and sometimes as long as six weeks.

Common Side Effects: Low blood pressure and dizziness after standing up fast; weight gain, sometimes as much as twenty pounds (in at least 10 percent of patients and probably more); swelling around the ankles from fluid retention; sleep disturbance, which can be insomnia for some people or sleepiness for others; trouble having an orgasm, for both men and women (in about 20 percent of patients). Tingling or shocklike sensations in the fingers and toes, nausea or diarrhea, and muscle twitching are also common side effects.

Less Common Side Effects: Hypertensive crisis is quite rare as long as the patient sticks to the dietary and medication restrictions. It is really not very hard to do this and very rarely does a patient object to these restrictions. Some of the side effects caused by the cyclic antidepressants—dry mouth, constipation, blurry vision, difficulty urinating—can also occur with Marplan but to a much smaller degree. Patients may experience a hypomanic (opposite of depression) high; they feel happy all the time, without a care in the world, and are very self-confident. They experience little need for sleep and have tremendous energy and a high sex drive. Some patients actually enjoy this effect, but those around them complain that they are irritable, intrusive, grandiose, and talk too much. Because patients may not identify hypomania as a problem, it is important to enlist the aid of a spouse, parent, sibling, close friend, or adult child to monitor the progress of the patient on phenelzine.

What to Do About Side Effects: Low blood pressure and dizziness— even younger people find these effects troublesome. The best remedies are to rise slowly from a lying or sitting position; avoid saunas and dehydration, which lower blood pressure further; and drink fluids throughout the day. Some doctors prescribe salt tablets or recommend extra salt intake during meals to keep blood pressure up. Special surgical stockings that compress the legs may also help, but most people hate to wear them. Finally, a pill called Florinef can be prescribed for a few weeks to keep blood pressure up.

Occasionally, this side effect is bad enough to warrant stopping the drug. Weight gain—like low pressure, this side effect sometimes limits the ability of people to use Marplan. Calorie restrictions and exercise help. Most people lose the weight once they stop the drug. Swelling—fingers and ankles sometimes swell as a result of water retention. The swelling usually goes down; a water pill (called a diuretic) may help, but it may lower blood pressure further and should therefore be prescribed cautiously. Sleep disturbances—these usually level out in time. One strategy in battling insomnia is to take the medication in the morning. If sleepiness is the problem, the drug can be taken at bedtime. The daytime sleepiness sometimes caused by Marplan is difficult to eliminate but usually lasts only an hour or two in the afternoon. It is best to be cautious about prescribing sleeping pills to counteract insomnia, but this can sometimes be the only solution; avoid drinking a lot of coffee to counteract sedation. Trouble with orgasm— both men and women frequently complain that the length of time to orgasm is longer. As this effect usually goes away with time, patience is important. If it persists, lowering the dose may help. Hypertensive crisis— this can be avoided by following the prescribed diet. If dietary restrictions are violated and the blood pressure suddenly increases, the first symptom is usually a severe, throbbing headache. In this medical emergency, the patient should go to an emergency room immediately because prompt treatment can bring the blood pressure back down before anything serious happens. Some psychiatrists give patients a medication called nifedipine (Procardia, Adalat) to carry with them at all times. The patient is instructed to place a capsule under the tongue at the first sign of a headache. This can bring the blood pressure down again very quickly (see Table 15 to learn what to do if you get a headache) but also has resulted in some serious medical complications. Therefore, I do not recommend it but rather make sure that patients understand fully the seriousness of strict adherence to the dietary restrictions. Hypomania—the dose of the drug should be lowered or the drug stopped. Sometimes, counteracting medications are prescribed. Tingling and shock-like feelings—as a decrease in vitamin B_6 causes this effect, vitamin B_6 pills are usually administered.

If It Doesn't Work: There are several strategies available to the person who does not respond to Marplan after six weeks. Thyroid pills and lithium are sometimes added to boost the response. Some of the atypical antipsychotic drugs, like Risperdal, Zyprexa, Seroquel, and Geodon, may also work, but unlike with other classes of medications it is not safe to add Wellbutrin or a psychostimulant (like Ritalin, Cogentin, Adderall, or Mirapex) to an MAOI. Very experienced psychiatrists may try to combine Marplan with other antidepressants, but this must be done with great caution. Patients should *never* do this on their own. Often, a failure to respond to Marplan means that more intense efforts at psychotherapy will be required.

If It Does Work: Marplan usually works, so the major issue is mainly coping with the side effects. Most patients find that the benefits of freedom from depression far outweigh the side effects. Patients on Marplan should be seen about once a month by the doctor and will usually need to raise and lower the dose many times to maintain as much freedom from side effects as possible without sacrificing the antidepressant effect. The usual rule of remaining on the drug at least six symptom-free months applies. Atypical depression, however, is often a chronic condition and some patients slump right back into depression when they try to stop the medicine. For that reason, many patients elect to stay on Marplan for years. There are no known long-term health risks.

Cost: Only the brand-name drug is available, making it fairly expensive.

Special Comments: Marplan has come back on the market only in the last few years. It is my impression that its side effect profile is a bit less burdensome than Nardil or Parnate, and although I have treated only a few patients with it, it seems to be as effective. My concern has always been supply: It is manufactured by a small company and sometimes patients have found it hard to find even after checking with several pharmacies. From the list of side effects, patients may wonder who would be bold enough to try Marplan. But for people who get relief after years of chronic depression, the side effects are usually tolerable. MAOIs should be prescribed cautiously but not avoided when necessary.

SELEGILINE PATCH

Brand Name: Emsam.

Used For: Depression. Emsam (selegiline transdermal or selegiline patch) is a brand-new drug. Hence, it is not yet clear whether it is effective for particular types of depression or for depression in general. Only time and its use by many patients and their doctors will clarify this.

Do Not Use If: You do not think you can stick to the diet and medication restrictions, use cocaine (which may precipitate a hypertensive crisis), or ever have to take the painkilling drug meperidine (Demerol). Theoretically, these cautions apply only to patients using the 9-mg patch or higher; patients using only the 6-mg patch every day do not need to adhere to the MAOI dietary and drug restrictions. It is possible that this will turn out to be too conservative and that in the future higher strength patches will also not require the MAOI diet, but for now it is best to adhere to these recommendations.

Tests to Take First: It is probably a good idea for the doctor to record your blood pressure before you start taking the drug to know how the drug affects it.

Test to Take While You Are on It: None.

Usual Dose: Emsam comes in three patch strengths: 6, 9, and 12 mg. The patient starts by applying the 6-mg patch daily, the only strength that does not require the special MAOI diet at this time. After two weeks, if the response is not satisfactory, the dose can be raised to application of the 9-mg patch every day, and after two more weeks another increase to the 12-mg patch can be made.

How Long Until It Works: Again, the relative newness of Emsam makes it difficult to know for sure because sometimes there are surprises (pleasant or otherwise) after a new drug has been around for a while. For now, we will say at least two weeks, usually four weeks, and possibly six weeks.

Common Side Effects: Weight gain, dizziness upon standing up, lowered blood pressure, diarrhea, insomnia, headache, and rash or irritation around the patch application site.

Less Common Side Effects: It is currently recommended that patients who use patches with more than 6 mg of Emsam adhere to the MAOI diet to avoid hypertensive crisis. Hypertensive crisis is quite rare as long as the patient sticks to the dietary and medication restrictions. It is really not very hard to do this and very rarely does a patient object to these restrictions. Patients may experience a hypomanic (opposite of depression) high; they feel happy all the time, without a care in the world, and are very self-confident. They experience little need for sleep and have tremendous energy and a high sex drive. Some patients actually enjoy this effect, but those around them complain that they are irritable, intrusive, grandiose, and talk too much. Because patients may not identify hypomania as a problem, it is important to enlist the aid of a spouse, parent, sibling, close friend, or adult child to monitor the progress of the patient on Emsam.

What to Do About Side Effects: Most side effects appear to be mild, but again the drug is new and this is not a certainty yet. Because Emsam may lower blood pressure, some people will experience dizziness, particularly if they get up quickly from a sitting or lying position. It is best to get up slowly. Also, dehydration will make this worse, so drink plenty of fluids and do not restrict salt while you are on Emsam. It is probably best to avoid saunas as well. In the studies leading up to approval of Emsam, most patients took it for only a few weeks or months. Most patients with depression usually need to take medication for at least six months, and if a drug is going to cause weight gain, this is the period of time in which it usually becomes a problem. The only remedy is to cut calories and exercise. Sleep disturbance is usually mild, but the problem can be dealt with by the cautious use of sleeping pills like trazodone (Desyrel), Ambien, or Lunesta. If the skin becomes irritated underneath or around the patch, try moving the patch to different locations from day to day. Diarrhea and mild headache usually go away on their own but can be treated with the usual home remedies. Hypertensive crisis can be avoided by following the MAOI diet when the dose is greater than 6 mg daily. If dietary restrictions are violated and the blood pressure suddenly increases, the first symptom is usually a severe, throbbing headache. In this medical emergency, the patient should go to an emergency room immediately because prompt treatment can bring the blood pressure back down before anything serious happens. Some psychiatrists give patients a medication called nifedipine (Procardia, Adalat) to carry with them at all times. The patient is instructed to place a capsule under the tongue at the first sign of a headache. This can bring the blood pressure down again very quickly (see Table 15 to learn what to do if you get a headache) but also has resulted in some serious medical complications. Therefore, I do not recommend it but rather make sure that patients understand fully the seriousness of strict adherence to the dietary restrictions. If hypomania occurs, the dose of the drug should be lowered or the drug stopped. Sometimes, counteracting medications are prescribed.

If It Doesn't Work: If Emsam doesn't work, the doctor and patient face the same question as is the case when any antidepressant fails: augment or switch? Augmenting means adding a second drug to the first. In the case of an MAOI like Emsam, this can be thyroid hormone, lithium, or an atypical antipsychotic drug like Zyprexa, Seroquel, or Geodon. If this doesn't work, it is usually time to switch to a different treatment, including psychotherapy.

If It Does Work: This will depend a great deal on the type and duration of the depression. In general, for patients experiencing a first episode of major depression, the rule of thumb is to stay on the drug for at least six months from the time of response, then taper and cautiously observe for any signs of recurrence. For someone with a history of multiple episodes of major depression or with chronic forms of depression like dysthymia and atypical depression, much longer periods of taking medication are often desirable.

Cost: As no generic is available, Emsam is not cheap.

Special Comments: Selegiline was first introduced many years ago as a treatment for Parkinson's disease, for which it is still sometimes prescribed. Because it is an MAOI and because it was theorized that it might have a better side effect profile than the existing MAOIs (like Nardil, Parnate, and Marplan), many of us tried to give it to patients with depression and anxiety disorders. In general, however, it didn't work. The idea of putting it into a patch or transdermal preparation is intriguing. The risk for hypertensive crisis from traditional MAOIs comes from their inhibiting the breakdown of tyramine, an amino acid found in specific foods, in the gastrointestinal tract. By administering selegiline in the patch, it bypasses the stomach and intestines and therefore should not affect tyramine and hence should carry much less risk of hypertensive crisis. That does appear true for Emsam, but to be on the safe side, the FDA ruled that the drug company could recommend giving the drug without the MAOI dietary restriction only for the lowest dose, 6 mg per day. It may well be that 9 mg could also be safe without the diet, but that is not recommended now. The problem is that if Emsam really works, and that remains to be seen as we get more experience with it, many patients are likely to need higher doses and therefore they will have to be on the diet. The advantage of Emsam over the traditional monoamine oxidase inhibitors will be more mild side effects; the disadvantages will be the patch, which can irritate the skin and may not be to every patient's liking, and most important, the possibility that it won't be all that effective.

SSRIs, SNRIs, AND OTHER "MODERN" ANTIDEPRESSANTS

The drugs in this category were introduced into the American market in the late 1980s, starting with Prozac (fluoxetine). They include the medications that have entirely replaced cyclic antidepressants and monoamine oxidase inhibitors as the first-line treatment for depression and most of the anxiety disorders (including panic disorder, social phobia, obsessive-compulsive disorder, and post-traumatic stress disorder). They are safer than the older drugs and work just as well for most people. There are still instances in which the older drugs are necessary, but for the most part the only reason cyclics are still used is for patients with severe depression who don't respond to one of the newer medications (see Table 16). The same is true for the monoamine oxidase inhibitors.

It is hard to come up with a name that can be used to categorize all of these drugs. With one exception—Wellbutrin (bupropion)—the newer antidepressants all influence the brain chemical serotonin. Serotonin is now believed to be involved in depression and anxiety, and the new drugs increase the effectiveness of serotonin in the brain. In fact, several genes that work in the serotonin system have been shown to influence the risk for developing depression. I tend to call this group of drugs "new" or "modern" because they

Table 16.

What Illnesses Do the Newer Antidepressants Treat?

ILLNESS	PROZAC	PAXIL	ZOLOFT	LUVOX	EFFEXOR XR	SERZONE	WELLBUTRIN SR	CELEXA	LEXAPRO	CYMBALTA
Dysthymia	✓	✓	✓	✓	✓	✓	✓	✓	✓	✓
Atypical depression	✓	✓	✓	✓	✓	?	✓	✓	✓	✓
Bipolar depression (with mood stabilizer)	?	✓	✓	✓	✓	?	✓	✓	✓	✓
Psychotic depression (with antipsychotic)	✓	✓	✓	✓	✓	✓	?	✓	✓	✓
Panic disorder	✓	✓	✓	✓	✓	?	x	✓	✓	✓
Obsessive-compulsive disorder	✓	✓	✓	✓	?	?	x	✓	✓	✓
Social phobia	✓	✓	✓	✓	?	?	?	✓	✓	?
Post-traumatic stress disorder	✓	✓	✓	?	?	?	?	✓	✓	?
Bulimia	✓	✓	✓	?	?	?	x	?	?	?

Key: ✓=yes, x=no; ?=not known

are the ones we use today, even though Prozac is more than twenty-five years old and many of these medications are now available in generic forms (and should be thought of as the first ones to try). These include fluoxetine (Prozac), paroxetine (Paxil, Pexeva), sertraline (Zoloft), citalopram (Celexa), mirtazapine (Remeron), and bupropion 12-hour tablets (Wellbutrin SR). Some of the new drugs work exclusively on the serotonin system; they are called SSRIs, which stands for "selective serotonin reuptake inhibitors." The SSRIs available in the United States are Prozac (fluoxetine), Zoloft (sertraline), Paxil (paroxetine), Celexa (citalopram), Lexapro (escitalopram), and Luvox (fluvoxamine). Most of them are approved for anxiety disorders in addition to depression. Prozac, Zoloft, and Paxil are officially approved by the FDA for the treatment of depression and obsessive-compulsive disorder. Paxil is also approved for panic disorder, social anxiety disorder, post-traumatic stress disorder, and generalized anxiety disorder. Zoloft is approved for all of the anxiety disorders as Paxil and also for premenstrual dysphoric disorder. Prozac is approved for panic disorder and Lexapro is approved for generalized anxiety disorder. Luvox is approved only for obsessive-compulsive disorder, but it works for the other conditions as well. Four other newer antidepressants also affect serotonin, but not exclusively: Effexor XR (venlafaxine), Serzone (nefazodone), Cymbalta (duloxetine), and Remeron (mirtazapine). These are all indicated for depression and may be useful for some of the anxiety disorders as well. Effexor XR is indicated by FDA for the treatment of social anxiety disorder, generalized anxiety disorder, and panic disorder. Wellbutrin stands alone as the only newer antidepressant with no direct action on serotonin. It works mainly on noradrenaline.

The newer antidepressants have revolutionized the treatment of depression. It is not that they work better than the older drugs. In fact, in most studies they work exactly as well for depression and maybe a bit better for panic disorder than cyclics. The cyclic antidepressants seem to work better than the SSRIs for severe depression but are still not used first because of their risky side effects. What is important, however, is that the newer drugs are safer. The cyclics all have important effects on the heart and blood pressure, which for some can be dangerous (see Table 12). None of the newer antidepressants have dangerous side effects, although the issue of whether they increase the risk for suicide is an important caution that is discussed in a special section below. In fact, it is impossible to commit suicide by taking an overdose of any of them, something that is all too easy with cyclic overdoses. Because of this, the newer antidepressants can be safely prescribed to many patients who cannot take the older drugs. That has meant an increase in the number of people who now take antidepressants. Many have asked if we are treating too many people for depression with drugs these days. I am sure it is true that there are people who have been prescribed Prozac or Zoloft who don't have depression or an anxiety disorder and don't really need it. However, study after study continues to show that the majority of people in the United States who are suffering with clinically defined and treatable depression are actually not getting the help they need. Hence, for every person taking an antidepressant who shouldn't be, there are at least two more people who need one and aren't getting it. Once again, it is important to emphasize that the major reason for the increase in antidepressant prescriptions is that the newer drugs are safer and can be given to people with depression who previously had to be left untreated and depressed. The old argument that the newer drugs are being prescribed so often because drug companies promote them to doctors heavily no longer holds water because several newer drugs, including Prozac, Zoloft, Celexa, Paxil, Luvox, Remeron, and Wellbutrin SR, are no longer patented and have become fairly inexpensive. In fact, I feel strongly that in the majority of cases of depression, one of these antidpressants now available in generic form should be prescribed before any of the more expensive drugs like Lexapro, Effexor XR, Emsam, or Cymbalta.

This does not mean that the newer drugs are free of side effects or that everyone should take them just to see how they work. These are serious medications intended to treat real illnesses. They do produce side effects, even though, with the possible exception of a very small increased risk for suicide in the first few weeks, these are rarely dangerous and require careful monitoring by a physician. They are not to be taken to improve grades or make an investment banker "get an edge." They do nothing for people who do not have depression or an anxiety disorder except cause a stomachache or headache.

FLUOXETINE

Brand Name: Prozac.

Used For: All types of depression and several anxiety disorders, including panic disorder, obsessive-compulsive disorder, and social phobia. Also effective for the eating disorder bulimia.

Do Not Use If: You are bothered by severe insomnia or your weight is dangerously low (even these conditions do not always preclude the use of Prozac, which is a very safe drug) or you are taking a cyclic antidepressant or monoamine oxidase inhibitor. There are better choices than Prozac for patients with bipolar disorder who become depressed.

Tests to Take First: None, because there are no known medical problems that make taking Prozac a risk.

Tests to Take While You Are on It: None usually required. Very rarely, Prozac can have an effect on the way the kidneys handle sodium. If you experience sudden and severe weakness and lethargy while on Prozac, alert your doctor, who may order urine and blood tests. This side effect is more common in elderly patients.

Usual Dose: Prozac comes in 10- and 20-mg capsules and in liquid form. The manufacturer says that most people get the maximum antidepressant effect from just one 20-mg capsule daily. Many clinicians find, however, that an occasional patient needs a higher dose, and people seem to tolerate at least 80 mg daily fairly well. Other people may experience more side effects, such as agitation, at the higher doses. The drug has a long length of action; it takes several days for a single capsule to be completely eliminated from the body and Prozac can still be present in blood weeks after stopping it. This means that the whole dose can be taken once a day, usually in the morning. If for some reason 20 mg a day is too much, the patient may do well on one pill every other day.

How Long Until It Works: Some patients may start to feel better after two weeks, but the full antidepressant effect takes about four weeks.

Common Side Effects: Prozac clearly has fewer side effects than the previously available antidepressants. The major common side effects are difficulty having an orgasm; insomnia (trouble falling asleep or frequent awakening during the night); nausea, diarrhea, or stomach cramps; headache; weight gain; and nervousness.

Less Common Side Effects: Drowsiness, serious weight loss, hypomania (opposite of depression; patients become hyperactive, overly optimistic, and extremely talkative), and increased risk for suicidal thinking and suicide attempts in the first few weeks.

What to Do About Side Effects: Most of Prozac's side effects are mild and go away completely after the first week or two on the drug. The best thing to do about all the side effects is to wait, because they will probably disappear. Sleep problems are made easier by taking Prozac in the morning. Sleping pills like trazodone, Lunesta, or Ambien can be used if insomnia becomes a serious problem. Some people think the weight loss it promotes is actually a plus, but overweight people should not count on Prozac for weight reduction; the most lost is usually about five pounds in the first few weeks and it is almost always regained. In fact, many patients actually gain weight on Prozac after taking it for more than two months. If Prozac makes a patient very anxious, it is best to take 10 mg a day or 20 mg every other day. Antianxiety agents like Valium, Xanax, or Ativan can sometimes be cautiously added to help with this problem. When hypomania occurs, the dose is lowered or the drug is stopped temporarily. Sometimes, counteracting medication is necessary. The sexual side effects can be very bothersome. At least 40 percent of men and women have trouble achieving orgasm with Prozac, which may later lead to a decrease in sex drive. This side effect often goes away and responds to lowering the dose. However, in some cases this becomes a persistent problem and seems worse to the patient than the original depression. Some studies have shown that adding Wellbutrin SR helps with sexual side effects. But for some patients, switching to a different drug that does not cause sexual problems is the only answer.

If It Doesn't Work: Attempts can be made to boost the antidepressant response by adding other drugs if Prozac hasn't worked by six weeks and the dose has been pushed to 80 mg. These are called augmenting agents and include thyroid hormone, lithium, Wellbutrin, psychostimulants (like Ritalin, Concerta, Adderall, and Mirapex), and atypical antipsychotic agents (like Risperdal, Abilify, and Geodon). After that, it is probably best to try a different antidepressant.

If It Does Work: A patient should remain on Prozac for six months after relief from depression and then try to stop it. A patient with a history of three or more episodes of depression may benefit from longer-term treatment. A patient on 20 mg a day can stop abruptly; those on higher doses should taper off, but there is not much of a problem with withdrawal.

Cost: Generic Prozac (fluoxetine) is available, is every bit as good and as safe as the brand-name drug, and should always be selected.

Special Comments: Prozac seemed like a wonder drug when it was introduced in this country in 1988. It is safe and most people find the side effects quite tolerable. Indeed, it is the first antidepressant introduced since the 1970s that represented any kind of an advance. It is, like all of the newer antidepressants, far from perfect, however. Some patients say it makes them feel like they have been drinking black coffee all day. Others find that the problem in having an orgasm makes the treatment worse than the disease. Finally, as with all of the newer antidepressants, there is the persistent claim, which I believe to be partly true, that Prozac increases suicide risk in a very small number of patients. A few years ago there were proposals to make Prozac an over-the-counter drug because it was deemed to be so safe that a doctor's supervision was unnecessary. No one would advocate for this now. Prozac is a very useful drug, but it is not aspirin and needs careful monitoring by a knowledgeable physician.

SERTRALINE

Brand Name: Zoloft.

Used For: All types of depression, panic disorder, obsessive-compulsive disorder, post-traumatic stress disorder, social phobia, and premenstrual dysphoric disorder.

Do Not Use If: You are bothered by severe insomnia or your weight is dangerously low. However, even under these circumstances, Zoloft is sometimes well tolerated. Do not combine with a cyclic antidepressant without careful supervision or take with a monoamine oxidase inhibitor. Grapefruit juice may also increase the blood level of Zoloft. In general, it is a very safe drug.

Tests to Take First: None.

Tests to Take While You Are on It: Very rarely, Zoloft can have an effect on the way the kidneys handle sodium. If you experience sudden and severe weakness and lethargy while on Zoloft, alert your doctor, who may order urine and blood tests.

Usual Dose: Zoloft comes in 25-, 50-, and 100-mg tablets that are scored and can easily be cut in half. The advantage here over Prozac is that it is easier to be flexible with the dose because a patient can readily take half a pill if necessary. A disadvantage is that it can be tricky to pick the right dose. Most patients with depression are started at 50 mg, taken once in the morning. Patients with panic disorder should start at 25 mg, because they tend to be very sensitive to medications. In my experience, the usual dose for response is 100 mg to 200 mg daily, again taken all at once in the morning. Therefore, after a week at 50 mg it is reasonable to try to raise the dose to 100 mg for most patients. After that, if there is no response after one or two more weeks, the dose can be increased to as high as 200 mg daily. Patients with obsessive-compulsive disorder who are treated with Zoloft typically need doses at the high end of the scale, while patients with depression and panic disorder usually do well at about 100 mg.

How Long Until It Works: The full antidepressant effect usually takes four weeks to begin, but response can take as long as six weeks. Therefore, patients should stick with Zoloft for at least six weeks before deciding to try another treatment.

Common Side Effects: In general, Zoloft is a very well-tolerated drug. It is very safe from a medical point of view, with almost no effect on the heart, blood pressure, liver, or kidneys. Even people with medical illnesses can usually tolerate Zoloft, although it must be taken under careful supervision of a doctor. The side effects of Zoloft are very similar to those of Prozac. Some people get an upset stomach with nausea and diarrhea. Trouble falling asleep, headache, and shakiness can also occur. Some people describe the initial feeling they get from taking Zoloft as resembling drinking too much black coffee. Probably the most troublesome side effect, which is also a major problem with all of the SSRIs, involves sexual function. Both men and women frequently complain that it takes longer to achieve orgasm while taking Zoloft. Often, while depressed, patients have little interest in sex. When Zoloft starts to work, they feel better and their sex drive returns, but they find that orgasm becomes difficult. The delay in time to orgasm is probably due to Zoloft's effect on the serotonin system. This side effect is highly variable; not everyone gets it and when it does occur it can involve anything from just a little increase in the time it takes to have an orgasm to a complete inability to have one, something called anorgasmia. Often, this side effect disappears on its own.

Less Common Side Effects: Occasionally, people experience drowsiness from Zoloft. An increase in cholesterol level can occur in some people, although it is usually not enough to worry about. Weight gain seems a little less common with Zoloft than other SSRI antidepressants, especially Paxil, but can occur after several months. Like most antidepressants, Zoloft can induce a state called hypomania, which is the opposite of depression. A person with hypomania becomes almost euphoric with hyperactivity, irritability, boundless energy, and unrelenting optimism. Although this may sound attractive, the hypomanic patient typically makes a mess of things because of poor judgment and reckless behavior. Finally, Zoloft, like all of the newer antidepressants, may increase suicidal thinking in a small number of patients in the first few weeks.

What to Do About Side Effects: The side effects of Zoloft tend to be mild and may go away without any intervention. To combat stomach cramps, nausea, and diarrhea, the dose can temporarily be lowered or over-the-counter stomach remedies like Pepto-Bismol can be used for a brief time. Some patients have found that acidophilus tablets, which can be bought in a health food store, are helpful. Insomnia also tends to be a temporary side effect, often made less troublesome by taking Zoloft in the morning. If insomnia proves to be longer lasting, many clinicians have the patient take a low dose of the antidepressant trazodone (Desyrel)—about 50 mg—at bedtime. Trazodone is quite sedating but not as habit-forming as sleeping pills like Lunesta and Ambien. On the other hand, Desyrel lasts longer in the body than those sleeping pills and therefore is more likely to make the patient feel sleepy the next day. If Zoloft causes drowsiness, the first thing to check is whether it is making you feel sleepy during the day because you aren't sleeping at night. If that is the case, trazodone or a sleeping pill can be added at bedtime as described above. If the drug is really making a patient sleepy, it can be taken at bedtime, which sometimes helps. The side effects of shakiness and headache also usually disappear after a week or two, but if they are bothersome the dose can be lowered to as little as 25 mg until the patient adjusts to the medication. The sexual side effects can be hard to deal with. Again, this problem sometimes disappears on its own, so one approach is merely to wait for a few weeks to see if things get better. Several drugs have been touted as antidotes for sexual side effects from antidepressants, but except for some studies of Wellbutrin, none of them held up to rigorous testing. Finally, the solution to hypomania is usually to lower the dose or stop the medication immediately.

If It Doesn't Work: If Zoloft has not worked by six weeks and the dose has been raised to 200 mg, there are still things that can be tried to get a response. The most common strategy nowadays is to add another drug. These are called augmenting agents and include thyroid hormone, lithium, Wellbutrin, psychostimulants (like Ritalin, Concerta, Adderall, and Mirapex), and atypical antipsychotic agents (like Risperdal, Abilify, and Geodon). If this fails, it is usually time to try a different antidepressant.

If It Does Work: The current recommendation is that a first episode of depression should be treated with antidepressant medication for six months following response. For people with recurrent depression, currently defined as three or more episodes of depression in a lifetime, continuous antidepressant medication therapy is recommended. Thus, Zoloft should be continued for at least six months after a depressed patient responds. The same is true for people with panic disorder, obsessive-compulsive disorder, or social phobia. For patients with recurrent depression, however, it is advisable to continue medication for years because this is the best way to prevent recurrences. When it is time to stop Zoloft, it is important to taper the dose over about two weeks to prevent withdrawal symptoms of dizziness and nausea.

Cost: Generic sertraline is just as good as brand-name Zoloft and just as safe. It is also considerably cheaper. There is no reason to prescribe the brand-name drug.

Special Comments: Zoloft was the second drug in the SSRI (selective serotonin reuptake inhibitor) class of antidepressants introduced into the United States, after Prozac. The main difference between Zoloft and Prozac is in something called half-life. The body takes a long time to break down and eliminate Prozac; after the patient stops Prozac, it can still be detected in the blood for weeks. Zoloft has a much shorter half-life than Prozac, so that it can be eliminated in days rather than weeks. This makes a difference in two ways: If something goes wrong, such as a patient developing a rash on Prozac because of a drug allergy and the drug is stopped, the rash will last for quite a while as the liver continues to eliminate Prozac. A rash from Zoloft will go away much more quickly when the drug is stopped. Similarly, if a patient develops hypomania on Prozac and it is discontinued, the hypomanic state can last for weeks, while less than a week is more typical with Zoloft after it is discontinued. On the other hand, withdrawal effects, which include anxiety, insomnia, and shocklike sensations throughout the body, are worse when Zoloft is stopped abruptly than when Prozac is stopped abruptly because the latter tapers itself with its slow elimination from the body. If things are going well, it is hard to find much of a clinical difference between Zoloft and Prozac; both have relatively few side effects and work well for a variety of conditions.

PAROXETINE

Brand Names: Paxil, Paxil CR, Pexeva.

Used For: Depression and the anxiety disorders including panic disorder, obsessive-compulsive disorder, post-traumatic stress disorder (PTSD), generalized anxiety disorder, and social phobia.

Do Not Use If: There are very few conditions that absolutely mean you cannot take Paxil, but do not take it in combination with a tricyclic or monoamine oxidase inhibitor.

Tests to Take First: None.

Tests to Take While You Are on It: Very rarely, Paxil can have an effect on the way the kidneys handle sodium. If you experience sudden and severe weakness and lethargy while on Paxil, alert your doctor, who may order urine and blood tests.

Usual Dose: Paxil comes in 10- , 20- , 30- , and 40-mg tablets. Depressed patients can usually be started at 20 mg, taken in the morning. This is usually the dose that depressed patients respond to, although some need to take 30, 40, or even 50 mg a day. I recommend waiting four weeks at 20 mg to see if there is a response and raising the dose only if the patient has not gotten better. Patients with obsessive-compulsive disorder usually need high doses of medication, so 40 or 50 mg a day is not unusual. Patients with panic disorder, on the other hand, tend to be very sensitive to medication and are usually started on 10 mg; this is raised to 20 mg after a week and to 40 mg if 20 mg doesn't work.

How Long Until It Works: As with all antidepressants, response usually takes four weeks, although it may take as long as six weeks. Patients should stay on Paxil for at least six weeks before deciding to try a different drug or treatment.

Common Side Effects: Except for weight gain, sexual problems, and withdrawal effects, side effects of Paxil are usually mild and very much the same as those of Prozac or Zoloft. The most common are nervousness, insomnia, shakiness, and upset stomach with nausea or diarrhea. Paxil seems a little less likely than Prozac or Zoloft to cause the "black coffee" activation type of side effects in which the patient initially feels agitated. Some patients get a mild dry mouth. The biggest problem, as with Prozac and Zoloft, is an increase in the amount of time it takes to have an orgasm, experienced by both men and women. Sexual side effects are generally more common and more severe with Paxil than with any other newer antidepressant except

Effexor XR. Although not everyone gets this side effect, when it occurs it is at the very least a nuisance. Often, delayed orgasm simply goes away on its own. It is believed to be caused by Paxil's effect on the chemical serotonin, which the nervous system uses for a variety of normal functions. For some patients, this side effect is worse than the original depression and Paxil turns out to be a poor choice. Similar to the sexual side effects, weight gain is more of a problem with Paxil than with the other SSRIs. Finally, like Effexor XR, withdrawal effects, including anxiety, agitation, insomnia and shock-like feelings through the body, are more of a problem with Paxil than with other antidepressants.

Less Common Side Effects: Occasionally, patients feel drowsy while taking Paxil. The drug can also cause hypomania, as can almost any antidepressant. This is the opposite of depression—the patient experiences a very elevated mood, boundless energy, little need for sleep, and rapid thoughts. Hypomanic patients can be irritable and they can get themselves into trouble because of relentless optimism that leads to poor judgment and reckless behavior. As with all antidepressants, Paxil may increase the risk for suicidal thinking in a small number of patients during the first few weeks. This issue is discussed in a separate section below.

What to Do About Side Effects: Many of Paxil's side effects go away on their own. If they are initially too troublesome, the dose can be lowered until the patient adjusts to the medication. Gastrointestinal side effects can be treated with over-the-counter remedies like Pepto-Bismol. Some patients have found that taking acidophilus tablets from the health food store helps with the diarrhea that is sometimes caused by Paxil. If insomnia occurs, many clinicians now add the antidepressant trazodone (Desyrel) in low dose (about 50 mg) at bedtime. Trazodone is quite sedating but not as habit-forming as sleeping pills like Lunesta and Ambien, but it is also more likely to cause daytime drowsiness than these sleeping pills. Sexual side effects are difficult to treat, although again they often go away on their own, so sometimes patience is the best approach. Several medications have been recommended as antidotes to delayed orgasm caused by Paxil, but only the addition of Wellbutrin has stood up to rigorous testing. As mentioned above, sexual side effects can be particularly severe with Paxil, sometimes forcing the patient to switch to a different antidepresant. Drowsiness from Paxil is sometimes the result of the drug disturbing sleep at night, making the person feel sleepy during the day. If that happens, the solution might be to add trazodone or a sleeping pill at night to improve sleep. If Paxil is truly causing sleepiness, it can be taken at bedtime, which sometimes helps. Hypomania is treated by immediately lowering the dose or stopping Paxil. Weight gain is especially a problem with Paxil, usually not showing up until the patient has been on the medication for at least two months.

Calorie reduction and exercise are the best remedies but are not always effective. This problem sometimes means that a different antidepressant is better.

If It Doesn't Work: If there is no response to Paxil after six weeks, most clinicians now attempt to increase the drug effect by adding another medication to boost the response. These are called augmenting agents and include thyroid hormone, lithium, Wellbutrin, psychostimulants (like Ritalin, Concerta, Adderall, and Mirapex), and atypical antipsychotic agents (like Risperdal, Abilify, and Geodon). If this strategy does not work, it is usually time to switch to a different antidepressant. However, it is very important *never* to stop Paxil abruptly. The drug must always be tapered slowly, usually over a period of weeks.

If It Does Work: The current recommendation is to stay on an antidepressant for at least six months after responding. However, for people with recurrent depression, usually defined as having had three or more episodes of depression in a lifetime, it is increasingly recommended that antidepressants be continued indefinitely. This is because the relapse rate is very high for people with recurrent depression, but treatment with antidepressants clearly reduces this risk. It is important to note that when Paxil is discontinued, it should be tapered slowly and never stopped abruptly.

Cost: Generic paroxetine is every bit as effective and safe as brand-name Paxil or Paxil CR and cheaper. In my opinion, there is no advantage of Paxil CR over ordinary paroxetine.

Special Comments: Paxil was the third SSRI antidepressant introduced to the United States, after Prozac and Zoloft. Paxil may be less activating than Zoloft or Prozac so that patients who experience initial agitation from Prozac or Zoloft sometimes do better on Paxil. However, Paxil is associated with particularly severe sexual side effects, weight gain, and withdrawal problems and therefore is not my favorite antidepressant in most cases. Paxil CR (continuous release) is supposed to have fewer initial nausea side effects than regular Paxil. In fact, although nausea sometimes occurs with all antidepressants that affect the serotonin system, it is rarely a significant enough problem to make a patient want to stop the drug and almost always goes away in a week or two. Many people have called the "CR," "XR," and "SR" additions to drugs "patent extenders." That is, when a drug is about to go off patent and a company is going to face competition from a cheaper generic version, the company making the drug develops a "new and improved" version that it can get a new patent for and claim superiority over the original drug. In a very few cases this is true and the new formulation is better (Effexor XR and Wellbutrin SR are examples). In most cases, however, this is just a gimmick to allow the company to continue to profit from its medication. Paxil CR, in my opinion, is one of those instances.

CITALOPRAM

Brand Name: Celexa.

Used For: All types of depression and, although without official FDA indication in the United States, for most anxiety disorders (it does have approval for some of them by the European authorities).

Do Not Use If: There are very few situations that automatically mean Celexa is not a possiblility for your depression or anxiety disorder. In general, it is a very safe drug, but do not take it in combination with a monoamine oxidase inhibitor.

Tests to Take First: None.

Tests to Take While You Are on It: Very rarely, Celexa can have an effect on the way the kidneys handle sodium. If you experience sudden and severe weakness and lethargy while on Celexa, alert your doctor, who may order urine and blood tests.

Usual Dose: Celexa comes in 10-, 20-, and 40-mg tablets and in a liquid that is 10 mg per teaspoon. Most patients with depression are started at 20 mg, taken once in the morning or evening. Patients with panic disorder should start at 10 mg, because they tend to be very sensitive to medications. In my experience, the usual dose for response is 20–40 mg daily, again taken all at once. After four weeks at 20 mg it is reasonable to try to raise the dose to 40 mg if the response has not been satisfactory so far. After that, if there is no response after one or two more weeks, the dose can be increased to as high as 60 mg daily. Patients with obsessive-compulsive disorder who are treated with Celexa typically need doses at the high end of the scale, while patients with depression and panic disorder usually do well at about 20–40 mg.

How Long Until It Works: The full antidepressant effect can occur as early as two weeks but usually takes four weeks to begin, and response can take as long as six weeks. Therefore, patients should stick with Celexa for at least six weeks before deciding to try another treatment.

Common Side Effects: In general, Celexa is a very well-tolerated drug. In fact, in my opinion it is about the best tolerated of all the SSRI drugs, which include Prozac, Zoloft, Paxil, Luvox, and Lexapro. It is very safe from a medical point of view, with almost no effect on the heart, blood pressure, liver, or kidneys. Even people with medical illnesses can usually tolerate Celexa, although it must be taken under careful supervision of a doctor. The side effects of Celexa are usually mild and go away on their own. Initial nausea and diarrhea can sometimes occur. Trouble falling asleep, headache, and shakiness can also occur. Probably the most troublesome side effect, which is a major problem with all of the SSRIs, involves sexual function. There was a rumor floating around when Celexa was first introduced that it might have fewer sexual side effects than other serotonin reuptake inhibiting antidepressants, but that turned out to be wishful thinking. Both men and women frequently complain that it takes longer to achieve orgasm while taking Celexa. Often, while depressed, patients have little interest in sex. When Celexa starts to work they feel better and their sex drive returns, but they find that orgasm becomes difficult. The delay in time to orgasm is probably due to Celexa's effect on the serotonin system. This side effect is highly variable; not everyone gets it and when it does occur it can involve anything from just a little increase in the time it takes to have an orgasm to a complete inability to have one, something called anorgasmia. Often, this side effect disappears on its own. After taking Celexa for several months, weight gain occurs in many patients.

Less Common Side Effects: Occasionally, people experience drowsiness from Celexa. An increase in cholesterol level can occur in some people, although it is usually not enough to worry about. Like most antidepressants, Celexa can induce a state called hypomania, which is the opposite of depression. A person with hypomania becomes almost euphoric with hyperactivity, irritability, boundless energy, and unrelenting optimism. Although this may sound attractive, the hypomanic patient typically makes a mess of things because of poor judgment and reckless behavior. Finally, Celexa, like all of the newer antidepressants, may increase suicidal thinking in a small number of patients in the first few weeks.

What to Do About Side Effects: The side effects of Celexa tend to be mild and may go away without any intervention. To combat stomach cramps, nausea, and diarrhea, the dose can temporarily be lowered or over-the-counter stomach remedies like Pepto-Bismol can be used for a brief time. Some patients have found that acidophilus tablets, which can be bought in a health food store, are helpful. Insomnia also tends to be a temporary side effect, often made less troublesome by taking Celexa in the morning. If insomnia proves to be longer lasting, many clinicians have the patient take a low dose of the antidepressant trazodone (Desyrel)—about 50 mg—at bedtime. Trazodone is quite sedating but not as habit-forming as sleeping pills like Lunesta and Ambien. On the other hand, Desyrel lasts longer in the body than those sleeping pills and therefore is more likely to make the patient feel sleepy the next day. The side effects of shakiness and headache also usually disappear after a week or two, but if they are bothersome the dose can be lowered to as little as 10 mg until the patient adjusts to the medication. If Celexa causes drowsiness, the first thing to check is whether it is making you feel sleepy during the day because you aren't sleeping at night. If that is the case, trazodone or a sleeping pill can be added at bedtime as described above. If the drug is really making a patient sleepy, it can be taken at bedtime, which sometimes helps. Sexual side effects and weight gain, although milder than with Paxil, are still very hard to overcome. The sexual side effects sometimes go away on their own or respond to lowering the dose (as long as that doesn't make the depression come back). Many antidotes to sexual side effects have been described, but only adding Wellbutrin has held up in a few studies to rigorous testing. Weight gain is highly variable; lowering calories and exercise help. Finally, the solution to hypomania is usually to lower the dose or stop the medication immediately.

If It Doesn't Work: If Celexa has not worked by six weeks and the dose has been raised to 60 mg, there are still things that can be tried to get a response. The most common strategy nowadays is to add another drug. These are called augmenting agents and include thyroid hormone, lithium, Wellbutrin, psychostimulants (like Ritalin, Concerta, Adderall, and Mirapex), and atypical antipsychotic agents (like Risperdal, Abilify, and Geodon). If this fails, it is usually time to try a different antidepressant. Although not as bad as with Paxil or Effexor XR, there can be withdrawal effects if Celexa is stopped abruptly; they include agitation, anxiety, insomnia and shocklike sensations through the body. Celexa should be tapered slowly when it is time to stop it.

If It Does Work: The current recommendation is that a first episode of depression should be treated with antidepressant medication for six months following response. For people with recurrent depression, currently defined as three or more episodes of depression in a lifetime, continuous antidepressant medication therapy is recommended. Thus, Celexa should be continued for at least six months after a depressed patient responds. The same is true for people with panic disorder, obsessive-compulsive disorder, or social phobia. For patients with recurrent depression, however, it is advisable to continue medication for years because this is the best way to prevent recurrences. When it is time to stop Celexa, it is important to taper the dose over about two weeks to prevent withdrawal symptoms.

Cost: Generic citalopram is just as good as brand-name Celexa and just as safe. It is also considerably cheaper. There is no reason to prescribe the brand-name drug.

Special Comments: Before being introduced to the United States, Celexa was a popular antidepressant with Europen physicians. They often claimed that it worked at least as well as the other SSRIs, with fewer side effects. Nevertheless, many people wondered why the company wanted to expend all the effort and money to bring it to the United States, where it would have to go up against the three commercial blockbusters Prozac, Zoloft, and Paxil and enter a fiercely competitive market. In fact, Celexa sales took off and it became a much prescribed antidepressant. Celexa is not really that much different from the first three SSRIs, but it is probably a bit better tolerated, certainly causes less weight gain and has fewer sexual side effects and withdrawal effects than Paxil, has a shorter length of action than Prozac so that if something goes wrong (like a drug allergy or hypomania) it can be stopped and doesn't last in the body for weeks, and may be a bit less activating than Zoloft. All things considered, now that an inexpensive generic preparation is available, I generally start almost all depressed and anxiety disorder patients on generic citalopram as the first choice.

ESCITALOPRAM

Brand Name: Lexapro.

Used For: All types of depression and generalized anxiety disorder (GAD).

Do Not Use If: There are very few situations that automatically mean Lexapro is not a possiblility for your depression or anxiety disorder. In general, it is a very safe drug, but do not combine it with a monoamine oxidase inhibitor.

Tests to Take First: None.

Tests to Take While You Are on It: Very rarely, Lexapro can have an effect on the way the kidneys handle sodium. If you experience sudden and severe weakness and lethargy while on Lexapro, alert your doctor, who may order urine and blood tests.

Usual Dose: Lexapro comes in 5-, 10-, and 20-mg tablets and in a liquid that is 5 mg per teaspoon. Most patients with depression are started at 10 mg, taken once in the morning or evening. Patients with panic disorder or GAD should start at 5 mg, because they tend to be very sensitive to medications. In my experience, the usual dose for response is 10–20 mg daily, again taken all at once. After four weeks at 10 mg it is reasonable to try to raise the dose to 20 mg if the response has not been satisfactory so far.

How Long Until It Works: The full antidepressant effect can occur as early as two weeks but usually takes four weeks to begin, and response can take as long as six weeks. Therefore, patients should stick with Lexapro for at least six weeks before deciding to try another treatment.

Common Side Effects: In general, Lexparo, which is just a variant of Celexa, is a very well-tolerated drug. It is very safe from a medical point of view, with almost no effect on the heart, blood pressure, liver, or kidneys. Even people with medical illnesses can usually tolerate Lexapro, although it must be taken under careful supervision of a doctor. The side effects of Lexapro are usually mild and go away on their own. Initial nausea and diarrhea can sometimes occur. Trouble falling asleep, headache, and shakiness can also occur. Probably the most troublesome side effect, which is also a major problem with all of the SSRIs, involves sexual function. It was thought when Lexapro was first introduced that it might have fewer sexual side effects than other serotonin reuptake inhibiting antidepressants, but that turned out to be wishful thinking, and both men and women frequently complain that it takes longer to achieve orgasm while taking Lexapro. Often, while depressed, patients have little interest in sex. When Lexapro starts to work they feel better and their sex drive returns, but they find that orgasm becomes difficult. The delay in time to orgasm is probably due to Lexapro's effect on the serotonin system. This side effect is highly variable; not everyone gets it, and when it does occur it can involve anything from just a little increase in the time it takes to have an orgasm to a complete inability to have one, something called anorgasmia. Often, this side effect disappears on its own. After taking Lexapro for several months, weight gain occurs in many patients.

Less Common Side Effects: Very occasionally, people experience drowsiness from Lexapro. An increase in cholesterol level can occur in some people, although it is usually not enough to worry about. Like most antidepressants, Lexapro can induce a state called hypomania, which is the opposite of depression. A person with hypomania becomes almost euphoric with hyperactivity, irritability, boundless energy, and unrelenting optimism. Although this may sound attractive, the hypomanic patient typically makes a mess of things because of poor judgment and reckless behavior. Finally, Lexapro, like all of the newer antidepressants, may increase suicidal thinking in a small number of patients in the first few weeks.

What to Do About Side Effects: The side effects of Lexapro tend to be mild and may go away without any intervention. To combat stomach cramps, nausea, and diarrhea, the dose can temporarily be lowered or over-the-counter stomach remedies like Pepto-Bismol can be used for a brief time. Some patients have found that acidophilus tablets, which can be bought in a health food store, are helpful. Insomnia also tends to be a temporary side effect, often made less troublesome by taking Lexapro in the morning. If insomnia proves to be longer lasting, many clinicians have the patient take a low dose of the antidepressant trazodone (Desyrel)—about 50 mg—at bedtime. Trazodone is quite sedating but not as habit-forming as sleeping pills like Lunesta and Ambien. On the other hand, Desyrel lasts longer in the body than those sleeping pills and therefore is more likely to make the patient feel sleepy the next day. The side effects of shakiness and headache also usually disappear after a week or two, but if they are bothersome the dose can be lowered to as little as 5 mg until the patient adjusts to the medication. If Lexapro causes drowsiness, the first thing to check is whether it is making you feel sleepy during the day because you aren't sleeping at night. If that is the case, trazodone or a sleeping pill can be added at bedtime as described above. If the drug is really making a patient sleepy, it can be taken at bedtime, which sometimes helps. Sexual side effects and weight gain, although milder than with Paxil, are still very hard to overcome. The sexual side effects sometimes go away on their own or respond to lowering the dose (as long as that doesn't make the depression come back). Many antidotes to sexual side effects have been described, but only adding Wellbutrin has held up in a few studies to rigorous testing. Weight gain is highly variable; lowering calories and exercise help. Finally, the solution to hypomania is usually to lower the dose or stop the medication immediately.

If It Doesn't Work: If Lexapro has not worked by six weeks and the dose has been raised to 20 mg, there are still things that can be tried to get a response. The most common strategy nowadays is to add another drug. These are called augmenting agents and include thyroid hormone, lithium, Wellbutrin, psychostimulants (like Ritalin, Concerta, Adderall, and Mirapex), and atypical antipsychotic agents (like Risperdal, Abilify, and Geodon). If this fails, it is usually time to try a different antidepressant. Although not as bad as with Paxil or Effexor XR, there can be withdrawal effects if Lexapro is stopped abruptly, including agitation, anxiety, insomnia, and shocklike sensations throughout the body. Lexapro should be tapered slowly when it is time to stop it.

If It Does Work: The current recommendation is that a first episode of depression should be treated with antidepressant medication for six months following response. For people with recurrent depression, currently defined as three or more episodes of depression in a lifetime, continuous antidepressant medication therapy is recommended. Thus, Lexapro should be continued for at least six months after a depressed patient responds. The same is true for people with GAD. For patients with recurrent depression, however, it is advisable to continue medication for years because this is the best way to prevent recurrences. When it is time to stop Lexparo, it is important to taper the dose over about two weeks to prevent withdrawal symptoms.

Cost: There is no generic for Lexapro, so it is quite an expensive drug.

Special Comments: Lexapro is a clever (both scientifically and commercially) variant of Celexa (citalopram). Only one half of the molecule that comprises Celexa is actually an active antidepressant (this is called the S-enantiomer). The other half (the L-enantiomer) may either do nothing or, according to some very well-conducted animal studies, may actually interfere with Celexa's antidepressant effects. So as Celexa neared the end of its patent life and the drug companies that are involved in selling it realized that they would soon face cheap generic competition, they split Celexa and isolated the pure S form, called escitalopram. This became the new antidepressant Lexapro. It is very hard to see any real difference between Celexa and Lexapro except that brand-name Lexapro, the only form available, is a lot more expensive than generic Celexa. The extra expense is hardly worth it for most patients and it is my opinion that citalopram (generic Celexa) should be prescribed before Lexapro is considered.

VENLAFAXINE

Brand Name: Effexor XR.

Used For: Depression, social anxiety disorder, panic disorder, and generalized anxiety disorder (according to official FDA approvals); also good for other anxiety disorders, for hot flushes associated with menopause, and for pain.

Do Not Use If: As explained below, Effexor can cause high blood pressure, so people who already have high blood pressure should use it cautiously. It is perfectly possible, however, that a person with high blood pressure who is satisfactorily treated with antihypertensive medication will do just fine on Effexor. Do not combine it with a monoamine oxidase inhibitor.

Tests to Take First: Have your blood pressure taken before you start Effexor.

Tests to Take While You Are on It: Blood pressure should be checked regularly.

Usual Dose: A starting dose of 37.5 mg daily is reasonable, but many psychiatrists start patients at 75 mg a day. If jitteriness occurs at the higher dose, it can always be cut to 37.5 mg until it subsides and then the dose increased. Patients with anxiety disorders, especially panic disorder, should be started at 37.5 mg. Effexor XR, which is taken once a day, is no different from the SSRIs like Celexa (citalopram) and Zoloft in terms of side effects and effectiveness until the dose is raised to at least 150 mg a day. At that point, it may become more effective than those drugs. Doses up to 225 mg are approved by the FDA, but the drug is safely administered to many patients at doses of 300 mg, 375 mg, or even higher, depending on side effects. This is where, in the opinion of many psychopharmacologists, Effexor XR becomes particularly strong, expecially when treating severe depression.

How Long Until It Works: Like all antidepressants, it usually takes about four weeks for Effexor XR to work, although it can take six weeks.

Common Side Effects: The most common side effects are nausea, nervousness, and loss of appetite (this occurs only at first; later, most patients gain weight). Most people also experience delayed orgasm and weight gain. These side effects are very similar to those experienced by patients taking the SSRI-type antidepressants like Paxil. This is no surprise, because one of the main actions of Effexor XR is to affect the serotonin system in the same way that those drugs do. The unique side effects of Effexor XR are sweating and its ability to cause hypertension (high blood pressure). This occurs in about 5 percent of patients and is more pronounced the higher the dose of the drug.

Less Common Side Effects: Sedation, dry mouth, dizziness, constipation. Effexor XR is like Paxil in causing very severe withdrawal symptoms if it is stopped abruptly. These include nausea, dizziness, agitation, anxiety, insomnia, and shocklike sensations throughout the body. As with all antidepressants, Effexor XR may increase the risk for suicidal thinking in the first few weeks.

What to Do About Side Effects: Most of the side effects caused by Effexor XR are dose-dependent, which means they get worse as the dose is increased. Therefore, if side effects are bothersome and persist, the dose can be lowered. Sexual side effects and weight gain may not, however, respond to dose reduction. Sexual side effects range from a small delay in orgasm to complete inability to have one (called anorgasmia). Many antidotes have been recommended, but only the addition of Wellbutrin, in a few studies, seems to work. Weight gain can respond to diet and exercise. If blood pressure is increased and remains high after starting Effexor XR, however, it is probably best to stop it and try something else. An exception to this is if Effexor XR has been the only drug to work for a serious case of depression. Then, rather than allow the patient to relapse into depression, it is fairly easy to lower blood pressure with antihypertensive medication and continue the patient on Effexor XR.

If It Doesn't Work: If Effexor XR does not work, the first step is to add another drug to boost the response. These are called augmenting agents and include thyroid hormone, lithium, Wellbutrin, psychostimulants (like Ritalin, Concerta, Adderall, and Mirapex, although care must be given not to make any increase in blood pressure worse), and atypical antipsychotic agents (like Risperdal, Abilify, and Geodon). If this doesn't work, and the dose has been pushed to as high as tolerated, it is probably best to try something else. Effexor XR should *never* be stopped abruptly; the dose should be decreased gradually over at least a two-week period and sometimes much longer.

If It Does Work: Stay on it for at least six months after your depression improves. It is now generally recommended that people who have had three or more episodes of depression should be treated with antidepressant medication indefinitely to prevent recurrence. Long-term treatment may also be recommended for patients with chronic depression (like dysthymia) and anxiety disorders.

Cost: No generic form of Effexor XR is currently available, so it is fairly expensive.

Special Comments: First a word about "XR." As discussed in the description of Paxil (paroxetine), the explosion of adding "XR," "CR," and "SR" to a drug and calling it "new and improved" is very often a gimmick by a drug company to continue to make money on a drug that is about to go off patent by getting a new patent even though the "new drug" has no advantage over the original. This is definitely not the case for Effexor XR. Although still available, original Effexor is not nearly as good as Effexor XR (it has to be given twice daily and has more side effects), and even though it costs more, Effexor XR is generally the only version prescribed today. Now, a more important issue: Is Effexor XR more effective than other antidepressants? My opinion is a definite yes, but it must be kept in mind that this issue is very controversial. A number of studies, but not all, showed that drugs that affect both the serotonin and norepinephrine (also called noradrenaline) systems in the brain are more powerful antidepressants than those that affect only the serotonin system. This was originally shown pitting old cyclic drugs like Elavil (amitriptyline) against SSRIs like Celexa (citalopram). Effexor XR was the first of the SNRI antidepressants—antidepressants that affect both systems (but only at doses of 150 mg a day or higher)—and to many of us it seems to be more potent than the SSRIs. The drug company that makes Effexor XR published a series of studies, all very legitimate in my opinion and checked by eminent scientists, also showing a small but consistent superiority of Effexor XR over Paxil, Zoloft, and Prozac. The FDA made the company stop using this in advertising to doctors, but this was mainly for technical legal reasons rather than scientific ones. So the issue remains: Are SNRIs more effective than SSRIs? I have already stated my opinion and I believe that Effexor XR is a good first-line drug for more severe depression and also very good for cases of depression that have not responded to SSRIs. Because it is more expensive than generic Celexa (citalopram) and not all that much better (if it is at all), I still start patients with mild to moderate depression who need antidepressants on citalopram. Effexor XR will go off patent fairly soon, and then I may change my mind and make generic venlafaxine my preferred antidepressant.

DULOXETINE

Brand Name: Cymbalta.

Used For: Depression and pain are its two official FDA-approved uses, but it is probably also helpful for the same range of anxiety disorders and hot flushes during menopause as Effexor XR.

Do Not Use If: As explained below, Cymbalta can cause high blood pressure, so people who already have high blood pressure should use it cautiously. It is perfectly possible, however, that a person with high blood pressure who is satisfactorily treated with antihypertensive medication will do just fine on Cymbalta. Do not combine it with a monoamine oxidase inhibitor.

Tests to Take First: Have your blood pressure taken before you start Cymbalta.

Tests to Take While You Are on It: Blood pressure should be checked regularly.

Usual Dose: Cymbalta comes in 20-mg, 30-mg, and 60-mg tablets. One minor controversy is whether it has to be taken twice a day in divided doses, or if once a day, the drug company's recommendation, is sufficient. I generally start patients on 20 mg once a day, morning or evening according to their preference, and increase to 20 mg twice daily in about a week. Then, if the response is not sufficient after four weeks of taking Cymbalta, it can be increased to 30 mg twice a day. Many psychopharmacologists, however, start at 20 mg or even 40 mg once a day and increase to 60 mg once a day if the response is inadequate. Initial nausea or jitteriness usually subsides on its own but sometimes merits temporary dose reduction.

How Long Until It Works: Like all antidepressants, it usually takes about four weeks for Cymbalta to work, although it can take six weeks.

Common Side Effects: The most common side effects are nausea, nervousness, and loss of appetite (this occurs only at first; later, most patients gain weight). Most people also experience delayed orgasm and weight gain. These side effects are very similar to those experienced by patients taking the SSRI-type antidepressants like Paxil and the SNRI drug Effexor XR. This is no surprise, because one of the main actions of Cymbalta is to affect the serotonin system in the same way that those drugs do. The unique side effect of Cymbalta, shared with its cousin SNRI Effexor XR, is its ability to cause hypertension (high blood pressure). For unclear reasons, this may be less common than with Effexor XR, but it is still a good idea to monitor.

Less Common Side Effects: Sedation, dry mouth, dizziness, constipation. Cymbalta can be associated with withdrawal symptoms if it is stopped abruptly. These include nausea, dizziness, agitation, anxiety, insomnia, and shocklike sensations throughout the body. As with all antidepressants, Cymbalta may increase the risk for suicidal thinking in the first few weeks.

What to Do About Side Effects: Most of the side effects caused by Cymbalta are dose-dependent, which means they get worse as the dose is increased. Therefore, if side effects are bothersome and persist, the dose can be lowered. Sexual side effects and weight gain may not, however, respond to dose reduction. Sexual side effects range from a small delay in orgasm to complete inability to have one (called anorgasmia). Many antidotes have been recommended, but only the addition of Wellbutrin, in a few studies, seems to work. Weight gain can respond to diet and exercise. If blood pressure is increased and remains high after starting Cymbalta, however, it is probably best to stop it and try something else. An exception to this is if Cymbalta has been the only drug to work for a serious case of depression. Then, rather than allow the patient to relapse into depression, it is fairly easy to reduce high blood pressure with antihypertensive medication and continue the patient on Cymbalta.

If It Doesn't Work: If Cymbalta does not work, the first step is to add another drug to boost the response. These are called augmenting agents and include thyroid hormone, lithium, Wellbutrin, psychostimulants (like Ritalin, Concerta, Adderall, and Mirapex, although care must be given to not making any increase in blood pressure worse), and atypical antipsychotic agents (like Risperdal, Abilify, and Geodon). If this doesn't work, and the dose has been pushed to as high as tolerated, it is probably best to try something else. Cymbalta should *never* be stopped abruptly; the dose should be decreased gradually.

If It Does Work: Stay on it for at least six months after your depression improves. It is now generally recommended that people who have had three or more episodes of depression should be treated with antidepressant medication indefinitely to prevent recurrence. Long-term treatment may also be recommended for patients with chronic depression (like dysthymia) and anxiety disorders.

Cost: No generic form of Cymbalta is currently available, so it is fairly expensive.

Special Comments: Cymbalta has an interesting history. The drug company that makes it once had it as a low priority for development until another drug they had under development as an antidepressant didn't pan out. Then they turned their attention to Cymbalta. It has turned out to be a useful drug. Like Effexor XR, it is a serotonin norepinephrine reuptake inhibitor (SNRI), which I believe will make it more effective than the selective serotonin reuptake inhibitors (SSRIs) like Prozac and Zoloft (but see my discussion of the controversy surrounding this statement in the Special Comments section for Effexor XR). It is said to be different from Effexor XR because the combined effect on serotonin and norepinephrine (also known as noradrenaline) does not occur with Effexor XR until the dose gets at least to 150 mg a day. Cymbalta, on the other hand, supposedly affects both brain chemicals even at the lowest dose. Scientists have not been able to confirm these claims yet, but Cymbalta is indeed much easier to dose than Effexor XR, which often takes several increases to get to a therapeutic level. Some experienced psychopharmacologists still insist that Effexor XR is more effective, but Cymbalta is very new and it will take some time to sort this out. In the meantime, were it not for the cost (which still makes me recommend citalopram [Celexa] as the best drug to start with for most depressed patients), Cymbalta could easily become the first-line antidepressant.

NEFAZODONE

Brand Name: Serzone. (Brand-name Serzone is no longer available in the United States, though some European countries still have it.)

Used For: Depression.

Do Not Use If: You will need to lower the dose of Xanax or Halcion before starting nefazodone and probably should stop taking any SSRI antidepressants like Prozac, Paxil, Zoloft, or Luvox. Do not combine it with a monoamine oxidase inhibitor.

Tests to Take First: Blood tests of liver function.

Tests to Take While You Are on It: Blood tests for liver function should be done periodically (there are no specific recommendations as to how often) and at the first signs of feeling sick or unusually tired.

Usual Dose: Start with 50 mg (half of a 100-mg pill) in the morning and at night. After about four days, increase to 100 mg twice a day and then to 150 mg twice daily in another four days. The usual effective dose is somewhere between 300 and 600 mg daily, and it may be necessary to take half in the morning and half at night.

How Long Until It Works: Four to six weeks.

Common Side Effects: Sleepiness, nausea, visual trails (a harmless sensation in which when you turn your gaze away from an object, it appears to persist in your view for a second or two; this occurs at higher doses of nefazodone).

Less Common Side Effects: Although nefazodone was touted as the newer antidepressant least likely to cause anxiety or agitation, if a patient is switched too quickly from an SSRI (like Prozac, Paxil, or Zoloft), a drug interaction may occur that results in the patient actually developing fairly high levels of anxiety. For this reason, it is best when possible to get off the SSRI before starting nefazodone. After Serzone had been on the market for several years, there were reports of a very small number of patients developing liver problems and some even dying from this. Although it appears to be a rare side effect, the fact that the drug was not that popular among psychiatrists anyway made this side effect enough to convince the manufacturer of brand-name Serzone to stop making it.

What to Do About Side Effects: In the package insert for nefazodone, a starting dose of 100 mg twice a day is recommended. Although this is fine for some people, most find that they are too sleepy during the day if they start at that dose. Hence, it is probably best to start with half that dose. If that causes sleepiness, some people start with just the nighttime dose and add the daytime dose a few days later. Nausea usually goes away on its own. The visual trails sensation usually ceases to bother people after a few days. In terms of the liver problems, it is probably wise to get liver function blood tests every few months and at the first sign of feeling sick or unusually tired.

If It Doesn't Work: Drugs can be added to try to boost the response. These are called augmenting agents and include thyroid hormone, lithium, Wellbutrin, psychostimulants (like Ritalin, Concerta, Adderall, and Mirapex), and atypical antipsychotic agents (like Risperdal, Abilify, and Geodon). If this doesn't help, switch to a different drug, probably from the newer antidepressant class.

If It Does Work: Remain on it for at least six weeks. People with a history of recurrent depression should stay on it even longer.

Cost: Generic nefazodone is inexpensive.

Special Comments: Serzone affects the serotonin system in much the same way as the SSRIs like Prozac but has an added feature or two that seem to completely change its side effect profile. Whereas the SSRIs sometimes cause insomnia and anxiety in the first few days of treatment, Serzone often improves sleep quality and decreases anxiety. Furthermore, Serzone does not cause the sexual side effects that are common to the SSRIs. Hence, from a side effect point of view, Serzone has advantages over the SSRIs. On the other hand, some people complain that it makes them feel sleepy during the day and others say it doesn't work as well as the SSRIs or Effexor XR. My own observation is that it rarely works and it not worth the risk of liver problems, however rare.

TRAZODONE

Brand Name: Desyrel.

Used For: Major depression. However, it is now mostly used as a sleeping pill.

Do Not Use If: You have certain heart rhythm abnormalities (which your doctor will tell you about).

Tests to Take First: An electrocardiogram may be required by your doctor.

Tests to Take While You Are on It: None required.

Usual Dose: Starts at about 50 mg a day and may be increased to between 200 and 400 mg. Occasionally, a doctor will prescribe as much as 600 mg. The dose is usually taken at night after a meal or a light snack. When used as a sleeping pill, its most common use nowadays, the dose is usually 50 mg, or if that doesn't work, 100 mg about an hour before bedtime.

How Long Until It Works: About four weeks for depression but after the first dose for insomnia.

Common Side Effects: Sleepiness, dizziness after standing up quickly, and nausea and vomiting.

Less Common Side Effects: Priapism, or sustained erection of the penis, has been reported in some patients taking trazodone. It is estimated to occur in between one in one thousand and one in ten thousand men who take the drug. This is a serious emergency because severe damage can occur to a penis that has been erect for several hours. One-third of the men who develop priapism require surgery. Disturbances in heart rhythms can occur in people with underlying heart disease.

What to Do About Side Effects: For the sedation caused by trazodone, it is best to take the medicine in one dose before bedtime. Dizziness can be controlled by standing up slowly. Nausea usually goes away on its own. Sustained erection of the penis is an emergency and you should call your doctor immediately. Patients with heart disease should probably not be given trazodone in most cases.

If It Doesn't Work: Switch to a different drug.

If It Does Work: Remain on it for six months and then try to discontinue use. Longer for people with recurrent depression.

Cost: Generic trazodone is as safe and effective as brand-name Desyrel and considerably less expensive.

Special Comments: Desyrel is rarely used as an antidepressant any longer because it is of limited effectiveness and makes patients sleepy. The latter side effect, however, turned into a benefit as more and more doctors started using it as a treatment for insomnia. Unlike sleeping pills like Lunesta and Ambien, there does not seem to be any risk of getting hooked on trazodone when taken to improve sleep. However, it is not always felt to be better than sleeping pills because it lasts a fairly long time in the body and many patients complain that they still feel sleepy the next day. Lunesta and Ambien, on the other hand, are cleared from the body rapidly and do not generally cause daytime sleepiness. So trazodone has a place as a sleeping pill but is not automatically the best one.

AMOXAPINE

Brand Name: Asendin. (No longer available as brand-name drug.)

Used For: Major depression.

Do Not Use If: You are very anxious along with being depressed, have a lot of trouble sleeping, or have a history of seizures (epilepsy). Do not combine it with a monoamine oxidase inhibitor.

Tests to Take First: None required.

Tests to Take While You Are on It: None required.

Usual Dose: Starts with 100 mg two or three times daily and can be increased to between 300 and 600 mg to obtain an antidepressant effect. Usually taken early in the day.

How Long Until It Works: There are claims that amoxapine works very quickly, in about a week, but some patients may not feel the full effect for about three weeks.

Common Side Effects: Nervousness, agitation, and insomnia are the most troublesome, but 14 percent of patients experience drowsiness.

Less Common Side Effects: Alone among the antidepressant drugs, amoxapine has the potential to produce a serious and sometimes permanent side effect called tardive dyskinesia (TD). This involves involuntary movements of various muscles, usually beginning with chewing and lip smacking. TD is a potential side effect of most drugs used to treat schizophrenia, but amoxapine is the only antidepressant known to produce it.

What to Do About Side Effects: Taking the medication early in the day may counteract some of the insomnia. Lowering the dose can reduce the agitation but may also reduce the chance of the drug working. Because of its potential to cause tardive dyskinesia, amoxapine should not be taken longer than six months and should be stopped at the first sign of abnormal body movements.

If It Doesn't Work: Try a different antidepressant.

If It Does Work: Take it for about six months and then taper off over about two weeks.

Cost: Only the generic form of amoxapine is now available and it is fairly inexpensive.

Special Comments: Because amoxapine energizes people, it may make a sluggish depressed patient feel better in a week; it also makes some patients feel anxious and irritable. The risk of developing tardive dyskinesia is probably small, but because this effect is so serious and there are so many other drugs that work just as well, amoxapine is rapidly losing favor.

BUPROPION (AND BUPROPION 12-HOUR TABLETS)

Brand Names: Budeprion SR, Budeprion XL, Wellbutrin, Wellbutrin SR, Wellbutrin XL, and Zyban (for smoking cessation).

Used For: Major depression, bipolar depression, attention-deficit/hyperactivity disorder, smoking cessation. Also added to other antidepressants to augment response or to reduce sexual side effects.

Do Not Use If: You have a history of seizures (epilepsy) or bulimia, suffer from severe insomnia, or are very underweight. Do not combine it with a monoamine oxidase inhibitor.

Tests to Take First: None recommended.

Tests to Take While You Are on It: None recommended.

Usual Dose: When using regular bupropion or Wellbutrin, start with 75 mg twice daily and increase to 100 mg three times a day after several days. If there is no response in three to four weeks, the dose can be raised to a maximum of 450 mg per day, given in three doses of 150 mg each. Never take more than 150 mg in any one dose. A sustained-release formulation (bupropion 12-hour tablets or Wellbutrin SR) makes it possible to take Wellbutrin twice a day, starting at 150 mg once or twice a day to a maximum of 200 mg twice daily. Finally, Wellbutrin XL can be taken once a day, starting a 150 mg in the morning and going to a maximum of 450 mg in the morning.

How Long Until It Works: About four weeks.

Common Side Effects: Restlessness, agitation, and insomnia may occur in one-third of patients treated with Wellbutrin. About one-fourth of patients lose as much as five pounds (almost no one gains weight). Some patients also experience headache, nausea and vomiting, and rashes.

Less Common Side Effects: The major worry is the precipitation of seizures. Approximately four of one thousand people treated with the first preparation of Wellbutrin had a convulsion during the testing phase of the drug. The occurrence is probably less likely than that, particularly at doses of 300 mg or less. Furthermore, this is a very rare side effect of the newer forms of the drug, Wellbutrin SR and Wellbutrin XL. With those, only people with a history of epilepsy who are not taking adequate anticonvulsant medication are likely to have a problem.

What to Do About Side Effects: Restlessness and insomnia usually disappear on their own after a few weeks; some clinicians may add small amounts of an antianxiety benzodiazepine drug (like Xanax) to reduce these problems. Most patients welcome the small amount of weight loss. The risk of seizures should be explained to the patient, but with the SR or XL version is probably not something to worry about. Patients with a history of seizures should generally not take Wellbutrin.

If It Doesn't Work: Try a different antidepressant.

If It Does Work: Remain on it for six depression-free months. The medication should then be tapered. Withdrawal symptoms should not be a major problem. People with recurrent depression should be treated longer.

Cost: The many different forms of Wellbutrin are confusing, but straight Wellbutrin is usually no longer prescribed. Wellbutrin SR is now available in generic form, officially called bupropion 12-hour tablets. The generic is my preferred preparation because it is just as effective and safe as Wellbutrin SR and considerably less expensive. Wellbutrin XL is not available in generic form, so it is expensive. Some patients like it best of the different preparations, particularly because it can be taken once a day, but I see no advantage over generic bupropion 12-hour tablets (if the doctor writes the prescription for Wellbutrin SR and does not specify brand-name drug, pharmacists in most states automatically dispense bupropion 12-hour tablets, the version that most managed care pharmacies will pay for with the smallest co-pay). I have actually found that in many patients, Wellbutrin XL does not work as well as SR.

Special Comments: When Wellbutrin was about to be released on the market, several cases of convulsions were reported in patients with bulimia. The release was halted until the FDA was satisfied that the risk of precipitating a seizure is acceptable at the 0.4 percent level. After its release, however, the risk of seizure seemed considerably less than this, particularly at doses of 300 mg or less. It was a nuisance, however, taking Wellbutrin three times a day, and the subsequent release of the SR form, which needs to be taken only twice a day, was most welcome. In its generic form, that is what I recommend. Wellbutrin XL, although having the advantage of needing to be taken only once a day, is not, in my opinion, worth the added cost. Wellbutrin worked as well as the other antidepressants in clinical studies of depression, but most clinicians believe it is not as potent as the SRIs and SNRIs and is usually reserved for mild depression. Its big advantages over drugs in those classes of antidepressants, including Paxil, Celexa, and Effexor XR, is that it doesn't cause weight gain or sexual side effects. Wellbutrin is probably most often added to another antidepressant either to boost response when the first drug does not work well enough or to reduce sexual side effects caused by all of the SSRIs and SNRIs. Wellbutrin is said to have less tendency to produce hypomania and mania than other antidepressants and therefore may be especially useful in patients with bipolar depression who often get high when treated with antidepressants. However, many psychopharmacologists, including me, are very skeptical of this claim. Wellbutrin has also been shown to be somewhat effective for children and adults with attention-deficit/hyperactivity disorder. For children, it does not seem to be as effective as the other available agents, like Strattera, long-acting Ritalin (Concerta, Focalin, Metadate, and others), and Adderall. For adults, however, it is a very good place to start. Finally, bupropion (Zyban) works for smoking cessation. In conjunction with nicotine substitutes like the nicotine patch, and often with behavioral psychotherapy, it works.

FLUVOXAMINE

Brand Name: Luvox. (Brand-name Luvox is no longer available in the United States.)

Used For: Obsessive-compulsive disorder (its only official FDA-approved indication), panic disorder, depression.

Do Not Use If: You will have to lower the dose of Xanax or Halcion if you are taking one of these drugs, and be cautious about combining with other antidepressants. Do not take if you are on a monoamine oxidase inhibitor. Grapefruit juice can also increase the blood level of fluvoxamine.

Tests to Take First: None required.

Tests to Take While You Are on It: None required. An exception is the infrequent instance in which fluvoxamine lowers the body's sodium level. This is a bit more common in older patients. The symptoms are extreme lethary and fatigue, which should be reported to your doctor immediately so he or she can order a blood test to see if sodium level is too low.

Usual Dose: Most patients are started at 50 mg at bedtime, with subsequent dose increases to a range of 100–300 mg daily. When the dose gets above 100 mg, it is usually best to split it and take half in the morning and half at night.

How Long Until It Works: Four to six weeks.

Common Side Effects: Like all SSRIs, fluvoxamine can cause nausea, diarrhea, headache, insomnia, and anxiety, particularly when you first start to take it. Down the line, the main problem is sexual side effects, which mainly mean difficulty for both men and women achieving orgasm. This then sometimes leads to loss of sexual interest. Weight gain can occur, although it seems a little less likely than with the other SSRIs.

Less Common Side Effects: A few people get sleepy from Luvox. Sometimes, antidepressants including fluvoxamine cause too much elevation in mood and the patient becomes hyperactive, too talkative, irritable, and out of control. This is called hypomania and is not a desirable outcome from antidepressant treatment. As with all antidepressants, fluvoxamine may increase the risk of suicidal thoughts in the first few weeks.

What to Do About Side Effects: Most of the common side effects subside with time, and Luvox is fairly well tolerated. Lowering the dose can be helpful at first for nausea, diarrhea, headache, insomnia, and anxiety. The sexual side effects are more difficult to deal with. All SSRIs cause them. Sometimes they just go away. Patients have tried stopping the medication for the weekend, which sometimes restores sexual function, but going off for too long means a relapse of depression or obsessive-compulsive disorder. There are a number of antidotes that have been reported to work, but only Wellbutrin, in a few studies, has held up to rigorous testing.

If It Doesn't Work: For a partial responder when fluvoxamine is used for depression, physicians may add a second drug to boost the response. These are called augmenting agents and include thyroid hormone, lithium, Wellbutrin, psychostimulants (like Ritalin, Concerta, Adderall, and Mirapex), and atypical antipsychotic agents (like Risperdal, Abilify, and Geodon). If this is unsuccessful, it is best to try another drug. However, fluvoxamine should never be stopped abruptly because a withdrawal syndrome characterized by nausea, dizziness, agitation, anxiety, insomnia, and shocklike sensations throughout the body will occur. When stopping fluvoxamine, it should be tapered slowly over several weeks.

If It Does Work: Stay on it for at least six months, longer if you have recurrent depression or are being treated for obsessive-compulsive disorder.

Cost: Only the generic form is available and therefore it is relatively inexpensive.

Special Comments: It was difficult to decide where to place fluvoxamine in this book. Officially, the Food and Drug Administration has approved it only for the treatment of obsessive-compulsive disorder (discussed in Chapter 8). On the other hand, fluvoxamine is in fact no different from the other SSRIs, Prozac, Zoloft, and Paxil. It works for depression and panic disorder just as they do.

MIRTAZAPINE

Brand Names: Remeron, Remeron Sol-Tab.

Used For: Depression.

Do Not Take If: You are already very sleepy or overweight. Do not combine it with a monoamine oxidase inhibitor.

Tests to Take First: None.

Tests to Take While You Are on It: If you develop symptoms of the flu or get a fever, sore throat, or a cough while on Remeron, your doctor will probably recommend that you have a blood count.

Usual Dose: Remeron is usually started with one 15-mg pill at night. The final dose is between 30 and 45 mg, again taken at night.

How Long Until It Works: Four to six weeks.

Common Side Effects: Many people get sleepy and gain weight from Remeron.

Less Common Side Effects: Remeron can increase cholesterol levels. It may have an effect on the liver, although this is very rare and not a reason to avoid taking Remeron. While being tested, 3 out of 2,796 patients taking Remeron developed a serious and potentially fatal decrease in the production of cells needed for the immune system to fight infection. However, in the ten years it has been on the market, there have been no cases of this problem, called agranulocytosis, and it is no longer considered an issue.

What to Do About Side Effects: Some patients get over the sleepiness caused by Remeron if they take it for a while, and can live with the weight gain. If signs of an infection occur, it is imperative to call the doctor right away and follow instructions.

If It Doesn't Work: First, your doctor may have you add a second medication to boost the response of Remeron. These are called augmenting agents and include thyroid hormone, lithium, Wellbutrin, psychostimulants (like Ritalin, Concerta, Adderall, and Mirapex), and atypical antipsychotic agents (like Risperdal, Abilify, and Geodon). If this fails, it is time to switch to a different antidepressant.

If It Does Work: Stay on it for at least six months. Many patients with chronic depression or more than two previous episodes of major depression are advised to stay on it much longer.

Cost: Remeron is available as generic mirtazapine, which is cheaper and just as safe and effective as the brand-name drug. Remeron Sol-Tabs is a melt-in-your-mouth version that was supposed to be useful for people who cannot swallow a pill. It is expensive and not many people have this problem.

Special Comments: Remeron is one of the most overlooked medications in psychiatry. It has a unique way of working in the brain, which fascinates neuroscientists and psychopharmacologists. Remeron essentially increases the output of both norepinephrine and serotonin from brain cells (neurons) and therefore has the same ultimate effect as the SNRIs like Effexor XR (venlafaxine) and Cymbalta (duloxetine). This means that it may be more effective than the SSRIs like Zoloft and Celexa. It also does not cause most of the typical SSRI side effects: There is no insomnia, nausea, anxiety, or sexual side effect problem with Remeron. Unfortunately, it is very sedating and causes weight gain, which are difficult to tolerate. Nonetheless, it is a very effective antidepressant and for certain types of depressed patients, particularly those with a lot of anxiety, insomnia, and loss of appetite, it can be ideal. Because it can decrease nausea, whereas many of the other antidepressants cause it, it is particularly helpful for patients undergoing chemotherapy for cancer, who are often anxious, nauseous, and depressed, have trouble sleeping, and lose their appetites.

Summary of Newer Antidepressants

We have been in a new era of antidepressant treatment since the introduction of Prozac. A substantial number of drugs have been released in the last fifteen years that are safe and effective. Drug companies are fighting fierce battles to convince doctors and patients that a particular new drug is the best. In fact, it is hard to decide which the best are. Cost is also now a consideration because many of the newer drugs, like Prozac (fluoxetine), Zoloft (sertraline), Paxil (paroxetine), Celexa (citalopram), and Wellbutrin SR (bupropion 12-hour tabs), are off patent and available as generics. So here are my suggestions: For mild to moderate depression, generic Celexa (citalopram) is hard to beat. As an alternative, generic Wellbutrin SR may be used because it does not have sexual side effects or cause weight gain, but I believe it is less effective. For more severe depression, Effexor XR is a better place to start. Remeron is an excellent antidepressant for patients with anxiety, insomnia, and significant loss of appetite. Cymbalta may become a drug of first choice, although it will be many years before it goes off patent and is available as a generic drug. Beware, however, of all those television advertisements claiming that just by adding "SR," "CR," or "XR" to a drug it becomes vastly better than the original. In some cases this is true (Effexor XR is better than Effexor and Wellbutrin SR is better than Wellbutrin) but in many it is not (Paxil CR is not better than Paxil and Wellbutrin XL is not better than Wellbutrin SR).

STIMULANT ANTIDEPRESSANT DRUGS

Depression may also be treated with drugs called psychostimulants. Use of such drugs is reserved for four situations: (1) patients who have failed to respond to at least two other antidepressants and psychotherapy and who are seriously depressed; (2) patients with serious and usually terminal medical illnesses such as cancer who are depressed and too sick to take other kinds of antidepressants; (3) patients for whom an antidepressant has only partially worked and the doctor attempts to boost the response by adding a second drug, a practice known as augmentation; and (4) people with the adult version of attention-deficit/hyperactivity disorder (ADHD) (note that medications for children are not discussed in this book).

The reason for these restrictions is that many of the stimulant drugs are addictive and can cause high blood pressure, severe insomnia, psychotic symptoms (like seeing things or visual hallucinations), and heart problems. They include amphetamines, sometimes called speed or uppers (Dexedrine and Adderall are examples), methylphenidate (Ritalin, Concerta, Focalin, and Metadate are examples), and pemoline (Cylert). Three other drugs that do not exactly fit into this category but have very similar uses and are substantially safer than the ones just mentioned are Strattera (atomoxetine), Provigil (modafinil), and Mirapex (pramipexole). Amphetamines and methylphenidate produce a short-term mood elevation even in people who are not depressed. College students take them to stay awake all night and finish term papers. Adderall has become a major drug of abuse among teenagers and young adults and needs to be much more carefully monitored.

In most people, the effects of these stimulant drugs are short-lived and there is often a letdown or "crash" after they wear off (Stattera and Mirapex are generally not as prone to this problem). During this crash, the patient can feel very depressed, sleepy, and sluggish. Furthermore, and very much unlike the other drugs discussed so far in this chapter, stimulant drugs have the potential to induce tolerance. People who abuse amphetamines and other stimulants—usually in attempts to lose weight or stay awake for prolonged periods—often find that a dose that had worked for a while is suddenly ineffective and they need a higher dose. They then become tolerant to the higher dose and have to increase the dose again. Soon, the person is addicted to the drug. Stopping it suddenly leads to a severe withdrawal reaction characterized by serious depression and extreme fatigue. Suicides have been reported in people who suddenly stop taking amphetamines.

Given all these problems, why even mention the stimulant drugs? Simply because they are the only drugs that work for some depressed patients and for adults with ADHD (Wellbutrin SR, generic bupropion 12-hour tabs, is probably the safest way to begin treating the adult ADHD patient, however). A very small group of usually chronically depressed patients seems to be resistant to every other treatment for depression. These people usually function at a fairly low level relative to their ability and they feel sad and blue all of the time. They complain of fatigue, low interest in life, and inability to concentrate. Many say they have been depressed since childhood.

Another small group of patients with very serious medical problems also develops depression. Sometimes their medical problems make other antidepressant drugs unsafe, or the medical problems so magnify the side effects of the other antidepressants that the dying patient is made even more uncomfortable. Stimulant drugs may actually be the safest choice in this situation.

Perhaps the most common use of psychostimulants is to boost or augment the response of another antidepressant that has worked inadequately.

For these groups of patients stimulant drugs may be the only answer, even if the patient becomes addicted. This is not to be taken lightly. The decision to place a patient on a stimulant drug for depression is serious and must be done only after all other efforts are declared either unsafe or ineffective. The patient must understand that he or she will probably become addicted to the medication and that he or she should never stop taking it abruptly.

AMPHETAMINE

Brand Names: Dexedrine, Adderall, Adderall XR, Biphetamine, Desoxyn, Vyvanse.

Used For: Officially, for three conditions: (1) narcolepsy, a condition in which the patient falls asleep suddenly during the day; (2) obesity; and (3) attention-deficit/hyperactivity disorder (ADHD). Unofficially, it is sometimes used for chronic depression that fails to respond to all other treatments and for very ill medical patients with depression. It is also used to augment the response of a more traditional antidepressant like an SSRI or SNRI.

Do Not Use If: You haven't tried other antidepressants and psychotherapy, have high blood pressure or any form of heart disease, are very nervous or have severe insomnia, have a history of addiction to drugs or alcohol, or have Tourette's syndrome. Do not combine with monoamine oxidase inhibitors.

Tests to Take First: You should probably have an electrocardiogram to be sure nothing is wrong with your heart, and your blood pressure should be recorded.

Tests to Take While You Are on It: Blood pressure and pulse should be taken every day for the first week, then once a week for a month, and then at least every month.

Usual Dose: For amphetamines like Dexedrine (often also referred to as dextroamphetamine), dose usually starts with 5 or 10 mg per day and can be raised, sometimes to 50 mg or higher. Adderall is usually started at 5 mg in the morning and then increased by 5 mg to a maximum of 40 mg a day, usually taken in two divided doses. Adderall XR is the extended-release version of Adderall—each dose of regular Adderall lasts only a few hours whereas the XR version lasts most of the day. The higher the dose of any of these versions of amphetamine, the worse will be the side effects and the chance for addiction. Amphetamines should not be taken at bedtime.

How Long Until It Works: Usually almost immediately, sometimes an hour after the first dose. The effect also wears off quickly, lasting only a few hours. Each dose of Adderall XR taken in the morning works for most of the day. Therefore, the shorter-acting drugs are usually taken in divided doses two or three times daily, whereas Adderall XR is usually taken just once in the morning. After it has worked for a while, the effect may wear off and the patient may require a higher dose. This is called tolerance. At this point a decision must be made whether to keep raising the dose or to stop the drug because it is not working adequately.

Common Side Effects: Nervousness, insomnia, loss of appetite, addiction.

Less Common Side Effects: High blood pressure, rapid pulse rate, tolerance (constant need to raise the dose), feelings of suspicion and paranoia, visual hallucinations—seeing things that aren't there.

What to Do About Side Effects: The last dose of the drug every day should be taken several hours before bedtime to prevent insomnia. Nervousness usually goes away and appetite returns so that weight loss is rarely dangerous. Nothing can be done about the addiction except to remember not to stop taking amphetamines abruptly. If high blood pressure, rapid pulse, paranoia, or tolerance becomes a problem, the drug is usually stopped.

If It Doesn't Work: The drug should be slowly tapered. Fortunately, the withdrawal symptoms are psychological and not medical.

If It Does Work: Some people decide to stay on the drug indefinitely. A very sick medical patient may legitimately stay on it for the rest of his or her life.

Cost: Dextroamphetamine is a generic drug that is relatively inexpensive. Of all the different versions of amphetamines, Adderall XR is probably the best because it doesn't have to be taken multiple times a day, thus avoiding crashes during the day. Unfortunately, Adderall XR is not available as a generic preparation and is therefore expensive.

Special Comments: Amphetamines are given to adults only in special situations by very experienced psychiatrists. They are medically safe but usually produce addiction. There is also a good chance they will provide only temporary help. However, in the treatment of ADHD for children and young adults, Adderall XR is now prescribed frequently, often as the first-line drug. This, in my opinion, is a very serious mistake. Adderall is now abused throughout college campuses, where it is bought, sold, stolen, borrowed, snorted, and injected. It is a very powerful drug that undoubtedly works for ADHD, but there are alternatives with less abuse potential that should be tried first.

METHYLPHENIDATE

Brand Names: Ritalin, Ritalin LA, Ritalin SR, Concerta, Metadate CD, Metadate ER, Focalin, Methylin, Methylin ER.

Used For: Officially, for children with attention-deficit/hyperactivity disorder (ADHD) and for narcolepsy. Unofficially, Ritalin is sometimes prescribed for depression when nothing else has worked, or is added to other antidepressants when they have worked only partially, or is given to very medically sick people with depression. Adults with ADHD are also frequently given one of the many preparations of methylphenidate.

Do Not Use If: You have high blood pressure or heart disease, are very nervous, have severe insomnia, or have a history of addiction to drugs or alcohol. Do not combine it with a monoamine oxidase inhibitor.

Tests to Take First: Your pulse and blood pressure should be recorded. Some doctors will want an electrocardiogram (ECG, EKG).

Tests to Take While You Are on It: Pulse and blood pressure should be monitored frequently.

Usual Dose: There are so many versions of methylphenidate that I will restrict myself to the generic version (brand name Ritalin) and one of the long-acting versions, Concerta. For regular methylphenidate (Ritalin), dose begins at about 5 mg twice daily and may go as high as 60 mg to obtain a response. It should not be taken at bedtime. The problem with regular Ritalin is that its effect wears off after a few hours, so that it must be taken two or three times a day to avoid crashes. The many longer-acting versions, like Concerta, can be taken once in the morning and generally work until about dinnertime. Concerta is started at 18 mg in the morning and increased by 18 mg every week to a maximum of 72 mg in the morning.

How Long Until It Works: The antidepressant effect may be felt immediately, after the first dose.

Common Side Effects: Nervousness, insomnia, loss of appetite, addiction (although it is less addicting than amphetamines).

Less Common Side Effects: High blood pressure (but less likely with Ritalin than with amphetamines), rapid pulse rate and other heart problems, tolerance (constant need to raise the dose), feelings of suspicion and paranoia (but less likely than with amphetamines).

What to Do About Side Effects: The last dose of the drug every day should be taken several hours before bedtime to prevent insomnia. Nervousness usually goes away and appetite often returns so that weight loss is rarely dangerous. Nothing can be done about the addiction except to remember not to stop taking any version of methylphenidate abruptly. If high blood pressure, rapid pulse, paranoia, or tolerance becomes a problem, the drug is usually stopped.

If It Doesn't Work: The drug should be slowly tapered. Fortunately, the withdrawal symptoms are psychological and not medical.

If It Does Work: Some people decide to remain on the drug indefinitely. A very sick medical patient may legitimately stay on it for the rest of his or her life.

Cost: Generic methylphenidate is cheap, but most doctors prescribe the longer-acting versions, which are more expensive.

Special Comments: Methylphenidate (Ritalin) is best known as the somewhat controversial but highly safe and effective treatment for ADHD.

Ritalin calms children with ADHD and improves their attention spans, usually leading to significant improvements in behavior and school performance. A large study sponsored by the National Institute of Mental Health showed that Ritalin works better than psychotherapy for ADHD, but there are constant fears that methylphenidate may retard growth, have rare but important adverse effects on the heart, and lead to addiction in children. Overall, when it is prescribed for a child (usually a boy) who has carefully diagnosed ADHD, it is one of the most effective treatments in medicine. In adults, Ritalin has more complicated effects. For adults with ADHD, it mainly improves attention, but for adults with depression it has mainly a stimulant effect. It is less powerful than amphetamines and therefore somewhat less addicting. The market for methylphenidate is huge and therefore many drug companies have developed versions of the drug, each attempting to convince doctors that its version is the best. Focalin is a chemical variant of methylphenidate, dextro- or dexmethylphenidate, and also comes in an XR version. Naturally, the manufacturer insists it is better than all the versions of regular methylphenidate, but that claim is met with skepticism by many psychopharmacologists.

PEMOLINE

(The FDA revoked its approval of this drug in October 2005 and, therefore, it is no longer available in the United States.)

Brand Name: Cylert.

Special Comments: Pemoline is very similar to methylphenidate (Ritalin) except that it works longer and therefore needs to be taken only once daily. It is not used in adults very often. Liver function tests should be done periodically. It often takes weeks before pemoline works.

ATOMOXETINE

Brand Name: Strattera.

Used For: Officially for attention-deficit/hyperactivity disorder (ADHD), but also used as an augmenting agent to boost the effectiveness of standard antidepressants.

Do Not Use If: There are very few reasons why a person absolutely should not take Strattera. Do not combine it with a monoamine oxidase inhibitor.

Tests to Take First: It is not a bad idea, although not absolutely necessary, to check blood pressure before starting.

Tests to Take While You Are on It: None are required, but checking blood pressure after a few weeks and then every few months is a good idea.

Usual Dose: Strattera comes in a wide range of pill strengths. The standard dose schedule is to begin at 40 mg in the morning and slowly increase to a maximum of 100 mg in the morning. When adding to an antidepressant as an augmenting agent, however, it is better to start much lower, usually at just 10 mg, and to then increase the dose slowly as needed. If Strattera is added to Prozac (fluoxetine) or Paxil (paroxetine) as an augmenting agent, dose increases should be done very carefully because of interactions between those antidepressants and Strattera.

Common Side Effects: Dry mouth, insomnia, sexual side effects, nausea.

Less Common Side Effects: Strattera can cause high blood pressure and very rarely increased heart rate.

What to Do About Side Effects: Most of the side effects go away on their own, or with lowering of the dose. If hypertension (high blood pressure) or changes in heart rate occur, the dose is also usually lowered and sometimes Strattera is discontinued.

If It Doesn't Work: When used for ADHD, if Strattera doesn't work, the next stronger drug is usually used instead, generally one of the versions of methylphenidate (Ritalin). When used to augment an antidepressant that hasn't worked well, the doctor may elect to try a different augmenting agent or try an entirely new antidepressant.

If It Does Work: For ADHD, the treatment usually lasts for several years. As an antidepressant augmenting agent, there are as yet no clear guidelines as to how long it should be continued but generally it should be for as long as the antidepressant it is augmenting is continued.

Cost: No generic version is yet available, so Strattera is fairly expensive.

Special Comments: Strattera isn't really a "psychostimulant," but it fits well into this group of drugs that have very similar uses. Its mechanism of action is solely on the norepinephrine (also called noradrenaline) system in the brain. This makes it a selective norepinephrine reuptake inhibitor or SNRI. Several of the older cyclic antidepressants, like desipramine and nortriptyline, are also SNRIs. This means that Strattera ought to be an antidepressant, but for some reason it didn't beat placebo when put to the test as an antidepressant. Its main function is to treat ADHD in children and adults. It is also sometimes used to augment the response to an antidepressant that hasn't worked sufficiently. Strattera is arguably safer than methylphenidate and certainly less addicting than amphetamines like Adderall. Whether it is as effective for ADHD as methylphenidate (Ritalin) is questionable, but many physicians feel it is worthwhile to try it first.

MODAFANIL

Brand Name: Provigil.

Used For: Officially for narcolepsy and excessive sleepiness associated with things like shift work, sleep apnea, and multiple sclerosis, but also used as an augmenting agent to boost the effectiveness of standard antidepressants or when antidepressants cause excessive daytime sleepiness as a side effect. It is also being tested for ADHD and some doctors already use it for that purpose.

Do Not Use If: You have heart disease or are taking birth control pills. Do not combine it with a monoamine oxidase inhibitor.

Tests to Take First: None are required.

Tests to Take While You Are on It: None are routine.

Usual Dose: The usual starting dose is 200 mg in the morning, which can be increased to 200 mg in the morning and 200 mg in the late morning or early afternoon. It is best to avoid taking it too close to bedtime.

Common Side Effects: Headache, nausea, diarrhea, nervousness, dry mouth, insomnia.

Less Common Side Effects: Very rarely, Provigil can cause heart problems. It is also potentially addicting, although this also seems to be uncommon.

What to Do About Side Effects: Most of the side effects go away on their own, or with lowering of the dose. If heart problems occur, the drug is usually stopped.

If It Doesn't Work: When used for ADHD, if Provigil doesn't work, the next stronger drug is usually used instead, generally Strattera or one of the versions of methylphenidate (Ritalin). When used to augment an antidepressant that hasn't worked well or to overcome sedating side effects of an antidepressant that is working, the doctor may recommend trying a different augmenting agent or an entirely new antidepressant.

If It Does Work: For ADHD, the treatment usually lasts for several years. As an antidepressant augmenting agent, there are as yet no clear guidelines as to how long it should be continued but generally as long as the antidepressant it is augmenting is continued.

Cost: No generic version is yet available, so Provigil is fairly expensive.

Special Comments: Provigil is a psychostimulant, but it works by an entirely different, and essentially unknown, mechanism than amphetamines and methylphenidate (Ritalin). It is most often used in psychiatry to reverse the sedative side effects of antidepressants like Remeron and some of the SSRIs like Paxil and Celexa. It is also used as an augmenting agent. There are reports of Provigil being abused and causing addiction, but this seems to be much less common than with the amphetamines or Ritalin.

PRAMIPEXOLE

Brand Name: Mirapex.

Used For: Officially for Parkinson's disease, but there is growing evidence that it works for depression that has not responded adequately to a standard antidepressant, either as an addition to the antidepressant or on its own.

Do Not Use If: There are very few reasons that would absolutely rule out Mirapex but do not combine it with a monoamine oxidase inhibitor.

Tests to Take First: None are required.

Tests to Take While You Are on It: None are routine, but if dizziness or fainting becomes problematic, blood pressure should be checked and monitored.

Usual Dose: Dosing for depression has not yet been finalized, but a reasonable approach is to start with 0.125 mg once or twice a day and slowly increase as needed to a maximum of 1.5 mg three times a day.

Common Side Effects: Tremors, weight loss, dry mouth, sexual problems, headache, constipation, insomnia or sleepiness during the day, dizziness upon getting up from a siting or lying position,

Less Common Side Effects: Fainting, very low blood pressure, hallucinations, involuntary movements.

What to Do About Side Effects: Most of the common side effects go away on their own or with lowering of the dose. If side effects persist or the more serious less common side effects emerge, however, Mirapex should be slowly tapered. It is important never to stop it abruptly.

If It Doesn't Work: When used to treat depression, the doctor will usually recommend tapering the dose and then discontinuing Mirapex.

If It Does Work: As an antidepressant augmenting agent, there are as yet no clear guidelines as to how long it should be continued but generally as long as the antidepressant it is augmenting is continued.

Cost: No generic version is yet available, so Mirapex is fairly expensive.

Special Comments: Mirapex is not a psychostimulant but is included here because it is used for some of the same reasons as the psychostimulants, such as augmenting antidepressant drug response. It stimulates the dopamine system in the brain, which is why it is used in Parkinson's disease. Recently, deficiency of the dopamine system has been implicated in depression, and several studies suggest that Mirapex may be useful to augment an antidepressant that hasn't worked satisfactorily or for patients with severe depression that hasn't responded to anything else. It is generally well tolerated and should be considered when other treatments are not working.

TO SWITCH OR TO AUGMENT

Let us say that you have a clear case of depression, regardless of the variety, and your doctor has prescribed a standard antidepressant, maybe an SSRI like Celexa or an SNRI like Cymbalta. You take the medication for four weeks and feel no better. The doctor increases your dose to the maximum, but two weeks later you still feel no better. What is the best next step? Here we have one of the biggest questions in psychopharmacology. Should the doctor and patient abandon the drug that hasn't worked and start all over with a new one? Studies consistently show that substituting a new antidepressant for one that hasn't helped sufficiently works about one-third of the time. In some instances, when an experienced psychopharmacologist picks the right second drug, that rate can be a little better. The real drawback to this solution, however, is that it means starting all over again with the four- to six-week waiting period, the amount of time it takes for most antidepressants to work. An alternative is to keep you on the antidepressant that hasn't worked well and add a second drug to it, a practice known as augmentation. Augmenting agents include thyroid hormone, lithium, atypical antipsychotics (like Zyprexa, Risperdal, Seroquel, Geodon, or Abilify), Wellbutrin SR (bupropion 12-hour tabs), and the psychostimulant drugs that include Provigil, Mirapex, Strattera, amphetamines (including Adderall), and methylphenidate (including Concerta). Again, this works in about one-third or more of cases. Which one of these augmenting agents to pick is not easy to say and depends a great deal on the exact profile of the patient. Thyroid hormone, usually the variety called T-3 (also called triiodothyronine or Cytomel), has virtually no side effects but seems to work better in research studies than the real world. Lithium is quite effective as an augmenting agent, even in depressed patients who are not bipolar, but itself takes at least two weeks to work and has notable side effects. The atypical antipsychotics are obvious choices for psychotic depression but seem to work also as augmenters for ordinary depression. They, however, have a number of side effects of consequence (described in the chapter on treating schizophrenia). Psychostimulants are effective, although many of them are either addicting (including amphetamines and methylphenidate) or not that well studied (including Provigil, Mirapex, and Strattera). Of all the choices, Wellbutrin SR (bupropion 12-hour tabs) is probably the most commonly picked choice. In most cases, it has minimal side effects when added to another antidepressant and in fact may reduce some of the side effects of SSRI and SNRI antidepressants, including sexual side effects, weight gain, and fatigue.

So which solution to choose? A huge study sponsored by the National Institute of Mental Health (NIMH), known as STAR-D, was supposed to answer this question, but although it has provided a great deal of information on treating depression, it did not offer any guidance on the switch-versus-augment question. Here are my own guidelines:

1. First, make sure nothing was missed when making the original diagnosis. Substance abuse is an example of something that doctors forget to ask about and patients would rather not reveal, making the treatment of depression more difficult.

2. Be sure the patient has really been taking all the pills as prescribed.

3. Revisit the possibility that psychotherapy is needed.

4. After the first three are considered, if the antidepressant has worked somewhat, but not enough, pick an augmenting agent and stick with it for another two weeks.

5. If the antidepressant hasn't worked at all by six weeks, switch to another antidepressant.

DO ANTIDEPRESSANTS INCREASE
THE RISK OF SUICIDE?

The idea that an antidepressant drug might actually make someone contemplate suicide seems absurd, and indeed that is what I thought when the suggestion was first made many years ago. Shortly after Prozac (fluoxetine) became a widely used antidepressant in the early 1990s, there were claims that the drug increased suicidal thinking in some patients. Similar claims have been made regarding most of the popular newer antidepressants, including Paxil (paroxetine) and Zoloft (sertraline), and lawsuits have been filed against the companies that make these drugs by families of patients who actually killed themselves while taking one of them. At first, most psychiatrists and scientists dismissed these claims as pure coincidence. First of all, they argued, depressed patients often wait until the very last minute to get help. Antidepressants take weeks to work and it might be that a very demoralized depressed person doesn't get any immediate relief and decides his or her situation is hopeless. Second, many analyses of large available databases from the clinical trials done by pharmaceutical companies to get the newer antidepressants approved by the FDA failed to show any increase in suicidal thinking or suicide. Finally, many of the initial claims that antidepressants cause suicidal thinking came from organizations or individuals that are traditionally opposed to the use of psychiatric medications or that stood to gain financially. Hence, organized psychiatry dismissed the possibility.

More recently, however, there is reason to revise this opinion. The impetus to change our minds began when a reanalysis of data from several clinical trials of SSRIs used in children showed that about 3 percent of the subjects in the research studies who took the actual drug had new onset of self-destructive thoughts, significantly more than among those children who were given a placebo. That of course means that this did not happen in 97 percent of the children, but 3 percent is still a high rate for such a serious problem. Warnings were sent to doctors and placed in the official description (known as the "label") of all antidepressants that they could increase the risk for suicidal thinking in children. It is important to note that no child actually committed suicide in any of these studies. My colleague at Mount Sinai in New York City, Dr. Jeffrey Weiss, and I also analyzed the data from these studies and showed that the risk of suicidal thinking occurred at a higher rate with drugs that last a relatively short time in the body (technically that have a short half-life) compared to those that last a long time. Thus, Effexor XR (venlafaxine), Paxil (paroxetine), and Luvox (fluvoxamine) had rates of suicidal thinking in children higher than placebo, but Prozac (fluoxetine) and Zoloft (sertraline) did not. The explanation for this is not clear, but it did convince me that the observation is not mere coincidence. More recently, an increase in suicidal thinking and even actual suicides has been found in the research studies done with adults who took antidepressants, especially the newer ones (like SSRIs). For this reason, all antidepressants now have the warning that they may increase the risk for suicidal thinking and self-destructive acts. It is totally unclear why this is so, especially why it should be the case that newer antidepressants are more prone to the problem than older ones. But there is no way around the data.

One of the accusations that has cropped up around this issue is that drug companies deliberately concealed data from the FDA and the scientific community that would have shown the suicide-enhancing effect a long time ago. I cannot opine on whether this is true or not, but a good thing has come out of the accusations: the new practice of making the drug companies make public *all* of their clinical trials, even ones that are ultimately not submitted to the FDA, as soon as they are completed.

It is important to put this all in perspective. First, as I stated earlier, my own opinion has radically changed in that I now believe that a side effect of antidepressants is to increase the risk of suicidal thinking and suicides. Second, this effect appears to be most apparent in the first few weeks of taking the drug. Patients who take them long enough to respond and whose depression gets better seem to have a lower risk of committing suicide than depressed patients who do not take antidepressants. Third, only a very small fraction of people, probably around 2 or 3 percent, who take antidepressants get suicidal. Fourth, there will now be a good deal of research on this topic and hopefully it will lead to important new insights into depression and antidepressants. At this point, I believe the drug companies, which have a lot to lose otherwise, will be fully cooperative. Finally, and most important, is that all medications that are effective for serious diseases have serious side effects. Depression is a very serious illness that is one of the leading causes of death in the United States. It is naïve to think that antidepressants, which are powerful drugs, would be free of serious adverse reactions. In this regard, antidepressants are no different from the drugs used to treat cancer, heart disease, and diabetes. The key is to use antidepressants only when absolutely necessary—that is, only for people with clearly diagnosed depression who are not candidates for or do not respond to psychotherapy. Once they are prescribed, the patient must be carefully monitored by doctor and by family for any sign of emerging suicidal thinking. If this happens, it should be treated as an emergency situation.

We have learned that antidepressants are not trivial medications and that taking them has serious consequences. On the other hand, we know that untreated depression ruins lives and kills people. Antidepressants work, but they are still medications and still need careful supervision.

ELECTROCONVULSIVE THERAPY, VAGAL NERVE STIMULATION, AND REPETITIVE TRANSCRANIAL MAGNETIC STIMULATION

"Shock treatment" easily ranks as the most controversial treatment in psychiatry. Many people have seen the movie *One Flew Over the Cuckoo's Nest* and have derived from it an image of what electroconvulsive therapy (ECT) involves. To most people, shock treatment means strapping a resistant patient to a stretcher, slapping electrodes on his or her head, and sadistically releasing a painful electrical current to the brain. The whole procedure is viewed as an exercise in mind control, like a lobotomy (which the "hero," played by Jack Nicholson in *One Flew Over the Cuckoo's Nest,* also received).

ECT is obviously not a drug, and therefore it would be easy to avoid talking about it in a book about psychiatric drugs. Somehow that seems a cowardly approach to a very heated and controversial area. So without undertaking a lengthy discussion, I will make a few statements about ECT,

Table 17.

Reasons to Administer Electroconvulsive Therapy to the Patient with Major Depression

- Patient is extremely suicidal and it is dangerous to wait the weeks it usually takes for medication to work.
- Patient refuses to eat and is severely malnourished; waiting for an antidepressant drug to work may be dangerous.
- Patient has psychotic depression.
- Patient has medical problems that make antidepressant medications risky (very occasionally true for elderly depressed patients).
- Patient with major depression has not responded to at least a six-week trial of at least two antidepressants, both with augmenting agents, and to psychotherapy.

as well as two new medical treatments for patients with depression who have not responded to medication: vagal nerve stimulation (VNS) and repetitive transcranial magnetic stimulation (rTMS).

First, it is an inescapable fact that for the treatment of major depression, ECT is by far the most successful method. The problem is that ECT does not work for most cases of atypical depression, anxiety disorders, or personality problems that involve occasional states of depression (Table 17). The diagnosis is again crucial. If the patient is properly diagnosed with major depressive disorder, there is approximately a 90 percent chance that ECT will cure him or her.

Second, ECT, as it is now performed, resembles what was depicted in *One Flew Over the Cuckoo's Nest* about as much as a game of chess resembles a heavyweight boxing match. People who observe ECT are usually surprised at how boring and routine the procedure really is. The patient must first agree to undergo ECT, and many hospitals now require the consent of both the patient and at least one family member. So there is no strapping of people by force onto stretchers. Next, an intravenous line is inserted and the patient is given a short-acting anesthetic that puts him or her to sleep. After this, a small dose of a drug that temporarily paralyzes the muscles is given and a bag is placed around the patient's mouth and nose so that air can be given mechanically until the muscle paralyzer wears off. These drugs are now administered by anesthesiologists. Complications from any of these procedures are almost nonexistent. Finally, the electrodes are placed on the scalp and a brief (less than one second) pulse of electrical current is administered. Increasingly, only one electrode is placed, on the right side of the head (called right unilateral ECT), and only if this doesn't work after a few treatments is the procedure switched to electrodes on both sides of the head (called bilateral ECT). The patient does not actually move or convulse physically; all that usually happens is an instantaneous twitching of the toes. After a few minutes, the patient wakes up. More and more patients are undergoing ECT as an outpatient procedure, without being admitted even overnight to the hospital.

Third, ECT is not mind control. The major side effect of ECT is memory loss. All patients forget what happened during the time immediately before each ECT treatment. After a few treatments, many patients develop varying degrees of amnesia; they forget things that have just happened or people they have just met. Most usually remember remote events, things that occurred months and years before the treatment began, without any problem. Numerous good scientific studies have shown that in the great majority of patients, any memory problems caused by ECT disappear in time, usually well within a month. Careful neuropsychological testing in a number of studies has failed to show any long-lasting memory problems in most patients who have received ECT. Memory loss is less of a problem with unilateral than with bilateral ECT.

Sometimes, memory problems can last longer, although six months is generally the upper limit. What about those who insist they have "permanent brain damage" from ECT? Once again, it must be stated that careful scientific studies have never found any evidence of permanent memory loss resulting from ECT. It may be that patients with preexisting memory problems, such as occur with certain neurological illnesses, blame their problems on their ECT treatments. Recurrences of depression or other psychiatric illness after ECT treatment can also interfere with memory, but the patient may nevertheless mistakenly associate the memory problem with ECT. Finally, we must always entertain the possibility that for a *rare* patient, ECT might produce long-term memory problems, but this has simply never been picked up by research studies. The risk of permanent memory defect from ECT seems so remote that individual patients should probably disregard it.

A few clinicians recommend maintenance ECT to depressed patients in which the patient receives a treatment every week or every other week as an outpatient. Some patients have received as many as one hundred ECT treatments using this procedure. The indications and effectiveness of this procedure have never been rigorously studied. Furthermore, it is possible that such a large number of treatments might produce more long-term memory loss than the standard six to twelve ECT treatments generally recommended.

Medically speaking, ECT is extremely safe. It is recommended for the occasional depressed patients who are too sick to take antidepressant medications and for extremely depressed pregnant women, in whom antidepressant drugs could conceivably harm the fetus. It may surprise some people that it is generally believed by clinicians that shock treatment is less likely to harm a fetus than is the administration of antidepressant drugs to the pregnant woman. It is known that women with epilepsy who have seizures during their pregnancies usually deliver normal babies. There are very few instances in which ECT is ruled out on medical grounds.

Thus, ECT is a treatment of great effectiveness and very small risk. Why, then, is it so controversial?

First, the treatment is admittedly mysterious. One of my colleagues, Dr. Stuart Yudofsky of Baylor College of Medicine, once likened it to kicking the television set when the picture is fuzzy. We still haven't the slightest clue why it works. All that is known is that causing a convulsion in the brain relieves depression. Interestingly, ECT also relieves mania and reduces psychotic symptoms in some patients with schizophrenia, although it is rarely used in these situations anymore.

Second, it is probable that ECT was abused in the past. It may have been administered to patients with a form of depression for which ECT is not effective. These patients generally do not respond, but sometimes clinicians continue to administer ECT treatments long after it is clear there is not going to be a response.

There are very specific instances in which ECT is a lifesaver: the patient who is extremely suicidal but does not respond to antidepressant drugs, the patient who refuses to eat because of depression and again does not respond to or will not agree to take antidepressant drugs, and the patient with psychotic depression. These people's lives are at risk. Nothing about ECT is bad enough to justify denying such patients an effective treatment.

For less urgent situations, most clinicians reserve the use of ECT for patients who have not responded to at least two antidepressant drugs, both with augmenting agents added. It goes without saying that ECT should not be attempted until it has also been determined that psychotherapy either is not an option or hasn't worked. Many of these drug refractory patients respond very well to ECT.

ECT is usually given in a series of six to twelve treatments, each treatment separated by at least one day. After completing ECT, the patient is generally placed on an antidepressant drug for several more months for maintenance of the normal mood.

Are there alternatives to ECT when medication and psychotherapy fail to help a depressed patient? An experimental (and hopefully soon FDA approved) procedure called repetitive transcranial magnetic stimulation (rTMS) might be that alternative. Instead of using electric current, rTMS uses a magnetic field current to stimulate the brain. This does not produce an actual convulsion and no anesthesia or muscle paralyzing agent is required. The patient sits up and a clinician aims a magnetic beam at a precise point so that specific brain structures are stimulated. This is done repetitively in each session. The only side effect is an occasional mild headache; rTMS has no adverse effect on memory. This procedure sounds almost too good to be true, except that it is not clear how well it works. Some studies have shown it to be just as effective as ECT, but in others it has not performed well. More evaluation is needed.

Finally, what do we recommend for a patient who does not get better even with ECT? Recently, the FDA approved a procedure called vagal nerve stimulation (VNS) for this situation. VNS has been used for several years to treat patients with epilepsy whose seizures do not respond to anticonvulsant medication. For a number of theoretical reasons, it seemed that VNS might work in depression as well. The procedure is done on an outpatient basis and involves a surgeon making a small incision in the chest and inserting a pulse generator and another incision in the neck and placing an electrode on the vagus nerve. This electrode can be stimulated by remote control. Each time the nerve is stimulated, electric current runs up the nerve to the brain. The patient does not feel anything, but there is very transient decrease in heart rate and hoarsness of the voice. Rarely, there can be permanent damage to the vocal cord and fainting if the heart rate goes too low. Overall, as shown in many epilepsy patients who have had VNS, the procedure is fairly simple and painless. It is still quite controversial, however, how well it works for depression. Testing VNS was difficult: Because it is reserved for only the most seriously depressed patients who have not responded to any other treatment, it was considered unethical to do the usual formal clinical trial in which the patient is not permitted to take anything else for depression. Furthermore, there is no ethical way to come up with a placebo or sham treatment. I am not entirely certain from looking at all the data if VNS works, but given its relative safety and the fact that it is reserved for desperate patients for whom there is really no alternative, I am pleased that it is available as an option.

Chapter 8

Drugs Used to Treat Anxiety

Anxiety is not only normal, it is necessary. Anxiety makes us run away from a burning building, bring our children to the doctor when they complain of earaches, check the bindings on our skis every winter, and declare all our income on our tax returns. Worrying is a part of everyday life, and although it may be unpleasant, it is a powerful mechanism to ensure that we avoid danger.

So why do we need drugs to make anxiety go away? Unlike depression, which seems to serve no useful purpose and therefore is best done away with, anxiety can be beneficial. Wouldn't drugs that eliminate anxiety do more harm than good? Do we really want to go through life entirely carefree without worries or fears?

These are absolutely legitimate questions. In fact, prescribing drugs to block anxiety can sometimes be very harmful. There is no question that unrestrained use of tranquilizers, street drugs, and alcohol to reduce life's normal cares and worries is dangerous.

Yet at least three extensive scientific surveys conducted by the National Institute of Mental Health surprised many professionals and laypeople alike by showing that anxiety disorders are the most common psychiatric illnesses in the United States today. In any six-month period, at least one out of every twenty Americans will suffer from an anxiety disorder that should be treated by a mental health professional. There are now excellent "evidence-based" psychotherapies, most of them varieties of cognitive behavioral therapy (CBT), that have been proved by rigorous scientific study to be effective for each of the anxiety disorders. Whenever possible, these should be the first approach to treating anxiety disorder. In those situations in which psychotherapy has not worked or the patient is adverse to being in psychotherapy, medication is the best and safest way to treat anxiety disorders.

THREE FORMS OF ANXIETY

The first and perhaps most important thing to know about anxiety is that it takes many forms; some require treatment and some are better left alone. I like to divide anxiety into three categories: (1) normal anxiety, (2) excessive anxiety, and (3) anxiety disorders. Let me explain a bit more what I mean.

Normal Anxiety

There are many good reasons to feel anxious, even though feeling anxious doesn't feel particularly good. If your daughter complains of a sore throat, you may well worry that it could be strep throat, that she might miss school, and that you may have to miss time from work to take her to the pediatrician. If you get into your car in the morning and the engine doesn't turn over, you will probably worry that the repair may be expensive, that you might have to do without the car for a few days, and that it could take hours for the tow truck to show up.

This kind of anxiety actually is helpful, because it will motivate you to take action. You worry about your daughter's sore throat, so you go to the phone and make an appointment to get a throat culture. The car may be in bad shape, so you start making arrangements for a tow truck and a rental car. In these situations the anxiety disappears when the stressful situation clears up. Once the pediatrician tells you nothing is seriously wrong with your child, you breathe a sigh of relief and stop worrying. When your mechanic says the only problem with your car is that the battery is old and he'll have a new one within an hour, you realize that it's only a minor inconvenience. So normal anxiety is related to a real-life event, motivates you to take appropriate action, and goes away when the stressful situation clears up. You shouldn't waste your money on psychiatrists for this and certainly shouldn't take drugs.

Excessive Anxiety

Sometimes a stressful situation arises that would make anyone feel anxious, but the anxiety grows out of proportion to the real threat involved. For example, many people feel anxious before meeting with their boss. They may worry several hours before the meeting about what the boss might say or do. Some may even have a little trouble getting their work done for a few hours. Once the meeting is over and nothing serious has happened, the person normally relaxes and goes on with things. Let's look, however, at an example in which such anxiety becomes exaggerated:

Allen, a thirty-three-year-old investment banker with a large firm, receives a call one morning from his boss's secretary, who says that the boss wants to meet with him at three that afternoon. "What is it about?" Allen asks the secretary. "I think it's about the car company deal you just finished," she answers, although she obviously isn't sure. Instantly, Allen is in a panic. The deal he worked on had been successfully completed for the firm, but now he wonders if he left something out that has just come to light. Maybe the boss thinks he didn't work hard enough on the deal. After all, one night last week he left work before midnight, right in the middle of a crucial part of the transaction. Allen is unable to work the rest of the day. He feels nauseous, gets a headache, and suddenly starts worrying that he may have cancer, that his wife might be having an affair, that his tax return is going to be audited, and so on.

The meeting with the boss actually goes well, although Allen shakes the whole time. The boss thinks he did a good job, makes a few suggestions of things he might have done better, tells Allen he is doing well with the firm, and then gets to the real purpose of the meeting: going over the next big deal he wants Allen to work on. But Allen's anxiety is unrelieved. He focuses only on the few suggestions for improvement the boss gives him, insisting to himself that unless he does better on the next deal, he will certainly be fired. He spends the next week unable to sleep, fighting with his wife, and constantly worried. Eventually, as he becomes involved in the new deal, he calms down. But his wife, who somehow puts up with all of this, points out to him that he seems to get into this state of high anxiety very often since he began working at the firm.

Obviously, Allen took normal anxiety about a meeting with his boss and blew it way out of proportion. He focused on the one slightly negative comment made by his boss and ignored all the praise. Instead of recognizing that the boss was obviously so satisfied with his work that he was putting him on another big deal, Allen turned things completely around to make it appear that he was on the brink of being fired. And Allen brought in all kinds of extraneous worries. Why should a meeting with his boss make him suddenly worry about his relationship with his wife, his physical health, or his income tax return? Finally, he suffered several physical signs of anxiety, like headache and upset stomach.

Excessive anxiety arises from a life stress but soon goes beyond what is called for. It serves no purpose and doesn't go away once the stress is over. Note, however, that Allen's anxiety eventually did go away; it lasted only about a week and did not really impair his ability to work too much. Mostly, it was unpleasant and unnecessary and probably annoying to his wife.

Excessive anxiety often requires treatment but rarely drug treatment. Various forms of psychotherapy are very useful for people like Allen to help them look at things more realistically and stop turning everyday life events into mental catastrophes. Sometimes people want to know more about what causes them to be so anxious and therefore may choose to have long-term psychotherapy that is based on psychoanalytic principles originally articulated by Sigmund Freud. Other people use short-term psychotherapies to learn how to cope better with stress and to think more logically about things that happen. Either way, medications are usually not necessary.

Anxiety Disorders

Anxiety disorders arise without any obvious life stress provocation. Then they persist, sometimes for life, if they are not treated. Unlike normal anxiety or excessive anxiety, anxiety disorders can have very great impact on the ability to function in day-to-day life. Although some doctors and scientists think that anxiety is nothing to be concerned about, some anxiety disorders can ruin a person's life.

In the last twenty-five years, scientists have made great progress in categorizing anxiety disorders and finding effective treatments. Some of these treatments do involve drugs. Like depression, anxiety disorders can almost always be treated successfully, and sometimes the symptoms can be completely eliminated.

THE ANXIETY DISORDERS

There are six main anxiety disorders, each with its own treatment requirement: generalized anxiety disorder (GAD), panic disorder (which can involve phobias including agoraphobia), the phobias (social and specific), obsessive-compulsive disorder (OCD), and post-traumatic stress disorder

(PTSD). A version of PTSD that lasts for only a month is called acute stress disorder. A description of each is necessary so that the patient with an anxiety disorder can understand the drug treatments that may be recommended. Let me emphasize once more, however, that I always explore with a patient who has an anxiety disorder the possibility of having cognitive behavioral therapy (CBT), a form of psychotherapy usually lasting between three and six months, before considering drug treatment. Research studies show that CBT works as well as medication (although it may take a bit longer to have a positive effect) and that the beneficial effects of CBT last much longer when the treatment is completed than do those of medication after the medication is discontinued. CBT also has no side effects.

Generalized Anxiety Disorder

A form of chronic anxiety, generalized anxiety disorder lasts at least six months. The patient is constantly anxious, tense, and worried. Usually it is difficult to fall asleep and there are lots of aches and pains like headache, stomachache, menstrual cramps, and backache. Although stressful events may make this condition worse, people with GAD are anxious even if everything is going great in their lives. Many drink excessively to try to calm down or fall asleep, so the risk of developing a problem with alcohol is high with GAD. Often, after many months or years with chronic anxiety, the patient develops a full-blown depression requiring antidepressant treatment. People with GAD usually have a lot of trouble at work. They don't have much fun because they are always on edge and usually very fatigued. The most common medications that work for GAD, if medication is elected, are antidepressants, like any of the SSRIs or SNRIs described in the previous chapter (including Paxil, Celexa, Zoloft, Effexor XR, and Cymbalta); the benzodiazepines, which include familiar names like Valium, Xanax, Ativan, and Librium; and a drug called buspirone (BuSpar). A drug called pregabalin (Lyrica) that is now available for the treatment of pain and for epilepsy may also be approved soon to treat GAD because research studies show it is effective.

Panic Disorder

The best way to describe panic disorder, which affects 3 percent of Americans at any given moment, is through a clinical example. Jane, a neurosurgeon, is driving to work one day over a bridge when traffic gets a bit heavy and she wonders for a moment if she will get to the hospital on time. All of a sudden her heart starts to pound, she feels as if she can't catch her breath, and she shakes, trembles, and is sure she must be having a heart attack. Convinced she is about to die or lose control of the car, she drives very slowly in the right-hand lane. When Jane gets to the hospital, her symptoms are relieved but she still goes to the emergency room and tells the nurse that she thinks she is having a heart attack. The nurse is skeptical; Jane is, after all, a perfectly healthy-appearing thirty-five-year-old woman. Nevertheless, she is seen immediately by an emergency room doctor, who orders an electrocardiogram and several blood tests. Everything is normal.

Jane feels relieved. Her symptoms are now gone. Perhaps she simply has been working too hard. Maybe she needs a vacation. Everything goes back to normal until two days later when, while sitting at home reading, it happens again. Her heart pounds, she breathes too fast, and she feels dizzy and light-headed. The symptoms last twenty minutes; by then Jane is back in the emergency room. This time a neurologist is called. Maybe it's a brain tumor. She is admitted to the hospital and undergoes many tests, but nothing abnormal is found. Jane is relieved to find she is not suffering from a deadly disease. But she keeps having attacks, each lasting about twenty minutes, and each terrifying. They happen in the car, at work, and at home.

Now Jane starts worrying about when the next attack might strike; we call this *anticipatory anxiety*. She also starts avoiding situations in which she might not be able to get help right away if an attack occurs. She doesn't want to drive across the bridge during rush hour for fear of being trapped in the car during a traffic jam; she turns down a chance to fly to Hawaii for a conference; she sits near the door in church and the movies so she can get out fast. Soon, Jane becomes so afraid of getting an attack that she avoids going anywhere unless accompanied by a close friend.

Jane has developed panic disorder. The attacks are called panic attacks. Unlike a person with generalized anxiety disorder who is more or less always anxious, the patient with panic disorder becomes anxious in sudden and unpredictable bursts. Scientists believe that the cause of this disorder is partly medical and partly psychological. It is believed that panic disorder has a biological basis but that stressful life events contribute to the severity of the illness. Some patients get so fearful of having attacks that they avoid places where help will not be immediately available; this is called *agoraphobia*.

Medications have been known for more than twenty years to be very successful in blocking panic attacks. Most of these medications are antidepressants.

Although the cyclic antidepressants (like imipramine) were the first to be proven to work for panic disorder, the newer serotonin reuptake inhibitors (SSRIs) and serotonin norephineprine reuptake inhibitors (SNRIs) have become the first-line treatment for panic. One of them, Paxil (paroxetine), received FDA approval in 1996 for the specific treatment of panic disorder; after that, several other medications in these classes also received FDA approval (including Zoloft, Prozac, and Effexor XR). However, studies show that all of the drugs in these classes (including Celexa) are also effective. Xanax (alprazolam) and Klonopin (clonazepam) are benzodiazepine antianxiety drugs that have also been shown to be effective in treating panic attacks, but they are generally used only when one of the antidepressants does not work well enough. Desyrel, Asendin, and Wellbutrin are not generally effective for panic disorder. BuSpar is almost certainly not an antipanic drug even though it is effective for generalized anxiety.

Phobias (Specific and Social)

Phobias are irrational fears of things or situations that become so extreme the person avoids them. To be classified as a phobia, the avoidance must seriously interfere with the ability to function. A person who is afraid of skydiving does not have a phobia, because most of us live very nicely without jumping out of airplanes.

Specific phobia is a fear of a specific situation or object, for example, fear of heights, fear of closed-in spaces (claustrophobia), and fear of animals. Specific phobias are very normal in childhood. There are no drug treatments for specific phobias, which usually respond nicely to behavioral psychotherapy.

Social phobia is a fear of social situations. People with this disorder have severe anxiety attacks if they have to talk in front of a group, speak up in class, call someone for a date, or even sign a check when the bank teller is watching. Whenever they feel they are being watched or have to perform, people with social phobia become extremely anxious, have palpitations, shake, blush, and tremble. Then they think people can see them shaking and blushing and they get even more nervous. Let me give an example of social phobia:

Jonathan was a very popular and outgoing teenager until one day when he had to give a speech in front of his high school class. As he approached the podium he noticed that his heart was pounding. Previously, this stage fright had disappeared once he began, but this time it just got worse as he began talking. In addition to the pounding heart, Jonathan started shaking, felt his voice was going to crack, and began to sweat. He feared that everyone in the audience could see his nervousness and that he would be thoroughly embarrassed. Somehow he got through the speech, but he was convinced he did a terrible job. Afterward, he refused to speak in front of the whole class ever again. Next, it became difficult for him to raise his hand in class because he would experience similar symptoms whenever the teacher called on him. Finally, he started to avoid parties and other social events. Almost any social interaction precipitated an anxiety attack. Now, as an adult, Jonathan rarely attends social events. Although he is very intelligent, he has never advanced in his career because he cannot make presentations or withstand job interviews. He feels lonely and frustrated and often gets drunk if he cannot avoid a social encounter.

Social phobia is obviously more than stage fright. Once again, both medications and psychotherapies can relieve the condition to a considerable extent. Effective medications include the SSRIs (Prozac, Paxil, Celexa, Zoloft), SNRIs (Effexor XR, Cymbalta), benzodiazepines (Klonopin), and monoamine oxidase inhibitors (Nardil, Parnate). However, whenever possible, cognitive behavioral psychotherapy, often conducted in group format, is the best first step, with medications reserved for people who either don't want or don't respond to therapy.

Finally, there is agoraphobia, which is a complication of panic disorder and is treated as such.

Obsessive-Compulsive Disorder

Formerly thought to be a rare condition, OCD is now felt to affect as many as one in one hundred people. It is the subject of intense scientific study, with some scientists claiming that they have developed an animal model of OCD, and some reasonably effective treatments are available. Cognitive behavioral therapy (CBT), pioneered by Dr. Edna Foa of the University of Pennsylvania among others, and several medications, help in many cases. The drugs include all of the SSRIs and SNRIs, plus the cyclic antidepressant clomipramine (Anafranil). Unfortunately, OCD is the toughest anxiety disorder to treat. In research studies, the definition of an effective treatment is usually not more than a 50 percent improvement in 50 percent of the patients in the study. That means that many OCD patients wind up having to combine CBT with medications, take high doses of medication, and stay on medication indefinitely in order to get relief of their symptoms.

Patients with OCD have one of two problems, or both. An excellent place to read about patients with OCD is in *The Boy Who Couldn't Stop Washing* by Dr. Judith Rapoport of the National Institute of Mental Health. Some examples follow:

If you met Clark at a party or business meeting, you would think he was a pretty ordinary person. He might tell you he works as an accountant, that he is married but has no children, and that he likes watching sporting events on television. You probably wouldn't notice that he refused to eat any food offered to him at the party and that he quietly disappeared to the bathroom five times in the course of only a few hours. And you might not observe that Clark's hands are red, raw, and blistered. He has had a compulsion to wash his hands as many as forty times a day since he was sixteen years old. Anytime he thinks his hands might be dirty, say from touching a piece of food, taking out the garbage, or dusting his apartment, he immediately gets an irresistible urge to wash them. He knows that this kind of dirt is not dangerous and that his hand washing is excessive.

For entirely mysterious reasons, however, the urge to wash his hands is overwhelming; if he doesn't do it he feels intolerable anxiety. Once he washes he immediately relaxes, until the next time. He can't travel or sit in a movie theater long because he has to know that a sink and soap will always be available nearby. Needless to say, he can hold only certain kinds of very restricted jobs where no one will notice. Sometimes he gets so sick of his compulsion that he becomes extremely depressed, but depression is clearly not the major problem. No matter how hard he tries, he cannot stop washing his hands.

Clark has classic *compulsions* as part of his obsessive-compulsive disorder. Like many people with this illness, he has had symptoms from adolescence—some people get this as young children—and is tortured by the compulsions. He does not really want to wash his hands, he does not think the hand washing is necessary, but he cannot stop. Others have different compulsions, for example, scrubbing their homes over and over to be sure there is no dirt or checking more than one hundred times that the gas on the stove is turned off before leaving home. Some compulsions seem bizarre to others. At times, it is not so clear that the person really knows that the compulsions are irrational and appears to believe, for example, that everything really is contaminated so that excessive hand washing is necessary. At this point, the line between having a compulsion and having a delusion becomes thin. This type of OCD with a delusional component often requires the addition of an antipsychotic medication (like Zyprexa, Risperdal, or Trilafon) to the antidepressant in order to get a response.

Another example, of a slightly different kind, is Janet, who is a secretary in a law firm. She does fairly good work but is slow and sometimes doesn't complete her assignments on time. This puzzles her bosses because they think she is unusually intelligent, dedicated, and very organized. Yet sometimes she seems to do everything in slow motion. The reason is that Janet cannot type a document until she first counts all the words in the document. Sometimes she gets almost to the end of counting when she suddenly fears she has made a mistake and must start all over again. If she is interrupted in the middle of counting, she also must begin again. At home, before Janet starts to read a magazine article, she counts all the words. She never throws out an article she has read because at any time she may suddenly doubt she has counted the words correctly and feel compelled to go back and count again.

Like Clark, Janet hasn't the slightest idea why she needs to conduct these counting rituals or why she has obsessive doubts that she has counted correctly. The obsessive doubts can be terrifying to her; once she thinks she has counted wrong she can think of nothing else until she counts again. At night she may lie awake with various obsessions, like trying to remember how many words were in a document she typed two weeks earlier. Janet has a combination of compulsions—needing to count over and over—and *obsessions*—thinking in her mind over and over about the number of words in various documents. No one else is aware of her behavior; the bosses simply think she is slow. Indeed, procrastination is a common symptom for people with OCD. Janet has never married or conducted a long-term relationship, so no other person has seen the piles of magazines on the floors of her apartment. Janet would do anything to stop her compulsions and obsessions, but no amount of effort ever works.

Many people with OCD also have tics and/or Tourette's syndrome, in which they have both tics and uncontrollably utter sounds and words, sometimes profanities. The combination of OCD and tics often calls for a combination of antidepressant and antipsychotic medications. Several scientific groups have linked OCD in childhood to strep infections (infections of the throat and other parts of the body with the common bacteria streptococcus). They advocate antibiotics as treatment. This is much debated in the scientific community.

Post-Traumatic Stress Disorder

Post-traumatic stress disorder is unique among anxiety disorders in that by definition it occurs only after a real-life event. Contrary to popular belief, most people with phobias and panic attacks did not get them after having a real-life frightening experience. Traumatic life events are probably involved in many if not most cases of anxiety disorder and depression, but the relationship is generally complicated and the stressful life events usually occur months to years before the event. PTSD, on the other hand, follows a clear-cut real event. That event must be life threatening. About one-third of people who experience awful traumatic situations—fatal car accidents, torture, earthquakes, concentration camps, ship sinkings, airplane crashes, war—develop the syndrome of PTSD. The person may have experienced or witnessed the life-threatening event, but it must include either death or bodily harm to others and/or the true fear that the person himself or herself will be seriously physically harmed or killed. Events after which which someone subsequently feels emotionally hurt or aggrieved, like being jilted by a girlfriend or getting fired from a job without good reason, are unfortunate but do not qualify as events capable of causing PTSD.

In order to meet the *DSM-IV* criteria for PTSD, the symptoms begin one month or more after the traumatic event. If symptoms occur immediately after the event, the condition is called acute stress disorder and the diagnosis of PTSD is not made until the one-month period following the event has occurred. The cardinal feature of PTSD is a reliving of the traumatic experience. People with PTSD, both in dreams and while awake, have frequent episodes in which they feel as if they are living through the awful experience all over again. For example, a Vietnam War veteran who witnessed his three closest friends blown up in front of him feels he is in the middle of a battlefield years later when he hears a car backfire. Or a Nazi concentration camp survivor feels herself back in Dachau upon encountering a uniformed security guard in a museum. In addition to reliving a traumatic experience, people with PTSD lose the ability to experience a wide range of emotions; there is a sense of emotional "blunting." They also feel on edge and are easily startled. They avoid things or places associated with the original traumatic event. Hence, the rape victim will not walk on the street or even go into the neighborhood in which she was raped, even if it is generally known as a safe neighborhood. Or someone who survived a fatal car crash will not get into a car again. Finally, there are associated symptoms of anxiety and depression.

Only about one-third of people exposed to a qualifying traumatic event actually develop PTSD. Others develop other psychiatric illnesses, predominantly depression, panic disorder, and substance abuse, but most people are able to get through a terrible event without getting psychiatrically ill. Some of the risk factors for getting PTSD are a prior history of a psychiatric illness, a family history of psychiatric illness, and little social support. There may be, therefore, a genetic predisposition to respond to traumatic events by getting PTSD. Social support can reduce the risk for getting PTSD. This may be why there are fewer cases of PTSD than originally expected among people who survived the 9/11 attacks and why a relatively high rate of rape and sexual abuse victims, who often receive the opposite of social support from law enforcement authorities and even friends and family, develop PTSD. In most cases, PTSD goes away on its own, so that ten years after the event only about 10 percent of people still have PTSD. However, treatment is often required because the suffering is great and the waiting period for a spontaneous recovery often too long to tolerate.

WHEN SHOULD YOU SEEK HELP
FOR ANXIETY?

We have now identified three broad categories of anxiety—normal anxiety, excessive anxiety, and anxiety disorders—and within these broad categories several subgroups. It may sound complicated: How can anyone figure out where he or she belongs? Here are some guidelines to help you decide when you should consult an expert and when you should consider taking medication:

1. First, try to figure out if there is an obvious reason why you are feeling nervous. Don't grasp at straws; you shouldn't be staying awake all night because you failed a math exam thirty years ago. Ask yourself if the reasons you think you feel nervous would make other people feel nervous and if it is likely that your life will calm down soon.

2. Next, try to decide if this is an isolated episode of anxiety or if you are always an anxious person. Do you have a history of letting little setbacks put you into a panic for months?

3. Finally, consider whether the anxiety is helping you stay on top of the situation and take effective action, or is impairing your ability to function.

If there is no obvious reason for the anxiety (or it follows a clear-cut life-threatening event), if you are constantly plagued by anxiety or anxiety-related symptoms, and if anxiety makes it hard for you to function, you should consult a psychiatrist for evaluation.

And even more important, if you find yourself abusing alcohol, tranquilizers, or any drug to calm yourself down, you should seek a consultation immediately. Anxiety disorders can cause alcohol and drug abuse.

What should the consulting psychiatrist tell you? First, the psychiatrist may help you recognize that there is a perfectly good reason for you to be anxious and that you should expect to feel better when things calm down. Let me give an example:

A forty-five-year-old woman asked me if I would give her a prescription for Valium. She had been feeling very nervous and anxious for several weeks, had difficulty sleeping, and was less able to concentrate at work. It turned out that two of her most trusted assistants had just resigned to take other jobs, and she now had to work sixty-hour weeks without much sympathy from either her boss or her husband. Her elderly mother had recently had a stroke and called her daily from the nursing home with new complaints. I felt that this woman, who liked to believe she could cope with anything and resented any emotional problem that might interfere with her usually high performance, had good reason to feel anxious. Giving her Valium would only make her sleepy during the day. Instead, I suggested she was overlooking how much stress she was under and worked out a plan for her to reduce the tension in her life. This included explaining to her boss and husband what the problems were, insisting that she get new assistants, taking a few days off, and asking her sister to help out more with their mother.

In this case, the psychiatrist was expected to hand out a prescription but he didn't. Sometimes, patients are disappointed or angry when told medication is not the right choice; how many internists prescribe antibiotics to patients suffering from viruses just so they can satisfy the patient's wish to get any drug?

On the other hand, there are opposite cases in which the patient may think there is enough stress to explain the symptoms when in fact he or she is avoiding the fact that a real psychiatric problem exists.

When I first saw Quincy, for example, he told me about his recurrent panic attacks. He had to have his wife in the car with him at all times, and even so refused to drive over bridges or through tunnels. He hadn't been in an airplane for five years and couldn't stand shopping malls because the exits are hard to find. So his life was constricted to being driven to his office every day and then driven home. Still, he had a full-blown panic attack at least once a month and was well-known to every emergency room and general practitioner in his hometown. Quincy insisted that he was merely suffering from "stress." Things had been hard at work lately, he told me. Sometimes he had fights with his wife. His college-age son was not getting very good grades. All of that might be true, I explained, but it really sounded like pretty routine stress to me. He had been suffering from panic attacks for five years, but his son started college only six months ago, he had had exactly four arguments with his wife in that period and their marriage seemed solid, and he had been at the same job for almost fifteen years. Quincy did not want to face the fact that he was suffering from panic disorder and that mere stress reduction was unlikely to help him. He needed treatment directed toward cessation of the panic attacks and then reduction of his phobias. He had a course of cognitive behavioral psychotherapy with a colleague that helped but did not completely eliminate the symptoms, so I prescribed Celexa. Four weeks later, he noticed that his panic attacks had stopped and he was making much more progress with CBT overcoming his fear of driving and flying on airplanes.

The psychiatrist, then, must first make a diagnosis. A patient with normal anxiety should be reassured that things will clear up in time. A patient with excessive anxiety should be told that he or she is overreacting and may need psychotherapy to learn how to keep things within bounds. Occasionally, a very short course of medication is used. A patient with an anxiety disorder requires either CBT or medication or both. Thus, an understanding of the nature of the anxiety problem is very important: The treatment must be tailored to the diagnosis.

THE BENZODIAZEPINES: ARE THEY REALLY DANGEROUS?

I have often joked that someday I will start a support group for physicians who prescribe benzodiazepines. It would be organized along the lines of an Alcoholics Anonymous group and I would begin by saying, "Hello, my name is Jack and I still prescribe Valium and Xanax." Then we would go around the room, and each doctor—surgeons, internists, primary care doctors, and psychiatrists alike—would confess to being a benzodiazepine prescriber.

When Valium (diazepam) was introduced in the United States in the early 1960s as the first member of the benzodiazepine class, followed shortly by Librium (chlordiazepoxide) and Klonopin (clonazepam), it was heralded as a virtual miracle drug. Unlike its predecessors for treating anxiety, like barbiturates and Miltown (meprobamate), Valium and the other benzodiazepines appeared to be medically safe, not addicting, and actually worked. But in the 1970s, when benzodiazepines became among the most often prescribed medications in the Western world, there was a strong backlash. The drugs were accused of being addicting and of "drugging" people who were really just bored or under mild stress. Even as new benzodiazepines were introduced, like Ativan (lorazepam) and Xanax (alprazolam), fierce debates arose about whether in fact they are safe and effective or addicting and virtual "mind control."

The benzodiazepines provoke so much heated debate that the average patient taking a benzodiazepine may wonder what is in them and physicians have come to feel like drug pushers when they prescribe them. Millions of benzodiazepine prescriptions are in fact actually written in the United States every year, but most doctors feel a little guilty about administering them. Nowadays it seems there are only two schools of thought: the school that says benzodiazepines are perfectly harmless and the school that says they are disasters. Listen to the first group and you'll think benzodiazepines are as safe as a warm glass of milk before bed. Listen to the second group and you'll think heroin is better.

It is appropriate for experts to fight it out on these issues. But they aren't the ones who are supposed to swallow the pills. So let me try to make some sense of this.

First, the positive side. From a physical medical standpoint, benzodiazepines are extremely safe. You cannot commit suicide even by taking a truckload of benzodiazepines, unless they are combined with other substances. Benzodiazepines don't hurt the brain, heart, liver, or kidneys. They also work very well to relieve anxiety. It is rare that a truly anxious person won't get some help from taking them, and the benefit may be realized after a day or two. Once a stable dose is established, most patients continue to realize benefit from benzodiazepines without needing to increase the dose. Contrary to popular belief, several excellent scientific studies show convincingly that tolerance to benzodiazepines—the need to constantly increase the dose to maintain the therapeutic effect—is extremely rare. And stopping use of benzodiazepines has no life-threatening consequences like stopping the use of barbiturates. Benzodiazepines are also anticonvulsants, muscle relaxants, and hypnotics (that is, they can be used as sleeping pills).

BENZODIAZEPINE DEPENDENCE

So benzodiazepines are medically safe, very effective drugs. What could be better?

Here are the negatives. Even though you won't die when you try to stop taking benzodiazepines, you won't enjoy the experience very much, either. A definite withdrawal syndrome is associated with coming off benzodiazepines. At least 50 percent of patients experience some degree of withdrawal when stopping benzodiazepines. The symptoms are listed in Table 18.

You can read more about withdrawal in general in Chapter 6. As far as the benzodiazepines are concerned, it is important to remember that the severity of the withdrawal symptoms depends directly on several factors:

• The higher the dose of the benzodiazepine, the worse will be the withdrawal once the drug is stopped.

• The longer the person has taken benzodiazepines, the worse will be the withdrawal once the drug is stopped.

• Short-acting benzodiazepines (Xanax, Serax, Ativan) may produce more severe withdrawal symptoms than long-acting benzodiazepines (Valium, Librium, Tranxene), but the difference is very small.

Table 18.
_____

Symptoms of Withdrawal from Benzodiazepines

MOST COMMON
Nervousness
Insomnia
Loss of appetite
Metallic taste
Tingling feelings
Headache
Lack of coordination
Perspiration
Noises sound very loud
Muscle aches
Lack of energy

LEAST COMMON
Poor concentration
Seizures

• Very potent benzodiazepines (Klonopin, Xanax, Ativan) may provide more severe withdrawal symptoms than less potent benzodiazepines (Valium, Librium, Tranxene).

• Withdrawal symptoms can be reduced a great deal by slow tapering of the medication. Almost all patients experience strong withdrawal symptoms if the medication is stopped suddenly.

• Withdrawal symptoms usually last two weeks and rarely longer than four weeks after the drug is stopped. They are not life-threatening and hospitalization is almost never required.

• People who abuse other drugs, especially alcohol, generally have a harder time stopping benzodiazepines than non–drug abusers.

• Withdrawal from benzodiazepines is far easier than from drugs formerly used to treat anxiety, such as barbiturates, meprobamate (Miltown, Equanil), Placidyl, Doriden, and Noludar.

In a sense, patients get hooked on benzodiazepines. The term _addiction,_ however, should not be applied to benzodiazepine use. Addiction implies a lifestyle totally consumed with obtaining and taking a drug even if it results in severe injury to the addicted person or others. A cocaine addict will kill to get cocaine and is willing to die for his or her coke. People who take Valium do not rearrange their lives or steal or murder to get Valium, and they do not disregard their own health. It is medically correct to say that benzodiazepines produce physical and psychological dependence evidenced by the withdrawal syndrome that occurs when they are stopped.

There are a few other problems with benzodiazepines. Their biggest side effect is sleepiness. That's okay if your problem is insomnia, but not so good if you have to drive your car. Some experts say that benzodiazepines are associated with traffic accidents. Also, they may cause memory problems and confusion in elderly people and there is some evidence that benzodiazepines, like a lot of drugs, can increase the risk of an elderly person falling and fracturing a hip.

As in any other debate on a medical topic, the truth about benzodiazepines lies between the two sides. Benzodiazepines are medicines with side effects and potential complications. They are not perfect and are prescribed to many patients who would be better off without them. Once you take them, it is important to try to keep the dose low and to stop as soon as possible. But it would be tragic for the person suffering from an anxiety disorder who barely gets through the day to be denied these safe and effective drugs. Aspirin causes far more physical harm than benzodiazepines if taken for long periods, and steroid drugs sometimes prescribed for problems as trivial as poison ivy can produce more serious psychological complications.

Let me give some examples of how to use and how *not* to use benzodiazepines:

A recently married woman visits her general practitioner, complaining of stomach cramps, diarrhea, and nausea over the last four weeks. All of the medical tests turn out to be normal. The woman admits to her doctor that she has been worrying a little bit lately about how happy she will be with her marriage. So the doctor gives her a prescription for a one-month supply of Xanax, with automatic renewals up to six months (automatic renewals of benzodiazepines are not permitted in some states). He tells her to try and stop worrying.

This is the classic case of overprescription of benzodiazepines. First, the woman could conceivably take the drug every day for six months without ever seeing a doctor. Second, it is unlikely that Xanax will make her marriage any better. Maybe the marriage is fine, but she is having trouble making the adjustment. Maybe the marriage is terrible and the couple should seek counseling. Maybe the marriage isn't the problem at all and the woman has a different psychiatric problem. By the time this woman's prescription runs out she will probably have a hard time getting off Xanax without experiencing withdrawal symptoms.

It is proper for nonpsychiatric doctors to prescribe short courses of anxiety medication. They often know their patients very well, and some people confide more in a trusted family doctor or gynecologist than in anyone else. Psychiatrists have made other physicians feel very guilty about prescribing benzodiazepines, but they themselves frequently prescribe them for one reason—they work. But the primary care physician is not specially trained in psychiatric disorders. Remember the rule: Don't take benzodiazepines prescribed by a nonpsychiatric physician longer than a couple of weeks. If you need drugs for anxiety that badly, a short-term prescription won't be enough; you should be seeing a psychiatrist.

Now let me relate an opposite situation. A forty-year-old woman has been taking small doses of the benzodiazepine antianxiety drug Klonopin for ten years. About once a month she sees her psychiatrist for a prescription renewal. She is working well as an executive at a bank and maintains good social relationships. She has gotten some benefit from psychotherapy but now wants to go on with life without having to see a therapist on a regular basis. She does not abuse alcohol and reports no side effects from taking Klonopin.

One day the patient is having a routine checkup by a new internist. When taking her history, he seemingly becomes aghast when she tells him that she has been taking Klonopin. The internist tells her that she is probably addicted to Klonopin, that the "modern" way to treat anxiety is with antidepressants, and, without consulting her psychiatrist, convinces her to get off the Klonopin and start Zoloft (sertraline). So the woman stops the Klonopin. After two weeks of undergoing a withdrawal syndrome, the insomnia, ringing in the ears, and upset stomach go away, but over the next month, all her old anxiety problems return. She worries incessantly, feels jumpy and tense all the time, and can't concentrate at work. Zoloft is a very good medication for most anxiety disorders, but for this patient it does not seem to help nearly as much as Klonopin did. Finally, she sees her psychiatrist (her managed care company permitted only monthly visits, even though the psychiatrist had told her that in case of urgent situations like this one he would gladly see her for free), who recommends restarting Klonopin. Within a week, she is back to normal. The psychiatrist contacts the internist and asks him to please in the future not tell a patient to stop medication prescribed by another doctor without first consulting with him.

In the case of the bank executive, it is very hard to figure out what harm is done by having her take low-dose Klonopin on a regular basis. Without it, she suffers from generalized anxiety disorder to the point that her life is miserable. With it, she functions well and has no side effects.

Obviously, the two cases presented represent extremes. Yet they are entirely realistic and reflect the daily state of affairs. Benzodiazepines should

Table 19.

Long- and Short-Acting Benzodiazepines

LONG-ACTING	SHORT-ACTING
Valium	Ativan
Librium	Serax
Tranxene	Xanax
Klonopin	
Centrax	

be taken by people who need them for as long as they are needed. They should not be prescribed casually, and attempts to stop them should be made at regular intervals, but only with slow tapering, never abruptly. They should not be withheld from suffering patients.

When it is time to stop benzodiazepines, the rule is to do it slowly. This is especially important if benzodiazepines have been taken for more than a month. A patient who has taken 15 mg of Valium for two months should reduce the dose to 10 mg for a week and then 5 mg for a week before stopping. In some cases it may even be necessary to taper off in smaller increments. A patient treated for panic disorder with Xanax for six months, for example, usually feels most comfortable if the medication is slowly tapered over four to six weeks. It is important to work out a tapering schedule with your doctor when the time to stop medication comes.

TREATMENT OF GENERALIZED ANXIETY DISORDER

Three types of drugs are used, the SSRI and SNRI antidepressants (such as Paxil, Zoloft, Celexa, Lexapro, Effexor XR, and Cymbalta), benzodiazepines (Valium, Xanax, Klonopin, and Ativan), and a drug in a class of its own called buspirone (BuSpar), to treat GAD.

Although perhaps not as well studied yet as psychotherapies for some of the other anxiety disorders, there are good, effective, evidence-based psychotherapies for GAD. These include cognitive behavioral therapy, in which the patient is taught to make a more realistic evaluation of triggers for anxiety in his or her environment and to challenge worries and anxious thoughts, and applied relaxation, in which many of the CBT techniques are combined with a technique to learn how to relax muscle groups in the body. Whenever possible, these psychotherapies should be the first approach to treating GAD.

If the patient does not want psychotherapy or does not do well with psychotherapy, then medication may be the answer. Most experts now recommend trying one of the antidepressants first, supposedly because they are less likely to be habit-forming than the benzodiazepines. Interestingly, psychiatrists have convinced primary care doctors, who treat a lot of GAD in their practices, that this is the case, but themselves prescribe a lot of benzodiazepines. This is probably because they know that benzodiazepines work. Also, the side effects of the SSRI and SNRI antidepressants include sexual problems and weight gain, and many of them have withdrawal symptoms when they are discontinued abruptly, especially Paxil and Effexor XR. Benzodiazepines also have the problem of withdrawal symptoms upon discontinuation but do not cause sexual side effects or weight gain. Hence, it is really not clear which class of drug is better.

One thing that is clearly in favor of the antidepressants is that GAD is often accompanied by some level of depression and almost always leads to depression; antidepressants can be helpful for this side of things, but benzodiazepines are not. The characteristics of the SSRI and SNRI antidepressants are given in the chapter on treating depression. Prozac alone among these drugs may not be a good choice for GAD, but all of the others are effective. As is the case with depression, I usually choose Celexa (citalopram) because it is well tolerated, effective, and available in a generic form, making it less expensive than the drugs that are still on patent and therefore available only in brand-name preparations. In this chapter, then, I will give details only about benzodiazepines and buspirone (BuSpar). A drug called pregabalin has been found effective for GAD and may be approved by FDA for this purpose and/or for social anxiety disorder in the next few years. It has already been approved by FDA for treatment of seizures and some types of pain and is available under the brand name Lyrica.

Of the benzodiazepines, no one stands out among the others, and in terms of effectiveness and side effects they are pretty much identical. Psychiatrists tend to like to prescribe Klonopin (clonazepam) and primary care doctors Xanax (alprazolam) or Ativan (lorazepam). Valium (diazepam) in my opinon is a perfectly good drug that is not prescribed much any longer, probably because when the others first came out Valium and Librium were considered "old news," and while their successors were still on patent, drug companies convinced doctors that somehow they were better. All of the benzodiazepines are available in cheap generic forms. Recently, new versions of Xanax (Xanax XR and Niravam) and Klonopin (Klonopin Wafers) have been brought out and touted as superior by the manufacturers. However, I am convinced that except in very occasional cases they are definitely not worth the added cost.

Benzodiazepines can be divided into two groups, *long-acting* and *short-acting* (see Table 19). Long-acting benzodiazepines remain in the body days after the last pill is swallowed. This means that when they are stopped, the amount in the body slowly decreases to zero. This may make withdrawal symptoms less severe because in effect the drug tapers itself. Short-acting benzodiazepines are completely eliminated from the body a few hours after they are consumed, resulting in an abrupt on-off situation. If a short-acting benzodiazepine is taken before bedtime, by the time the patient wakes up, none will be left in the body. This may be desirable if the patient wants to be completely alert during the day, but it also means that withdrawal symptoms may be worse if the drug is suddenly stopped. Descriptions of all the benzodiazepines and of BuSpar follow.

DIAZEPAM

Brand Name: Valium.

Used For: Generalized anxiety disorder, sometimes for a condition called night terrors that occurs in children.

Do Not Use If: You have a history of alcohol abuse or other misuse of addictive drugs, have liver disease, or are nursing.

Tests to Take First: None required. Valium can be given to patients with very serious medical problems. It has no bad effects on the heart, lungs, or kidneys.

Tests to Take While You Are on It: None.

Usual Dose: Valium is a long-acting benzodiazepine, so one 5-mg dose often lasts the whole day. Patients usually take between 5 and 20 mg daily; the dose can be divided and taken in the morning and evening or taken all at once.

How Long Until It Works: Valium works more quickly than any other benzodiazepine, so relief from anxiety can be felt within thirty minutes to an hour after taking the first pill. For people with generalized anxiety disorder who take it regularly, there usually is a substantial improvement within one week. Once the dose of Valium that controls anxiety is found, most patients remain on that dose indefinitely without experiencing new anxiety symptoms.

Common Side Effects: Drowsiness, increase of the effects of drinking alcohol, withdrawal symptoms if the drug is stopped abruptly.

Less Common Side Effects: Disinhibition—some patients lose control of their impulses after taking drugs like Valium and do things they wouldn't ordinarily do, like shoplifting, arguing with the boss, or driving the car recklessly; dizziness; confusion and forgetfulness (especially in the elderly).

What to Do About Side Effects: The biggest problem is sleepiness, which usually goes away after a while. Lowering the dose or taking it only at bedtime helps. In general, patients taking Valium should drink very little alcohol, if any, and should never have anything to drink within hours of driving a car. Withdrawal symptoms are reduced by gradually tapering the dose, usually over two to four weeks. It should never be stopped suddenly, especially if it has been taken longer than two weeks. Patients who become disinhibited should probably not take Valium. Dizziness, confusion, and forgetfulness are particular problems in elderly patients, who should be given very small doses of Valium and checked carefully for these side effects. Elderly people should never be put on Valium without being seen regularly by a physician.

If It Doesn't Work: Failure usually means that the diagnosis was wrong and that the patient's main problem isn't generalized anxiety disorder. Sometimes a depression has been missed; Valium doesn't help depression much. Sometimes the real problems are difficulties in the patient's life that are better dealt with by psychotherapy. Changing from one benzodiazepine to another sometimes helps.

If It Does Work: The principle of using the smallest amount of drug for the shortest period possible holds. There is no known medical risk associated with remaining on Valium for life, but the longer a person takes such a drug, the harder it is to stop. After a few weeks, an attempt should be made to lower the dose. Every month or so, an attempt should be made to stop the drug entirely and see what happens. While a patient is on Valium, every effort should be made to find solutions to anxiety-provoking situations in his or her life.

Cost: The generic form is as safe and effective as the brand-name drug and much cheaper.

Special Comments: Valium is one of the all-time best-selling medications. There is no better benzodiazepine antianxiety drug. It is safe, works quickly, and helps most patients with anxiety problems a great deal. It is definitely habit-forming, and this must always be taken into account before use.

CHLORDIAZEPOXIDE

Brand Name: Librium.
Used For: Generalized anxiety disorder, alcohol withdrawal.
Usual Dose: 25–50 mg two to three times daily, but many people get by with less.

Cost: The generic form is as safe and effective as the brand-name drug and much cheaper.

Special Comments: Librium is in almost every respect similar to Valium (diazepam) and therefore I have not repeated all of the information that can be found in the Valium section above. Some people find Librium less sedating. It is a long-acting benzodiazepine. Besides being used for anxiety, it is sometimes used to help detoxify alcoholics. The side effects are similar to those of Valium. Librium is available in combination with another drug in a preparation called Librax for treatment of upset stomach. Librium also comes combined with the antidepressant drug amitriptyline in preparations called Limbitrol and Limbitrol DS. I usually recommend staying away from pills that combine different medications, so it is best to take antianxiety drugs and drugs for upset stomach or depression separately.

CLORAZEPATE

Brand Name: Tranxene.

Used for: Generalized anxiety disorder.

Usual Dose: Starts at 7.5 mg once or twice daily and usually levels off at about 30 mg a day. Some patients take 60 mg daily.

Cost: The generic form is as safe and effective as the brand-name drug and much cheaper.

Special Comments: The benzodiazepine Valium is turned into Tranxene by the body. It is almost identical to Valium and therefore a fuller description can be found in the Valium section. Tranxene is not prescribed very much any longer, but it is a perfectly good benzodiazepine.

HALAZEPAM

Brand Name: Paxipam

Used For: Generalized anxiety disorder.

Usual Dose: Starts at 20 mg once or twice a day to a maximum of 80–160 mg a day.

Cost: It is available in the generic form and thus is not expensive.

Special Comments: Once again, Paxipam is a long-acting benzodiazepine indistinguishable from Valium.

LORAZEPAM

Brand Name: Ativan.

Used For: Generalized anxiety disorder, calming agitated patients with mania or schizophrenia, assisting in detoxification of alcoholics.

Do Not Use If: You have a drinking problem or misuse any other addictive drugs, have serious liver disease, or are pregnant or nursing.

Tests to Take First: None required.

Tests to Take While You Are on It: None required.

Usual Dose: Ativan is a short-acting benzodiazepine, so a single dose is eliminated from the body in less than one day. Most patients start with 0.5 mg twice a day. This can then be raised if necessary to a total of 2–4 mg daily. Ativan can also be given by injection, although this is rarely necessary when treating patients for anxiety problems. It is frequently used as the injectible form in psychiatric emergency rooms and inpatient units to calm patients with schizophrenia or the mania phase of bipolar disorder in the unusual, but very urgent, situations when they became violent and dangerous.

How Long Until It Works: Some relief from anxiety is usually experienced about an hour after the first dose. Patients who need to take it regularly for severe generalized anxiety disorder will find the illness much relieved in the first week. They also find that they need to take the drug at least twice daily, because the effect doesn't last longer than eight to twelve hours.

Common Side Effects: Drowsiness, increases the effects of drinking alcohol, withdrawal symptoms when the drug is stopped, especially if stopped abruptly. There is some evidence that short-acting benzodiazepines like Ativan cause even worse withdrawal symptoms when they are stopped than long-acting benzodiazepines.

Less Common Side Effects: Disinhibition—some patients lose control of their impulses after taking drugs like Ativan and do things they wouldn't ordinarily do, like shoplifting, arguing with the boss, or driving the car recklessly; dizziness; confusion and forgetfulness (especially in elderly patients).

What to Do About Side Effects: The biggest problem is sleepiness, which usually goes away after a while. Lowering the dose or taking it only at bedtime helps, although the latter strategy won't help your daytime anxiety. In general, patients taking Ativan should drink very little alcohol, if any, and should never have anything to drink within hours of driving a car. Withdrawal symptoms may be even more severe than with Valium, and it is crucial that the dose be gradually reduced over two to four weeks if the patient has taken Ativan longer than two weeks. Patients who become disinhibited should probably not take Ativan. Dizziness, confusion, and forgetfulness are particular problems in elderly patients, who should be given very small doses of Ativan and checked carefully for these side effects. Elderly people should never be put on Ativan without being seen regularly by a physician.

If It Doesn't Work: This usually means that the diagnosis was wrong and that the patient's main problem isn't generalized anxiety disorder. Sometimes a depression has been missed; Ativan doesn't help depression much. Sometimes the real problems are difficulties in the patient's life that are better dealt with by psychotherapy. Changing from one benzodiazepine to another sometimes helps.

If It Does Work: The principle of using the smallest amount of drug for the shortest period possible holds. There is no known medical risk associated with remaining on Ativan for life, but the longer a person takes such a drug, the harder it will be to stop. After a few weeks, an attempt should be made to lower the dose. Every month or so an attempt should be made to stop the drug entirely and see what happens. While a patient is on Ativan, every effort should be made to find solutions to anxiety-provoking situations in his or her life. If Ativan is discontinued, however, it is essential to taper it slowly to avoid withdrawal problems.

Cost: The generic form is as safe and effective as the brand-name drug and much cheaper.

Special Comments: Ativan is used when a short-acting drug is desirable. Some patients like to have a pill they can take only occasionally when their symptoms get very bad, knowing that they won't feel sedated more than a few hours. If medication for generalized anxiety is needed longer than a week or two, a long-acting benzodiazepine is probably better. However, for elderly people with liver problems, the short-acting benzodiazepines are generally better than the long-acting benzodiazepines.

OXAZEPAM

Brand Name: Serax.

Used For: Generalized anxiety disorder.

Usual Dose: Serax is one of the shortest acting of all benzodiazepines, so it should be taken three times a day to avoid breakthrough anxiety symptoms. The dose ranges from 10 to 30 mg three to four times daily.

Cost: The generic form is as safe and effective as the brand-name drug and much cheaper.

Special Comments: Serax is very similar to Ativan, except that it is even shorter acting. For a fuller description of Serax, see the section on Ativan above. The effects of the drug usually last only about five hours. Serax is not prescribed very often any longer, although it is a perfectly good antianxiety drug.

ALPRAZOLAM

Brand Names: Xanax, Xanax XR, Niravam.

Used For: Generalized anxiety disorder, panic disorder.

Do Not Use If: You have a problem with alcohol or other addictive drugs, have very advanced liver disease, or are pregnant or nursing. Grapefruit juice may increase the blood level of alparazolam.

Tests to Take First: None required.

Tests to Take While You Are on It: None required.

Usual Dose: For regular alprazolam (Xanax), dose usually begins at 0.5 mg two or three times daily and can be increased to a total of 10 mg per day, divided equally in two or three doses. The top dose of 10 mg per day usually doesn't help that much, so 4–6 mg a day is a better maximum. Xanax XR can be taken once daily, with the same starting and maximum dose recommendations. Niravam is a melt-in-your-mouth preparation of alprazolam for people who have trouble swallowing pills. It is generally started at 0.25 mg two to three times a day and advanced to a maximum of 0.5 mg three times a day. Most patients find they have to take Xanax in the regular or Niravam preparations several times a day; it is very powerful but also short acting. Eight to twelve hours after the last dose, sometimes even earlier, a patient may start to feel some withdrawal symptoms and increased anxiety. Some patients even find that the effect of Xanax XR wears off too quickly and have to take it more than once a day.

How Long Until It Works: Like all benzodiazepines, Xanax offers some relief within an hour of taking the first pill. After a week of regular use, patients with generalized anxiety disorder feel much better. Panic disorder patients also start feeling better after the first week, but it may take two to four weeks until all of the panic attacks are blocked.

Common Side Effects: Drowsiness, increases the effects of drinking alcohol, and withdrawal symptoms (as with all of the short-acting benzodiazepines, especially if stopped abruptly).

Less Common Side Effects: Disinhibition—very rarely, some patients lose control of their impulses after taking drugs like Xanax and do things they wouldn't ordinarily do, like shoplifting, arguing with the boss, or driving the car recklessly; dizziness; confusion and forgetfulness (especially in the elderly). There have been a few reports of drug withdrawal seizures, but only in patients who had taken alprazolam for long periods and then stopped abruptly.

What to Do About Side Effects: The biggest problem is sleepiness, which usually goes away after a while. Lowering the dose helps. In general, patients taking Xanax should drink very little alcohol and should never have anything to drink within hours of driving a car. This drug must absolutely never be stopped abruptly by anyone who has taken it regularly for more than a week. Slow tapering, over about four weeks, is necessary for safety and to decrease withdrawal symptoms. Patients who become disinhibited should probably not take Xanax. Dizziness, confusion, and forgetfulness are particular problems in elderly patients, who should be given very small doses of Xanax and checked carefully for these side effects. Elderly people should never be put on Xanax or any other antianxiety drug without being seen regularly by a physician.

If It Doesn't Work: For patients with generalized anxiety disorder, if Xanax doesn't work, usually the original diagnosis was wrong. The true nature of the psychiatric problem should be reconsidered. About 20 percent of panic disorder patients fail to respond to Xanax; most are then switched to one of the other antipanic drugs (like Celexa, Effexor XR, Zoloft, or Paxil) discussed in the next section.

If It Does Work: Generalized anxiety disorder patients who are placed on Xanax are probably best served by trying to get off it as soon as possible. Many GAD patients do best taking it for indefinite amounts of time, but if it must be continued longer than a few weeks, a switch to a longer-acting drug to minimize breakthrough symptoms and decrease later withdrawal problems should be considered. Panic disorder patients are usually treated for six months after becoming panic free; then the dose is tapered slowly, over four to six weeks. (Treatment of panic disorder is discussed in the next section.)

Cost: Regular Xanax is available as the generic alprazolam, which is much cheaper than the brand-name drug and just as safe and effective. In my opinion, there is rarely a need to prescribe the expensive versions of Xanax XR and Niravam, which are not available as generics and offer very little advantage over regular Xanax.

Special Comments: Xanax is a marvel within the drug industry because of the rapidity with which it became the best-selling antianxiety drug in the 1970s and 1980s. It was marketed very heavily by the manufacturer while it was still on patent, and even today, especially among primary care doctors (but less so among psychiatrists), it is fairly frequently prescribed. It is very powerful and very safe. In general, patients like taking it and doctors don't worry that it will cause any harm. Nevertheless, very powerful and very short-acting antianxiety drugs (like Xanax) also seem to be the hardest to stop taking, and there has been some backlash against Xanax because of the withdrawal symptoms patients experience upon discontinuation. It is best to keep the dose low and to keep trying to get the patient off the drug. Some people with generalized anxiety disorder need to take Xanax for months or years, and patients with panic disorder should stay on it for at least six panic-free months. They need to understand beforehand that although this drug is medically safe, it is not always easy to stop using it. The patient can then decide if he or she wants to worry about future withdrawal problems, which are uncomfortable but not dangerous.

CLONAZEPAM

Brand Names: Klonopin, Klonopin Wafer.

Used For: Generalized anxiety disorder, panic disorder, seizures (rarely), and some types of pain.

Do Not Use If: You have a problem with alcohol or other addictive drugs, have very advanced liver disease, or are pregnant or nursing.

Tests to Take First: None required.

Tests to Take While You Are on It: None required.

Usual Dose: For regular clonazepam (Klonopin), the dose usually begins at 0.25 mg once or twice daily and can be increased to a total of 4 mg per day, divided equally in two doses. Klonopin Wafers are a melt-in-your-mouth preparation of clonazepam for people who have trouble swallowing pills. Dosing guidelines are the same as for regular Klonopin.

How Long Until It Works: Like all benzodiazepines, Klonopin offers some relief within an hour of taking the first pill. After a week of regular use, patients with generalized anxiety disorder feel much better. Panic disorder patients also start feeling better after the first week, but it may take two to four weeks until all of the panic attacks are blocked.

Common Side Effects: Drowsiness, increases the effects of drinking alcohol, and withdrawal symptoms (as with all of the benzodiazepines, especially if stopped abruptly).

Less Common Side Effects: Disinhibition—very rarely, some patients lose control of their impulses after taking drugs like Klonopin and do things they wouldn't ordinarily do, like shoplifting, arguing with the boss, or driving the car recklessly; dizziness; confusion and forgetfulness (especially in the elderly).

What to Do About Side Effects: The biggest problem is sleepiness, which usually goes away after a while. Lowering the dose helps. In general, patients taking Klonopin should drink very little alcohol and should never have anything to drink within hours of driving a car. This drug must absolutely never be stopped abruptly by anyone who has taken it regularly for more than a week. Slow tapering, over about four weeks, is necessary for safety and to decrease withdrawal symptoms. Patients who become disinhibited should probably not take Klonopin. Dizziness, confusion, and forgetfulness are particular problems in elderly patients, who should be given very small doses of Klonopin and checked carefully for these side effects.

Elderly people should never be put on Klonopin or any other antianxiety drug without being seen regularly by a physician.

If It Doesn't Work: For patients with generalized anxiety disorder, if Klonopin doesn't work, usually the original diagnosis was wrong. The true nature of the psychiatric problem should be reconsidered. About 20 percent of panic disorder patients fail to respond to Klonopin; most are then switched to one of the other antipanic drugs (like Celexa, Effexor XR, Zoloft, or Paxil) discussed in the next section.

If It Does Work: Generalized anxiety disorder patients who are placed on Klonopin should take it for the shortest time possible but often do well taking it indefinitely. Dose should, of course, be kept as low as possible. Panic disorder patients are usually treated for six months after becoming panic free; then the dose is tapered slowly, over four to six weeks. (Treatment of panic disorder is discussed in the next section.)

Cost: Regular Klonopin is available as the generic clonazepam, which is much cheaper than the brand-name drug and just as safe and effective. In my opinion, there is rarely a need to prescribe the more expensive Klonopin Wafer. Most people figure out how to swallow a pill and avoid the higher co-pay.

Special Comments: Klonopin is the most popular benzodiazepine among psychiatrists. It does have an advantage over Xanax and Ativan, more popular among primary care physicians, because it is long acting and therefore not as prone to periods of breakthrough anxiety between doses during the day. It is not clear that it is better than Valium, but since it also is available as a generic, it does not cost more. It is the most potent of the available benzodiapines and therefore it is particularly important not to stop it abruptly in order to avoid withdrawal symptoms. Slow tapering over several weeks is recommended. It is best to keep the dose low and to keep trying to get the patient off the drug. Some people with generalized anxiety disorder, however, need to take Klonopin for months or years, and patients with panic disorder should stay on it for at least six panic-free months. They need to understand beforehand that although this drug is medically safe, it is not always easy to stop using it. The patient can then decide if he or she wants to worry about future withdrawal problems, which are uncomfortable but not dangerous.

BUSPIRONE

Brand Name: BuSpar.

Used For: Generalized anxiety disorder.

Do Not Use If: You are taking a high dose of a benzodiazepine, because buspirone probably won't work in this case. Grapefruit juice may increase the blood level of buspirone.

Tests to Take First: None required.

Tests to Take While You Are on It: None required. BuSpar has no known effects on physical health.

Usual Dose: Most people start taking one-half of the 15-mg pill (7.5 mg) two times a day. After about a week the dose is raised to 15 mg twice a day. After several weeks, if the response is not adequate, the dose can be increased to 45 mg (15 mg three times a day) and then to 30 mg twice daily.

How Long Until It Works: About four weeks. Unlike the benzodiazepines, BuSpar does not work right away. You can't take one and expect to feel relaxed in an hour.

Common Side Effects: Mild headache and nausea sometimes occur but usually go away in a few days.

Less Common Side Effects: Rarely, patients become more anxious.

What to Do About Side Effects: The side effects are so mild that nothing much usually has to be done, although lowering the dose can eliminate the headache and nausea.

If It Doesn't Work: Another medication is called for, usually a benzodiazepine or antidepressant.

If It Does Work: BuSpar is not habit-forming; patients can pretty much start and stop it at will without worrying about withdrawal symptoms. No one knows yet exactly how long someone should stay on BuSpar, but it is already clear that in at least one-third of anxious patients who respond to it, anxiety symptoms return once it is stopped. So, like the benzodiazepines, BuSpar is not a cure, only a treatment. As always, I recommend trying to stop use after a few months.

Cost: Generic buspirone is as safe and effective as brand-name BuSpar and cheaper.

Special Comments: BuSpar is very different from the benzodiazepines listed earlier. It has completely different effects on the brain. It doesn't make the patient sleepy and doesn't relax muscles. It doesn't increase the effects of drinking alcohol. Also, BuSpar is not habit-forming, and there are no withdrawal symptoms, even if stopped abruptly. All of these are obviously advantages over benzodiazepines. The disadvantages are that it takes about four weeks to work, which may seem an eternity to a severely anxious patient. Also, there is reason to believe that patients who have previously responded to one of the benzodiazepines will not be helped by BuSpar. BuSpar cannot be used to reduce the severity of the symptoms of withdrawal from benzodiazepines. Thus, a patient cannot simply stop a benzodiazepine and start BuSpar. Tapering the benzodiazepine is still necessary. Patients who need immediate relief will probably do better with benzodiazepines. Most important, many psychiatrists, me included, have not found BuSpar to be

Table 20.

Features of Panic Disorder

1. The panic attack. Sudden burst of palpitations, chest discomfort, difficulty breathing or catching breath, dizziness, lightheadedness, sweating, feeling faint, tingling feelings in hands and feet, nausea, extreme fear of impending death or going crazy or losing control.
2. Anticipatory anxiety. Worrying that a panic attack is going to occur at any moment.
3. Phobic avoidance (also called agoraphobia). Avoiding situations in which a panic attack may occur but help is not immediately available, for example, driving in a car (especially over a bridge), flying in a plane, sitting in the middle of the row in a movie theater.

all that effective. Although still prescribed, its lack of effectiveness, in my opinion, usually outweighs its lack of side effects.

Summary of Drug Treatment for Generalized Anxiety Disorder

If the patient can wait for relief (about four weeks), BuSpar (buspirone) can be tried first, but because it is not very effective this is probably worthwhile only in very mildly affected patients.

Most experts now recommend treating GAD with an antidepressant (an SSRI like Paxil, Celexa, Zoloft, or Lexapro, or an SNRI like Effexor XR or Cymbalta), but patients may balk at the sexual and weight gain side effects and prefer a benzodiazepine. If that is the case, Klonopin (clonazepam) or Valium are the best choices, except for elderly people with liver problems who might do better with Xanax or Ativan. Patients placed on benzodiazepines should always be warned that it can be difficult to stop them because of the withdrawal effects (antidepressants, especially Paxil and Effexor XR, have withdrawal effects, too, but are usually easier to discontinue with proper tapering than benzodiazepines). When immediate relief is needed, one useful strategy is to start the antidepressant and Klonopin simultaneously, then after four weeks, when the antidepressant is working, slowly taper and discontinue Klonopin.

TREATMENT OF PANIC DISORDER

Panic disorder has three components: the actual panic attack, the anxiety patients experience between panic attacks when they worry about the next one (called anticipatory anxiety), and phobias (Table 20). The phobias usually involve the fear of having a panic attack in a situation where help is not immediately available, such as in a car riding over a bridge or in an airplane. One could say there is also a fourth component, depression, which eventually occurs in at least half of patients whose panic disorder goes inadequately treated.

It is important to understand the difference between generalized anxiety disorder and panic disorder. In GAD, the patient is almost continuously worried, tense, and anxious. In panic disorder, the main problem is the sudden, episodic bursts of anxiety and physical symptoms (like palpitations, dizziness, and difficulty breathing) that generally last ten to thirty minutes. Although neuroscientists speculate that GAD and panic disorder may involve different problems in the brain and different vulnerability genes, many patients with panic disorder also have GAD, and many patients with GAD get panic attacks. Hence, as with most of the disorders in *DSM-IV,* comorbidity (having more than one condition at the same time) is frequently the case for anxiety disorders.

Medications are used mainly to block the panic attack itself. Once this is done, many patients no longer have anticipatory anxiety and also overcome their phobias quickly. They also seem less likely to develop depression, especially if antidepressants rather than benzodiazepines are used to block the panic attacks. Anticipatory anxiety can also be treated with one of the benzodiazepines (Valium, Xanax, Klonopin, or Ativan) while waiting for the antipanic drug to work. Once the attacks are eliminated, however, some panic disorder patients continue to have phobias. These patients may require bevhavioral therapy and usually respond well to a few sessions.

Excellent results can be obtained in panic disorder patients with cognitive behavioral therapy (CBT). Many studies have proved this to be an effective treatment for panic disorder. Several years ago, David Barlow of Boston University, M. Katharine Shear of Columbia University, Scott Woods of Yale University, and I showed that CBT worked as well as medication to treat panic disorder. There was a suggestion that a combination of medication and CBT might be slightly better than either alone, but once the treatments were discontinued in patients who had responded, those who received CBT, with or without medication, remained well for significantly longer than those who had received only medication. Hence, CBT given by a therapist specifically trained in using it to treat patients with panic disorder should always be considered as the initial treatment. If the patient does not wish to have psychotherapy or it does not work well enough, either antidepressants or benzodiazepines are then used. (Full descriptions of these drugs are found in Chapter 7 and in the section earlier in this chapter titled "Treatment of Generalized Anxiety Disorder.") The tried-and-true drug for treating panic disorder was the cyclic antidepressant drug imipramine (Tofranil). However, it has now been replaced by antidepressants of the serotonin reuptake inhibitor (SSRI) and serotonin norepinephrine reuptake inhibitor (SNRI) classes. All of the drugs in these two classes (that is, Prozac, Zoloft, Paxil, Luvox, Celexa, Lexapro, Effexor XR, and Cymbalta) are effective, so I usually pick Celexa to start because it is well tolerated and available in inexpensive generic form. The only difference between treating panic and treating depression with these drugs is that panic patients are sometimes very sensitive to the antidepressants and may become even more anxious at the start of treatment. For that reason, I usually prescribe a lower dose to start—10 mg a day of Paxil or Prozac, 25 mg of Zoloft, 10 mg of Celexa, for example—for panic patients. Then, after the patient is used to the drug, the dose is raised to the same top doses used by depressed patients. Panic attacks are usually blocked completely after an SSRI or SNRI antidepressant is taken for four weeks.

The benzodiazepine drugs alprazolam (Xanax) and clonazepam (Klonopin) are very effective in blocking panic attacks. Both are also used to treat generalized anxiety disorder and are described in detail earlier in this chapter. Xanax is usually started at 0.5 mg two or three times daily and then increased to between 2 and 4 mg a day to completely block panic attacks. Occasionally, the dose is increased to as much as 10 mg, but I do not recommend this. Xanax works to block panic attacks more quickly than antidepressants, in about one to two weeks. It has far fewer side effects but is more difficult to stop. Klonopin is favored over Xanax by psychiatrists because it has a longer length of action in the body so that there are fewer periods of breakthrough anxiety during the day between doses. Like Xanax, however, it is hard to stop. Although all SSRI and SNRI antidepressants, especially Paxil and Effexor XR, have withdrawal symptoms, especially if stopped abruptly, they are generally easier to discontinue than benzodiazepines, even with appropriately slow tapering. On the other hand, benzodiazepines do not cause sexual side effects and weight gain the way SSRI and SNRI antidepressants do. So a careful discussion of risks and benefits should be had with all patients before they are started on a drug for panic disorder.

The most powerful antipanic drugs are the antidepressant monoamine oxidase inhibitors (MAOIs), also described in detail in Chapter 7. Drugs like phenelzine (Nardil) and tranylcypromine (Parnate) work for almost all panic disorder patients. Because of the many side effects they cause and the need for a special diet, however, most psychiatrists first try the patient on one of the other antidepressants, including a cyclic antidepressant if an SSRI or SNRI doesn't work. Less than 20 percent of patients do not respond to one of these; they can then be prescribed an MAOI.

The treatment of panic disorder can be summarized as follows (also see Table 21):

1. Get the right diagnosis. This can be tricky with panic disorder. Patients with depression and generalized anxiety disorder sometimes have panic attacks, although usually not often enough to warrant an additional diagnosis of panic disorder. Careful evaluation by an experienced doctor is required to distinguish panic disorder from other psychiatric problems.

2. Rule out the physical medical causes of panic attacks. A physical examination, blood tests, thyroid tests, and an electrocardiogram can help confirm that the panic attacks are not caused by a physical illness.

3. Make sure you understand the difference among the three components of panic disorder: panic attacks, anticipatory anxiety, and phobias. The panic attacks should be the focus of treatment in the beginning. Eliminating them is the key to overcoming the problem of panic disorder.

4. Decide between an antipanic drug and panic-disorder-specific CBT. If you want psychotherapy for panic attacks, make sure you are referred to a licensed therapist who has had specific training in treatment aimed at panic disorder. Remember that even the best psychotherapy takes about three months (twelve weekly sessions) to work and requires that you do homework between sessions. Do not feel ashamed if you decide that you would rather solve the problem as quickly as possible and choose the medication. Remember, however, that on the other end of things, if you respond to medication, relapse after stopping it is common, whereas if you respond to CBT, relapse is much less common.

5. If you choose drugs, the doctor will probably prescribe an SSRI or SNRI antidepressant first. Some patients will decide to be treated with a benzodiazepine (Xanax or Klonopin) instead to avoid sexual side effects and weight gain. However, these are generally harder to discontinue than antidepressants because of withdrawal symptoms. Sometimes, in order to get a more rapid response, a benzodiazepine is started along with an antidepressant. After about four weeks, when the antidepressant has had enough time to work, the benzodiazepine is tapered and stopped.

6. If two or three drugs in the SSRI and SNRI classes are tried and fail, which occurs in less than 20 percent of patients with panic disorder, your doctor will ask you to consider a cyclic antidepressant (like imipramine)

and, if this doesn't work, an MAOI. These are all described in detail in Chapter 7. Almost all patients respond to one of the MAOIs (Nardil, Marplan, or Parnate), but these drugs must be prescribed carefully by a very experienced psychiatrist because of the many side effects.

7. Remain on the medication for six months once the panic attacks are blocked. This gives you the best chance of staying panic free once the medication is stopped. Unfortunately, relapse is common when medication is stopped and some patients do better staying on it for a year or more.

8. When the panic attacks stop, push yourself to confront situations you have become phobic about and avoid. Convince yourself that the panic attacks will not occur after the drug starts working, even if you get caught in your car in a traffic jam or fly in an airplane. If you are still phobic and avoid things even after the panic attacks have stopped, ask your doctor to help you with some exercises to overcome these phobias. CBT can be helpful in these situations.

Table 21.

Treatment of Panic Disorder

1. Rule out medical conditions that may be the real cause (physical examination and routine blood and thyroid tests if the medical history suggests there may be a physical medical problem).
2. Consider a focused, antipanic psychotherapy by an experienced cognitive behavioral therapist. This will take about three months to work. Or begin an antipanic drug. The usual first choices are an SRI (Paxil, Zoloft, Prozac, Luvox, Celexa, Lexapro) or SNRI (Effexor XR, Cymbalta), which takes about four weeks to work, or Xanax or Klonopin, which have few side effects, work in two weeks or less, but are more difficult to stop.
3. If psychotherapy is chosen, complete a full course and continue to do the exercises even after you stop seeing the therapist.
4. If medication is chosen, stay on it for six panic-free months. If psychotherapy doesn't work, try a first-line drug.
5. If a first-line drug doesn't work, try another first-line drug, then a cyclic antidepressant (like imipramine) and only then an MAOI (Nardil or Parnate). If phobias do not go away even when panic attacks are blocked, get behavioral therapy, which usually takes one to ten sessions.

9. Stay in touch with your doctor, even when you are off medication and feeling much better. Panic attacks sometimes return. Fortunately, the same treatment strategy that worked the first time usually works the second time, so there should be little problem getting better again.

Here are some examples of good and bad treatment for panic disorder.

Bad Treatment

When Mrs. Lewis described her anxiety attacks to her doctor, he felt she was under a lot of stress and prescribed 5 mg of Valium twice daily. He told Mrs. Lewis to take it for one month and then stop. He reassured her that everything would certainly be better by then. In fact, Mrs. Lewis kept having panic attacks for the whole month. The Valium made her sleepy and a little more relaxed, but that was all. After the month, she stopped taking Valium and for a full week felt more anxiety and had more trouble sleeping than ever before. The problem here is that such a low dose of Valium rarely blocks panic attacks. The doctor forgot to tell Mrs. Lewis that she might have withdrawal symptoms if she stopped taking Valium abruptly after regular use for a month. And if he thought she was under stress, why didn't he help her figure out how to make her life less stressful or refer her for psychotherapy?

Good Treatment

Mrs. Lewis contacted a psychiatrist through the local university-based medical school. The psychiatrist she selected was an expert in anxiety disorders. The psychiatrist felt that stress was not the problem; Mrs. Lewis was suffering from panic disorder with mild phobic avoidance. After thorough discussion of all the treatment options, Mrs. Lewis decided to try Celexa. She started with 10 mg every morning and increased this to 20 mg four days later. After four weeks, her panic attacks were gone. She began to force herself to drive longer and longer distances until she felt completely comfortable with this. Finally, she took a plane ride with her husband, without experiencing an attack.

Bad Treatment

Mr. Lewis also experienced panic attacks. They were so severe that he became completely afraid to ride the train to work. He quit his job and took a much less prestigious job because he could walk to work. He saw a psychotherapist who told him his problem was a deep-seated fear of success. The psychotherapist recommended twice-weekly therapy sessions and told Mr. Lewis it might take several years to get to the bottom of the problem.

Good Treatment

Fortunately, Mr. Lewis sought another opinion. He was referred to a therapist who specialized in panic disorder treatments and underwent a twelve-session cognitive behavior therapy (CBT) specifically tailored for the treatment of panic attacks and phobias. After three months his panic attacks were almost completely gone and he was able to ride the train again.

These examples highlight the importance of getting the right diagnosis, seeking out specialists, and not being afraid to question an individual doctor's recommendations.

TREATMENT OF SOCIAL PHOBIA (SOCIAL ANXIETY DISORDER)

Until the mid-1980s, American psychiatrists barely paid any attention to social phobia, also known as social anxiety disorder. Now we know it is quite common and often a serious problem. It comes in two varieties. So-called specific social phobia involves only one or two specific performance situations. For example, the individual who routinely gets anxiety attacks during public speaking and dreads or even avoids giving a speech to the point of jeopardizing his or her career has specific social phobia if no other area of life is affected. More than half of the population claims to be afraid of public speaking, actually a larger number than say they are afraid to die, and therefore it is arguable whether fear of public speaking is actually a psychiatric illness or just a normal variant. If necessary, it can be treated with CBT and/or medications (see below) given right before the feared performance situation. On the other hand, patients with generalized social phobia develop severe anxiety attacks anytime they are in any type of social or performance situation. This leads to tremendous impairment in the ability to work, get an education, or have any kind of social or romantic life. This is clearly a psychiatric illness; it is more than simply shyness and requires treatment.

Fortunately, very effective treatments are available for social phobia. First, CBT works for at least 70 percent of patients with social phobia, and patients will want to consider trying that first before considering medication. As pioneered by Richard Heimberg of Temple University, CBT for social phobia is often given in group format. It takes between three and four months for most patients to respond. In a study Heimberg conducted with Michael Liebowitz of Columbia University, group CBT was equally effective as medication for social phobia. Remember, however, that cognitive behavioral treatments are not "psychotherapy as usual" and require a skilled therapist who has special training in this area.

Among the medications used for social phobia, there is no question that the monoamine oxidase inhibitor Nardil (phenelzine) is the most effective. (Nardil is described in more detail with the other antidepressants in Chapter 7.) Because Nardil has so many side effects, however, it is never given as the first medication. All of the SSRI and SNRI antidepressants (Prozac, Paxil, Luvox, Zoloft, Celexa, Lexapro, Effexor XR, and Cymbalta) work for social phobia and one of them is generally the best drug with which to start. (They are also described in more detail in Chapter 7.) The benzodiazepine Klonopin (clonazepam) was also shown in one study to work for social phobia, although many clinicians are wary of prescribing benzodiazepines for patients with social phobia because of concerns that the patients will have difficulty discontinuing them when they want to stop. Lyrica (pregalabin) is a drug now available for the treatment of pain and seizures that worked for social phobia in research studies. It may be approved by the FDA for social phobia and for GAD.

A class of drugs called beta-adrenergic blockers (or beta-blockers for short) were at first thought to be effective for treating social phobia. In fact, they are not, but they do block the racing heart, shaking, sweating, and blushing that patients with social phobia (or people with any type of "stage fright") experience when they are in front of an audience. One beta-blocker, propranolol (Inderal), can be given about an hour before a performance, usually in a dose of 20 or 40 mg, to block those symptoms. A surprising number of professional musicians and public speakers use propranolol, most often secretly, for this purpose.

Here are some examples of different ways to treat social phobia:

Alfred, an English teacher at a small community college, is friendly, likable, and generally outgoing. He has no trouble at parties or in front of his class. Once a month, Alfred has to give a talk to about three hundred students as part of a special lecture series. On the night before a lecture, he can barely sleep. A few hours before the lecture, he feels his heart pounding and he envisions losing his voice and humiliating himself. During the lecture, his mouth becomes very dry and he feels himself tremble and shake. Although he generally gets through the lecture, he hardly inspires the audience and the experience is thoroughly harrowing for him.

Alfred has a very circumscribed problem. It doesn't affect his whole life, but it does have a negative impact on his career. For a professor to advance, he or she must be able to speak comfortably in front of large groups. Alfred can get significant relief by taking propranolol (Inderal) about an hour before the big lecture. He should also have at least a few sessions of cognitive behavioral therapy to help him stop paying so much attention to his nervousness before the lectures. The treatment is very simple and brief.

Sandra has a slightly more complicated problem. She had been a fellow graduate student of Alfred's. Sandra was viewed as the more promising student because her papers were outstanding. But somehow she never promoted herself very strongly and was overlooked for faculty appointments. The reason for this is that Sandra develops overwhelming anxiety whenever she is the center of attention. She dreaded speaking up in class or even having a casual conversation with a professor. She avoids parties and feels relaxed only with her closest friends and relatives. She works as an assistant librarian in a high school library and feels quite unfulfilled.

Sandra obviously needs more intense help than Alfred. She should first try a focused cognitive behavioral treatment program for her generalized social anxiety and phobia if she can locate a properly trained therapist. If this doesn't work, or works only partially, a trial of medication is indicated. The medication (usually an SSRI like Celexa, Paxil, or Zoloft, or an SNRI like Effexor XR or Cymbalta) will have to be given on a more continuous basis than Alfred's once-a-month schedule because Sandra's anxiety attacks occur in a larger number of social situations.

Finally, there is Richard, a high school friend of Sandra's and Alfred's. Richard was a very bright student and was a star on the football team. Around age seventeen or eighteen, he began feeling increasingly nervous and uncomfortable around people. He now feels that everything he does is inadequate or doomed to failure. Sometimes he becomes depressed and drinks too much. The most important feature of his problem is the constant feeling that he will make a complete fool of himself. When he calls a woman for a date, he stutters and stammers and usually can't get the words out. He hates going to restaurants because he sweats and blushes when he has to order. He doesn't even like telling taxicab drivers where to take him.

Richard at the very least requires formal cognitive behavioral psychotherapy and possibly medication as well. In addition, he may need long-term psychoanalytically based psychotherapy because his problems are complicated by a deep sense of inadequacy and constant pessimism. Patients with social phobia may have to try a few different treatment approaches to find what works for them. They should start with therapies that promise the quickest help to see if they work. In other words, they should consider medication, which works in two to four weeks, and cognitive behavioral therapy, which usually works in about three months. Long-term therapy should be reserved for situations in which these more immediate treatments do not prove helpful.

Table 22.

MAOIs and Social Phobia

Drug names	Nardil, Parnate
Most commonly used	Nardil
Usual dose	30 mg (two pills) to 90 mg (six pills) daily of Nardil
Side effects	*Common*—weight gain, dizziness after standing up quickly, trouble sleeping, swelling in ankles and fingers *Less common*—difficulty having an orgasm, getting high, shocklike feelings in fingers and toes *Rare*—hypertensive crisis (patients on MAOIs must stay on the special diet to avoid a sudden and very dangerous increase in blood pressure)
When it works	In about four weeks; effects can be dramatic

SSRIs and SNRIs appear to be effective for some patients with social phobia and are described in Chapter 7. The benzodiazepine Klonopin, described earlier in this chapter in the generalized anxiety disorder section, has also been shown effective. Finally, the MAO inhibitor Nardil, also described in Chapter 7, has been shown to be very effective for social phobia. Because of Nardil's many adverse side effects, however, it is usually reserved for patients with social phobia who fail to respond to an antidepressant and Klonopin. See Table 22 for a description of MAO inhibitors for social phobia.

PROPRANOLOL

Brand Name: Inderal.

Used For: Short-term relief of stage fright and symptoms of specific social phobia. Also used for many medical problems such as high blood pressure, angina, and migraine headaches.

Do Not Use If: You have an abnormally slow heart rate, asthma or allergies that regularly make you wheeze, or congestive heart failure.

Tests to Take First: Pulse and blood pressure should be recorded.

Tests to Take While You Are on It: Pulse should be taken the first few times you take it (the doctor can easily teach you how to do this) and should not drop below fifty beats per minute for most people (your doctor will give you individual guidelines).

Usual Dose: Most people take a 20- or 40-mg tablet about one hour before a stressful situation. It is taken only on an as-needed basis for this specific performance situation that routinely causes anxiety attacks.

How Long Until It Works: It should work in about one hour to block the physical signs of anxiety (heart pounding, sweating, blushing, and trembling).

Common Side Effects: Taken on this very occasional basis, Inderal has almost no side effects. Some people may feel a little light-headed or sleepy.

Less Common Side Effects: Again, taken occasionally, Inderal has few side effects. Patients with asthma should not take Inderal because it may induce an asthma attack.

What to Do About Side Effects: There really aren't many when the drug is taken only once in a while. If light-headedness or fatigue is a problem, the dose can be lowered to as little as 5 mg (half of a 10-mg tablet).

If It Doesn't Work: You will probably need more continuous medication treatment or psychotherapy.

If It Does Work: Take it when you need it. Remember, it is intended only as a once-in-a-while treatment before especially frightening performance-type situations.

Cost: Generic propranolol is as safe and effective as brand-name Inderal and is much cheaper.

Special Comments: Inderal is short acting (there are long-acting versions, Inderal XL and Inderal LA, which are not used for this purpose) and a very good choice for the treatment of occasional severe physical anxiety symptoms in patients with social phobia or with stage fright. Patients who take it must, of course, be able to predict what will be a frightening situation. Inderal is not useful after the social phobia patient experiences symptoms or as long-term treatment for generalized social phobia.

TREATMENT OF OBSESSIVE-COMPULSIVE DISORDER

Not so long ago, I would reserve the section on treating obsessive-compulsive disorder for the end of a lecture or chapter on anxiety disorders.

No treatment seemed beneficial for this condition, not long-term psychotherapy or behavioral psychotherapy or drug therapy.

The situation is substantially brighter now, although I still must concede that obsessive-compulsive disorder is one of the most difficult psychiatric conditions to treat. There are many psychological theories about the cause of this serious illness, but in my opinion it is one of the most biological of all mental disorders. Patients with OCD may seem perfectly normal to the casual observer. They have none of the odd behaviors or strange mannerisms common to some psychotic or schizophrenic patients. But they are prisoners to senseless thoughts and the need to repeat meaningless rituals. They wash their hands, check on things, clean the floors, and think about numbers for hours a day. Sometimes they become very depressed over this behavior, but patients with OCD rarely attempt suicide. They never believe that the obsessions and compulsions are necessary. They don't actually believe their hands are dirty enough to warrant incessant washing. They often swear they will stop. But they cannot. Something—a brain abnormality, perhaps—forces them to have the obsessions or act out the compulsions over and over.

Almost every psychiatric drug known has been used to treat OCD, including cyclic antidepressants, SSRIs, SNRIs, and other "newer" antidepressants, MAOIs, antipsychotic drugs, amphetamines, clonidine, tranquilizers, and electroshock treatment. Of all these medications, only those that work on the serotonin system appear effective. Thus, the SSRIs (Prozac, Zoloft, Paxil, Luvox, Celexa, and Lexapro) and the SNRIs (Effexor XR and Cymbalta) are all reasonable first-line treatments for OCD. Because these medications are all also used to treat depression and other anxiety disorders, they are already described in detail in Chapter 7. The most effective drug to treat OCD is a cyclic antidepressant called clomipramine (Anafranil). It is still a popular drug for treating depression and anxiety disorders in Europe, but in the United States its only official approved use, and for the most part its only actual use, is for the treatment of OCD. This is because it has more side effects than any of the other cyclic antidepressants. If one of the first-line drugs fails, however, clomipramine is usually tried.

CLOMIPRAMINE (ALSO CALLED CLORIMIPRAMINE)

Brand Name: Anafranil.

Used For: Obsessive-compulsive disorder. Has also been used successfully to treat major depressive disorder and panic disorder.

Do Not Use If: You have narrow-angle glaucoma, a very enlarged prostate, certain abnormal heart rhythms (your doctor will determine if this is an important consideration for you), or a history of seizures (unless your doctor takes special precautions).

Tests to Take First: You may need an electrocardiogram first, especially if you are over age fifty.

Tests to Take While You Are on It: None are universally required for all patients.

Usual Dose: You will probably be started on 25 mg per day and the dose will be raised over the next two weeks to 100 mg per day, usually taken in one dose. After that, the dose is raised over the next few weeks to 250 mg. Some patients have been treated with higher doses, up to 400 mg per day, but this is not recommended by the manufacturer because of a possible risk of causing seizures at higher doses.

How Long Until It Works: It will take about four weeks to have effect; sometimes six weeks or longer is required.

Common Side Effects: Dry mouth, constipation, nausea, difficulty urinating, weight gain, increased sweating, dizziness upon standing quickly, sedation, blurred vision, and difficulty having an orgasm. Anafranil will make you more sensitive to the effects of the sun.

Less Common Side Effects: There may be an increased risk of having a seizure on Anafranil, compared to other drugs of its class (the cyclic antidepressants), especially if the dose is raised too high. For that reason, the top recommended dose is now 250 mg. Elderly patients may experience confusion and memory impairment.

What to Do About Side Effects: Dry mouth—don't suck on hard candies containing sugar as you will ruin your teeth; try sugarless hard candies or mouthwash. Constipation—drink at least six glasses of water or juice daily. Laxatives may be prescribed. Blurry vision—normal vision usually returns in a couple of weeks, but a change in eyeglass prescription can help. Difficulty urinating—this problem is more frequent in men than women and can become a serious problem in older men. Usually it is only annoying. The drug bethanecol (Urecholine) can be prescribed to counteract this effect. Increased sensitivity to the sun—use very good sunblock with an SPF of at least 30 when out in the sun. Dizziness after standing up quickly—this is caused by a brief drop in blood pressure. The best remedy is to sit down and get up slowly. In elderly people this side effect can be more serious. Weight gain—this can range from just a few pounds to twenty or more pounds. No one knows why Anafranil does this and not a lot can be done except to diet. Sedation—the best approach is to take the medication as close to bedtime as possible. Difficulty having an orgasm—this problem often goes away on its own in a few weeks. Lowering the dose can sometimes help. Seizures—it is not clear just how much of a problem this is. It is safest to recommend keeping the dose at or below 250 mg and not giving Anafranil to patients with a history of seizures unless they are well controlled on anti-convulsant drugs.

If It Doesn't Work: After six to eight weeks, the drug should have some effect. It usually works best if combined with cognitive behavioral treatment. Sometimes, adding an antipsychotic drug (such as Trilafon, Risperdal, Geodon, or Abilify) can help, especially for patients who also have tics or who seem almost convinced that their obsessions are real and their compulsions actually necessary (that is, for patients who seem almost delusional). Zyprexa and Seroquel, other antipsychotics, can also be added, but they will increase the weight gain and put the patient at greater risk for all the complications of obesity, including diabetes.

If It Does Work: At least one study suggests that Anafranil treatment may be needed permanently to control obsessions and compulsions. The dose should be reduced after six months to the lowest possible dose that controls the symptoms, but the patient should be kept on the drug indefinitely.

Cost: Generic clomipramine is just as safe and effective as brand-name Anafranil and much cheaper.

Special Comments: Anafranil was the first drug approved for the treatment of OCD. It is usually used after the patient has not had a satisfactory response to a first-line drug (one of the SSRI or SNRI antidepressants). It is usually also combined with OCD-specific cognitive behavioral therapy.

With few exceptions, patients with OCD should usually have OCD-specific cognitive behavioral psychotherapy, either tried on its own before attempting medication treatment, or started immediately in combination with drugs. This is a very demanding psychotherapy that should be administered only by a therapist with specific training. CBT is more effective for compulsions than obsessions and the reverse is true for medication; hence the combination usually makes sense for most patients. CBT for compulsions involves two main techniques: exposure and response blocking. In the former, the patient is deliberately made to confront whatever stimulates him to carry out a compulsion. For example, the patient who thinks that his hands are dirty and must wash them over and over again is told to cover his hands with dirt. He must keep the dirt on his hands but cannot wash them. Eventually, after many trials of this procedure, the urge to wash declines. Response blocking involves making it impossible for the patient to carry out obsessions. In an extreme example, the taps are removed from sinks so that the patient cannot wash his hands. Obviously, this therapy requires a lot of cooperation from family members and has one of the highest dropout and failure rates of any form of CBT. Nevertheless, it is as effective as medication. Long-term psychoanalytically oriented psychotherapy does not appear to be helpful for OCD.

It is very important for psychiatrists and therapists who treat obsessive-compulsive disorder to be reassuring and supportive. Often, OCD patients are ashamed of their symptoms and burdened by repetitive thoughts that seem disgusting to them. The doctor must explain that these thoughts and actions are not the patient's fault and that they are no more repulsive than any other medical problem. Although we encourage patients to exercise as much control as possible over the symptoms, we want them to understand that they are not to blame and will not be condemned.

Some examples of treating OCD patients may be helpful.

Anna, an elementary school teacher who recently graduated from college, had a severe and incapacitating compulsion. At the time she first came for consultation she had been forced to go on a medical leave of absence because her compulsive rituals prevented her from getting to work on time. Often, she had to leave her classroom to wash. The rituals, she told the doctor, had been going on for almost five years. At first she had felt a bit uneasy about dirt and was merely fastidious about keeping clean. Over the years she became preoccupied with the worry that her hands might be dirty. If she believed there was the slightest chance her hands had come in contact with dirt, food, or another person, she would be tortured by anxiety until able to scrub.

Anna came to the consultation with her mother. The mother was worried because a doctor consulting for her daughter's school wrote on a disability form that Anna was schizophrenic. Schizophrenia, the mother knew, is a largely incurable psychiatric condition that usually leads to progressive incapacitation. So the consulting psychiatrist first asked questions relevant to schizophrenia. Had Anna ever heard voices or seen things? No. Did she believe the dirt she needed to wash from her hands was really dangerous? No. Was anybody, in her view, trying to harm her? No. Anna was not psychotic; there was no break from reality. She understood that there was no logical reason for the hand washing.

Next, because Anna was tearful and glum, the psychiatrist asked about possible signs of depression. But Anna had experienced no change in appetite, no trouble sleeping through the night, and no difficulty laughing during a funny movie or becoming absorbed in a good book. Although she felt her life was a mess, she had no wish to die and no intention of harming herself. Depression therefore seemed an unlikely diagnosis.

Finally, the doctor asked about possible medical problems that could produce this kind of psychiatric symptom pattern but found no physical illness involved. The diagnosis of obsessive-compulsive disorder was made.

After a thorough description of the illness and the different ways of treating it, the psychiatrist prescribed Luvox in its generic form (fluvoxamine), 50 mg at night. The dose was raised over the next few days to 100 mg twice daily. He also referred Anna to a colleague who specialized in cognitive behavioral psychotherapy. The psychiatrist spoke to his psychotherapy colleague and described the case.

Over the next four weeks, Anna met with the psychiatrist twice and spoke to him several times on the telephone. She experienced mild nausea for the first three days on Luvox, but this subsided.

Anna began the cognitive behavioral therapy. The therapist, a Ph.D. psychologist, began by taking a history. He then designed a program whereby Anna was asked to wait longer and longer before giving in to the urge to wash her hands. She was instructed to make a note in a diary of how long she scrubbed every time she washed. She was also instructed to record all of her thoughts as she got closer and closer to succumbing and washing. Over the next weeks and months, the psychologist helped Anna to control the thoughts that provoked her washing and to wait longer and longer before washing.

Four weeks after starting the drug, Anna's mother reported that she was washing her hands much less frequently. Over the next month, this behavior decreased to the point where Anna could get by with four ten-minute hand washings a day. Admittedly, she often felt anxious about dirt during the day and sometimes had to struggle to keep the hand washing in check, but she was now in much better control and much happier. She continued the therapy for a full six-month course but stayed on Luvox even longer. After six months Anna was able to return to work.

Anna obviously represents an example of optimal care and a fortunate result. The care she received is no more or less than what any patient should expect. But the result is not necessarily the outcome enjoyed by everyone with OCD, as the next example shows.

Bill had always been shy and nervous, and he suffered from a number of nervous facial tics. One day, shortly after getting his driver's license, he was driving in his car when he suddenly got the idea that he had hit a pedestrian. No, he thought, it can't be. There weren't any screams, no thud, nothing. What if he had just run over the person's foot? There might not have been much noise. Impossible. You don't run over someone's foot without knowing it. But it might be possible. So Bill turned the car around and retraced his route. No bodies on the road, no crowds, no flashing lights or ambulances. Everything seemed all right. But what if they had taken the victim to the hospital already? What if they saw his license plate number? He would be charged with hit-and-run. So Bill rushed to a pay phone and started calling hospitals to see if anyone who had had a foot run over had been admitted to the emergency room.

This went on for hours. Every time Bill believed he was just making up the hit-and-run story, he would have another doubt and start ruminating more. For days he had these obsessions. He told a few people—his parents, a friend, a teacher—what was on his mind and they thought he was either putting them on or taking drugs. After weeks of worrying to the point that he could no longer do his schoolwork, he was taken by his parents to the family doctor, who prescribed Valium. This only made Bill sleepy.

Bill's story from here on is very sad. He eventually was admitted to a psychiatric hospital, received shock treatments (which didn't help), and finally started psychotherapy. Despite twice-weekly sessions centered on his supposed anger at his parents and "unconscious homosexual feelings," he did not improve. From worrying about having hit someone with his car, he went on to worrying that he might stab his mother. Bill had never committed an act of violence in his life and had no conscious anger toward either of his parents, yet he developed a recurrent thought that he might pick up a knife and murder his mother. This is a typical obsession for patients with OCD. They never act on the thought and they know the thought is senseless. It is as if something forces them to entertain the most repugnant thing imaginable. Bill asked that all the knives in the house be put under lock and key and he developed a phobia of sharp objects.

Through the years, Bill had several psychiatric hospitalizations and was treated with many drugs. Ultimately, he was placed on Anafranil in its generic form (clomipramine), and this helped to some degree. The obsessions became less anxiety provoking and less intense. Bill found for the first time that he could read a book for as long as an hour before the obsessions took over. Despite the improvement, which was certainly more than any other drug had provided, Bill remained seriously burdened with obsessions. He also experienced many side effects from Anafranil, including a thirty-pound weight gain. Fortunately, he had a consultation with a specialist in OCD who was able to switch the medication to Effexor XR, which has fewer side effects than Anafranil, and added the antipsychotic drug Risperdal, which is particularly effective in combination with antidepressants for patients with OCD who also have tics. The specialist also began treating Bill with cognitive behavioral therapy. He now holds a job as a stockroom clerk and has a few friends. He enjoys bowling and having a few beers with his buddies, but he has not overcome the obsessions entirely.

Obsessive-compulsive disorder remains one of the challenges for psychiatric research. Medications and cognitive behavioral psychotherapy are now able to reduce some of the symptoms. Sometimes a patient is almost entirely cured. Most patients, however, have lingering pathology despite the best medical and psychological care. It is important to remember that many psychiatric conditions resist even the best treatment efforts.

POST-TRAUMATIC STRESS DISORDER

Post-traumatic stress disorder (PTSD) has become one of the most researched of all psychiatric illnesses. In part, this was prompted by a large number of Vietnam and first Gulf War veterans who began asking the Department of Veterans Affairs (VA) to grant them disability because of PTSD caused by traumatic events during these wars. The VA got involved in research trying to figure out what traumatic events really cause PTSD and what is the best way to treat it. Also, the 9/11 attacks on the World Trade Center and Pentagon increased interest in what are the risk factors for PTSD. Another reason behind the increased amount of research is the progress that has been made in the last decade in understanding the basic brain events that occur during fear. There are now good animal models for PTSD, allowing scientists to probe the brain and understand how a stressful event affects brain function. Many of the findings in animals have also been substantiated by brain-imaging studies in humans. Hence, PTSD stands as one of the psychiatric illnesses for which major breakthroughs are increasingly being realized in the laboratory.

By definition, PTSD cannot be diagnosed until one month after the traumatic event. As described earlier in this chapter, that event must be life threatening and the patient must either have witnessed or been the victim of events that threatened death or severe bodily injury. Symptoms of PTSD include reliving and reexperiencing the original trauma, avoiding situations reminiscent of the trauma, being very easily startled, losing the ability to feel deeply normal human emotion, and depression and anxiety. Only about one-third of people exposed to serious traumatic events develop PTSD, but that number is considerably higher in the case of rape and other forms of sexual abuse. Things that increase the risk of getting PTSD include a family history of psychiatric disorder, personal history of anxiety disorder, low levels of social support, being female, and having been exposed previously to traumatic events. High levels of social support decrease the risk of PTSD. If symptoms occur during the first month after the trauma, a diagnosis of acute stress disorder (ASD) is made. Patients with ASD often experience symptoms of dissociation, that is, feeling that things do not seem real and that they are separate from their own bodies. Whether dissociation predicts a higher rate of getting PTSD or is an important component of PTSD is controversial. If left untreated, most patients with PTSD and ASD recover spontaneously. However, once full-blown PTSD sets in, that recovery can take years and treatment is usually indicated.

Some studies have shown that treatment immediately following a traumatic event, especially if it is mandatory, actually makes people worse. For example, following a plane crash, it is best to let survivors and families of victims experience grief and mourning without intervention. Treatment should

Table 23.

Drug Treatment of the Anxiety Disorders

DISORDER	FIRST-LINE DRUGS	SECOND-LINE DRUGS
Panic disorder	Paxil, Zoloft, Prozac, Luvox	Xanax, Klonopin, Nardil
Generalized anxiety disorder	Valium, Librium, Tranxene, Centrax, Paxipam, Xanax, Serax, Ativan, BuSpar	None
Social phobia	Zoloft, Paxil, Prozac, Luvox	Klonopin, Nardil
Obsessive-compulsive disorder (OCD)	Luvox, Prozac, Paxil, Zoloft, Effexor XR, Cymbalta, Celexa	Anafril
Post-traumatic stress disorder (PTSD)	Prozac, Paxil, Zoloft, Effexor XR, Celexa, Cymbalta	None

be reserved for people whose symptoms develop into full-blown PTSD. Once PTSD occurs, several forms of psychotherapy have been proved effective and should be considered before medication. Of these, perhaps the best studied is prolonged exposure, pioneered by Dr. Edna Foa of the University of Pennsylvania. This involves exposing the patient, under the guidance of a specially trained therapist, to thoughts and places that evoke memories of the trauma. By doing this repeatedly, the patient becomes less anxious and avoidant and better able to cope with the memory of the traumatic event. Some therapists combine this with eye movements, called eye movement desensitization therapy, based on controversial evidence that moving one's eyes back and forth while remembering the traumatic event is particularly therapeutic. If psychotherapy is not sufficiently helpful, medications can be added. Those that have been shown to work are the SSRI and SNRI antidepressants (Prozac, Paxil, Zoloft, Celexa, Luvox, Effexor XR, and Cymbalta). These are discussed in more detail in Chapter 7. Benzodiazepines and sleeping pills like Ambien and Lunesta may make patients with PTSD worse and should be avoided if possible. For severe insomnia, trazodone (Desyrel) is a better choice. Table 23 summarizes drug treatment of the anxiety disorders.

Chapter 9

Drugs Used to Treat Bipolar Disorder (Manic Depression)

When we talk about depression and the anxiety disorders, we generally say that drugs aren't always needed. Sometimes no treatment is best, sometimes psychotherapy, sometimes drugs alone, and sometimes a combination of drugs and psychotherapy.

But when we talk about the illness psychiatrists now call bipolar disorder (formerly known as manic-depressive disorder), there is no debate: The patient should be on medication. The person with bipolar disorder is sometimes referred to as being manic depressive or having mood swings. Basically, the bipolar person is at times depressed, at times high, or manic, and at other times perfectly normal. Each person has his or her own natural cycle of the three states.

Bipolar disorder affects men and women equally and usually begins in the twenties. It can begin in childhood or adolescence, however. There is good evidence that this disease is genetic. This doesn't mean that a person with a bipolar parent will automatically develop bipolar mood disorder. Apparently, a host of unknown factors determine whether the gene for mood swings is actually expressed. It is probable, however, that without the inheritance of some abnormal genetic material, the likelihood of developing the illness is small.

Bipolar people experience some of the most severe depressions seen in psychiatry. Typically, these bipolar depressions are characterized by extreme loss of energy and the ability to concentrate, complete inability to enjoy anything, and suicidal ideas. Untreated bipolar people frequently commit suicide.

Sometimes, they have symptoms that are the opposite of what is seen in people with depression who are not bipolar. The depressed bipolar person may thus eat too much and sleep too much. All the antidepressant drugs discussed in Chapter 7 work for this phase, as does electroconvulsive therapy (ECT). A new medication for bipolar disorder, Lamictal (lamotrigine), is especially helpful for the depressed phase of bipolar disorder. But drawing the person out of the depression is only half the battle.

When high, or manic, bipolar people feel terrific. They talk constantly, need almost no sleep, and are continuously active. They spend more money than they have because they believe that they are so successful and brilliant that riches are around the corner. Manic people are also very irritable. They don't like anyone spoiling their fun or disagreeing with them. While high, they have an insatiable sex drive, and even the most faithfully married people may have affairs when manic. As the manic phase progresses, they may lose touch with reality and become increasingly psychotic. Voices tell them that they are wonderful, that they are going to be elected president, that God is taking a special interest. At this point a bipolar person may become very suspicious as irritability transforms into frank paranoia. He or she then resembles the person with schizophrenia and, indeed, until recently it was unfortunately very common for psychiatrists to misdiagnose bipolar disorder as schizophrenia. Many medications work for the manic phase of bipolar illness, including lithium, Depakote (divalproex sodium), and the antipsychotic drugs (Trilafon, Zyprexa, Risperdal, Seroquel, Geodon, and Abilify).

DIFFERENTIATION FROM SCHIZOPHRENIA

The main difference between bipolar disorder and schizophrenia is that the bipolar person usually passes through a normal phase between highs and lows. Sometimes, the normal period lasts a year or more, sometimes only a few days. Most bipolar people are able to resume their preillness level of functioning at several points. People with schizophrenia, on the other hand, rarely return to normal. After each psychotic break, they seem less motivated and less functional than before the break. As I discuss in more detail in Chapter 10, schizophrenia is usually a disease marked by progressive deterioration.

One of the main reasons for distinguishing bipolar disorder from schizophrenia is that treatment for the two conditions is different. Since the introduction of lithium thirty years ago, most cases of bipolar illness can now be controlled. Therefore, safe and effective treatment to prevent the highs and lows is available to most bipolar patients. The medications that are officially approved to prevent highs and lows in the bipolar patient—as opposed to treating the highs and lows when they occur—are lithium, Lamictal (lamotrigine), Zyprexa (olanzapine), and Abilify (aripiprazole). Many psychopharmacologists believe that Depakote (divalproex sodium) and possibly Tegretol (carbamazepine) are also effective as preventative agents, although research studies have not proved this to be true. Of all of these medications, lithium is still the best, but Lamictal, which is better for the depressed than for the manic side, is also an excellent drug.

One thing to always think about when dealing with a bipolar patient is the likelihood that substance abuse is also involved. Bipolar patients frequently abuse alcohol and illegal drugs as well. They may even use cocaine when they are manic, even though this makes the mania worse. Drug abuse makes treating bipolar patients particularly challenging, but often is overlooked. It must always be diagnosed and treated.

Once again, the importance of careful and accurate diagnosis cannot be stressed enough. Sometimes, the diagnosis of bipolar disorder is so easy that the elevator operator who transports the patient to the doctor's office can make it. Someone who is talking a mile a minute, believes that she and God are best friends, and just ran up a bill of $10,000 on her American Express card even though she makes only $30,000 a year is probably in the manic phase of bipolar disorder. The same person may show up two months later deeply depressed, insisting she is the cause of world hunger and deserves to die; she has "flipped" into the depressed phase of the illness.

Other times, however, the diagnosis is more difficult. When depressed, patients may have difficulty remembering their previous manic highs. They may say that they never felt well and that life has always been terrible. In this case, the psychiatrist may incorrectly diagnose major depressive disorder instead of the depressed phase of bipolar disorder. On the other hand, some chronically depressed patients misinterpret the few days a month when they feel a little less depressed as representing mania. They may say, "For a few days every month I feel really good, energetic, optimistic, talkative. . . ." What they are really describing is temporary relief from depression, not mania.

Mania itself comes in different varieties. I have described the full-blown type, in which the patient is wildly euphoric, spending money, having sex with everyone, full of self-confidence, and talking incessantly. A milder form of mania is called hypomania. In this situation, the patient becomes abnormally optimistic, talkative, energetic, and self-confident but is not as flagrant and does not do as many self-destructive things. When a patient has episodes of depression and full-blown mania, he or she is said to have bipolar I disorder.

When the patient has episodes of depression and hypomania, but never full-blown mania, he or she is said to have bipolar II disorder.

And of course, despite the great consciousness-raising that has occurred in the last two decades about psychiatric diagnosis, differentiating between mania and schizophrenia is still sometimes frankly impossible even for the most experienced clinicians. In fact, psychiatrists recognize a category of illness called schizoaffective disorder for patients who seem to straddle the line between schizophrenia and mood disorder or depression. Although a complete review of the differences between these conditions could be the subject of another book, some examples may be helpful. First, a very obvious case of bipolar disorder.

Charles, a twenty-five-year-old waiter and aspiring actor, had been admitted to a suburban hospital psychiatry ward in a floridly psychotic state. Over the previous six months, his roommate had started to notice changes in his behavior. Although usually sensible, Charles began talking about his brilliant career as an actor and the likelihood that he would soon be "discovered" for a big movie role. When his roommate pointed out that Charles had never succeeded at a single audition and had never been given any professional parts, Charles got annoyed and said his roommate was merely jealous of his ability.

Then Charles started staying up very late, supposedly reading scripts. His mother became alarmed when he started calling her asking for money to pay off his growing credit card bills. As the months passed, Charles became progressively more grandiose and irritable. One day he almost got into a fist-fight with a friend who disagreed with him about who was the best player in professional football. He also started drinking more and more, complaining that he could not fall asleep unless drunk. A week before being brought to the emergency room, Charles attempted to walk into the office of a major movie producer without an appointment, had sex with five different women, spent $2,500 in one afternoon on new clothes, and made six long-distance phone calls to an old girlfriend now living in Paris. Finally, his roommate called his parents one night in terror: Charles had been up all night drinking and making telephone calls. Now he was threatening to bomb the office of the producer for not "realizing I am the greatest actor living in the Western world today who can do Westerns and Easterns and make omelets and eat them faster than anyone else." In short, Charles was talking on and on without making sense and threatening everyone in sight.

The emergency room psychiatrist was able to make a diagnosis of bipolar disorder, manic phase, fairly easily after asking Charles's parents a few important questions. At age eighteen, they told the doctor, during his freshman year at college, Charles had developed a serious depression that required psychiatric treatment. Again, at age twenty-two, just after graduation, he became depressed, refused to look for a job, and made a suicide gesture by cutting his wrist superficially. He had been admitted to a hospital overnight and then released.

So Charles had had at least two episodes of serious depression and now a bout of mania. Between these periods he had functioned well, working hard, maintaining a relationship with a woman, and attending acting classes at night. During the long intervals between highs and lows, he behaved normally. Finally, it turned out that Charles's paternal uncle had a similar illness and had been treated with lithium for many years.

Several interesting features of Charles's case are worth pointing out. First, he had several bouts of depression before the episode of mania. This is usually the case with bipolar patients. Depression usually precedes mania, so at the beginning it is correct to treat only the depression, as if the patient is suffering from major depressive disorder. Occasionally, manic periods precede depressed phases. When depression occurs for the very first time at a very early age, before age twenty-one, and when there is a family history of bipolar disorder, there should be a very high index of suspicion that the depression is really part of bipolar disorder.

Second, as emphasized above, many manic patients drink alcohol excessively, probably in an attempt to calm themselves down. This makes the situation much worse, of course, because a drunk manic is even more disinhibited than a sober one. Often, the severity of the mania cannot be fully assessed until the patient is sobered up.

Third, without the history of previous depressions and normal functioning between episodes, Charles might have been diagnosed as schizophrenic when he was presented to the emergency room. At that moment he was violent, paranoid, and delusional (he believed he was in direct contact with God). So the presence of a relative or spouse who can provide the history is invaluable.

Now, a slightly less obvious case.

Patricia, a nurse, was seeing a psychiatrist for the first time at age thirty, complaining of depression. She had all the features of depression: loss of energy, decreased sex drive, waking up at 4 A.M. every morning, weight loss, and suicidal ideas. Years of psychotherapy had been very helpful in improving her relationships with men and her ability to get along with her supervisors at work. Her therapist had correctly noted that periods of depression lasting about four weeks seemed to occur regularly two to three times a year. The therapist wondered if medication might be needed to stabilize Patricia and prevent these regularly occurring depressions.

The depression part was easy to understand, but the consulting psychiatrist had difficulty figuring out what went on in Patricia's life when she

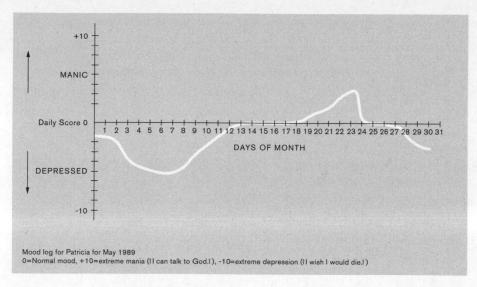

Mood log for Patricia for May 1989
0=Normal mood, +10=extreme mania (íI can talk to God.í), -10=extreme depression (íI wish I would die.í)

Figure 1.   **Patricia's Mood Log**

wasn't depressed. So the psychiatrist asked Patricia to keep a mood log like the one shown in Figure 1, a log that can be kept by anyone who suspects he or she might suffer from bipolar disorder. For one month the psychiatrist instructed Patricia to rate her mood daily and to have her husband rate it as well. On the mood log, a score of zero means normal mood, not too high or not too low. A score of −10 indicates that the patient is so depressed that she doesn't have the energy to do what she would most like to do: jump out the nearest window. A score of +10 is as manic as one can get; the patient thinks she can walk across water and might try to prove it. Some fluctuation around zero is okay, but the psychiatrist wanted to see how high Patricia was capable of reaching.

As it turned out, Patricia's two or three annual monthlong depressions were matched by similar periods of hypomania—not nearly as manic as Charles's, but still not normal. Patricia would recover from a depression, appear normal for a week or two, and then become talkative and provocative at work, behavior that often led to reprimands when she seemed like too much of a know-it-all. During these periods, she was extremely labile, that is, she would laugh raucously at the least funny joke and burst out in tears a few minutes later. She slept poorly, was jittery, and spent too much money. A couple of times during these highs she made sexual advances to doctors at the hospital and one time had an affair. This behavior was uncharacteristic of Patricia, who ordinarily felt very deeply about the need to remain faithful to her husband, whom she loved very much. She was filled with guilt about the affair, but when high, she felt her sexual urges were almost uncontrollable.

Unlike Charles, Patricia never became psychotically manic. She didn't hear voices or get delusional ideas or become paranoid. But her mood did become elevated above normal to the point where she did things that she herself believed were wrong.

After obtaining all the information, the psychiatrist was able to diagnose bipolar disorder and prescribe medication to level Patricia's moods.

Here again are important features that must be emphasized. Some might argue that it is wrong to interfere with a person's "good time." Maybe Patricia did know more than the other people at work. After all, nurses often are taken advantage of in hospitals and not treated with proper respect by doctors. Perhaps Patricia is really a liberated woman who should be allowed to have sex with anyone she wants to. People seem much more tolerant of husbands who cheat than of wives who do. Isn't treating Patricia's highs a form of psychiatric mind control, an attempt to turn her into a "socially acceptable" person? I have no doubt that psychiatry has been misused countless times in many countries, including the United States, as a form of social control. The concerns voiced in this area are legitimate; however, before assuming that prescribing lithium is an exercise in mind control, it is important to gain familiarity with what bipolar patients go through.

People like Patricia suffer just as much through the manic or hypomanic periods as they do through the depressed periods. Mania is often a disaster, even though for a while the patient may enjoy the good feeling. Manic patients have completely ruined themselves financially by reckless spending, only to face the consequences when the mania subsided. Manic patients ruin their marriages and are fired from jobs. They drink too much and always know that at the end of a manic period there looms the possibility of a severe depression.

Medications used to treat manic depressives do not affect their principles or political views. They do not make them incapable of experiencing sadness or joy. What they do is eliminate the extreme swings in mood that destroy lives. If Patricia wants to have affairs or assert herself more at work, lithium or other treatments for bipolar mood disorder will not stop her. The medications will enable her to make up her mind somewhat freer of the disabling and uncontrolled dips or elevations of mood.

Had lithium been available many years ago, it is possible that Virginia Woolf would never have drowned herself in 1941 and that Vincent van Gogh would never have cut off his ear and eventually killed himself in a French asylum in 1890. A study by the late Dr. Mogens Schou, the psychiatrist who first proved the effectiveness of lithium, showed that of twenty-four bipolar artists, six found that lithium reduced their creativity, six found no effect of lithium on creativity, and twelve found that lithium improved their creativity.

Another point to stress in Patricia's case is that it took some time to establish the diagnosis. Maintaining a mood log and obtaining information from as many people as possible can be very helpful.

Finally, I want to emphasize the good and close relationship between the psychiatrist and the therapist. Besides her bipolar disorder, Patricia had other problems that responded well to psychotherapy. Even after being placed on medication, Patricia continued her therapy and found it useful.

Finally, a case that presents great diagnostic difficulty.

Robert was a bright college student and graduate student, but always prone to moodiness. From time to time, he went for weeks without studying or contacting his friends. Few people aside from his family knew him well. His grades grew progressively worse and he never finished his graduate program. Instead he took a job and at first functioned well but then missed many days of work, complaining he didn't feel well or needed a rest. He finally was fired and took a new, less appropriate job.

At age twenty-six, Robert began the first of a series of psychiatric hospitalizations. Sometimes, he felt depressed and suicidal. Other times, he was psychotic, hearing strange voices and insisting that his food was poisoned; during these periods, he giggled and laughed inappropriately but didn't seem especially happy. Although the episodes seemed to occur in discrete periods, Robert never returned to normal when they were over. He went from job to job, finally ending up on disability and living alone in a cheap apartment.

Robert's case is hard to diagnose. Surely he suffered from highs and lows, but he also had a deteriorating course with more social isolation and less capacity to function over time. And the content of his psychosis was not that of the classically manic patient. The voices did not tell him he was great and wonderful; they said more frightening and sometimes very bizarre things.

Robert was diagnosed as having schizoaffective disorder and treated with both lithium and an antipsychotic drug also used for schizophrenia (Risperdal) (described in Chapter 10). Unlike Charles and Patricia, he never made a complete recovery and never worked again. The extremes of his depression and psychosis were controlled by the medication, however, and he no longer required multiple hospitalizations every year.

The drugs described in more detail in this chapter are used in psychiatry only for treating bipolar disorder (they are all also used to treat epilepsy): lithium, Depakote (sodium valproate), Tegretol (carbamazepine), and Lamictal (lamotrigine). Antipsychotic drugs that are used to treat both schizophrenia and bipolar disorder (Zyprexa, Risperdal, Seroquel, Geodon, and Abilify) are described in more detail in Chapter 10.

Table 24.

Treating the Bipolar Patient

- *If the patient is depressed:* Start an antidepressant (Wellbutrin is a good choice) and lithium or Lamictal. Stop the antidepressant about a week or two after the depression is over. Continue lithium or Lamictal.
- *If the patient is manic:* Start an antipsychotic (Trilafon, Zyprexa, Risperdal, or Seroquel). Start lithium. Stop the antipsychotic drug a few days after the mania is over. Continue lithium.
- *If the patient is euthymic (normal mood):* Start lithium or Lamictal.

TREATMENT OF BIPOLAR MOOD DISORDER

There are three states in which a person with bipolar disorder may present to the psychiatrist for the first time: depressed, manic, or normal. Each requires a different treatment approach (Table 24).

The Depressed Bipolar Patient

The first thing to do is get on top of the depression. Usually, one of the antidepressant medications described in Chapter 7 is prescribed. The risk of giving a bipolar patient an antidepressant is always that he or she will then develop mania. The chance of this happening is much reduced if the patient is also on one of the drugs that prevent highs and lows, called "mood stabilizers." These include lithium, Depakote (sodium valproate), atypical antipsychotics (Zyprexa and Abilify), and Lamictal (more about it later). Wellbutrin SR (bupropion 12-hour tabs) is thought by many to be the best choice because it appears to have the least chance of precipitating mania. However, others believe this is only because Wellbutrin SR (and its more expensive variant, Wellbutrin XL) is a relatively weak antidepressant. Several studies have shown that SSRI antidepressants, like Paxil, can be given to bipolar depressed patients without precipitating a manic episode, as long as they are also on a mood stabilizer. Cyclic antidepressants (like desipramine and nortripyline) seem to have the highest risk of flipping a depressed bipolar patient into mania and are not good first choices. Another concern has been that antidepressants may induce "rapid cycling" in bipolar patients, that is, the depression may resolve, but then the patient begins to go from high to low and back again even more rapidly than before. This is controversial. In my opinion, as long as the patient is on one of the mood stabilizers, it does not usually occur. The key, then, to treating a depressed patient in whom the diagnosis of bipolar disorder is also made is to start him or her immediately on both a mood stabilizer and an SSRI antidepressant. After the depression has resolved for several weeks, the antidepressant can often be tapered and discontinued and only the mood stabilizer is continued.

Another excellent stategy is to start the depressed bipolar patient on Lamictal (lamotrigine). Lamictal is one of the drugs approved by the FDA as a mood stabilizer, but it clearly works better for the depressed than for the manic side of the illness. Its virtue is that it treats depression without inducing mania. Its main drawback is that because of a potentially very serious and even life-threatening side effect that begins with a rash, the dose must be started very low and it then takes over a month to get to a therapeutic level. Hence, it is not ideal by itself if the depression is very severe because it will not usually resolve depression fast enough. It is also not ideal in combination with an antidepressant because it is not as strong as the other mood stabilizers in preventing a switch into mania. Lamictal is best for bipolar patients who present with relatively mild depression.

What about the patient who is already on lithium or another mood-stabilizing drug that is supposed to prevent high and lows but who becomes depressed anyway? Breakthrough depressions do occur, even to lithium-treated bipolar patients. They are usually much less frequent and less severe than those occurring in non-lithium-treated patients but are still worrisome. First, the doctor should check whether the patient is taking the mood-stabilizing medication as prescribed. Nonadherence, especially with a drug like lithium that must be taken daily even when the patient feels well, can cause the breakthrough depression. Second, the patient's levels of thyroid hormone should be monitored. Lithium can interfere with the thyroid gland, and low thyroid hormone levels can mimic depression. Finally, an antidepressant like Wellbutrin or an SSRI like Paxil may be prescribed but should be stopped soon after the depression is alleviated.

The Manic Bipolar Patient

The manic bipolar patient often feels so well that he or she is ambivalent about seeking treatment at all. Friends and relatives have usually had enough by the time they talk the patient into getting help. The acutely hypomanic (mildly manic) or manic patient may have a range of problems from simple overactivity, inability to sleep, and irritability to hallucinations, delusions, and a violent temper.

Friends and relatives are usually needed to establish that the patient is indeed bipolar, that is, that the patient has experienced episodes of depression in the past. Usually, an antipsychotic medication such as Zyprexa, Risperdal, or Seroquel is prescribed, although lithium or Depakote by itself is often effective for acute mania. These drugs work rapidly to calm the patient, reduce the overactivity, and stop psychotic symptoms like hallucinations and delusions. Antipsychotic drugs are complicated (they are fully described in Chapter 10). For bipolar patients, these drugs are usually taken for a week or two until the manic symptoms are cleared. In the emergency room or inpatient psychiatric hospital, when a manic patient becomes violent and threatening to himself or others, injections of the benzodiazepine Ativan (lorazepam) are given because they immediately quiet the patient with no adverse effects other than sleepiness.

Whether an antipsychotic or a benzodiazepine drug is prescribed, the patient is usually simultaneously started on a mood stabilizer. Lithium works too slowly to control very severe acute mania, just as it is not very good for relief of an acute depression. Nevertheless, it is a good time to start the patient on lithium, because when the mania subsides and the antipsychotic drugs are stopped, the patient will be protected by lithium from experiencing another manic outburst.

Not all manic patients can be treated on an outpatient basis. Mania is one of the psychiatric illnesses that often require hospitalization, because manic patients often refuse to comply with treatment or are so hyperactive they don't remember to take the pills properly. A manic patient can get into a lot of trouble, so sometimes it is best to offer him or her the protection of the hospital, where medication can be administered regularly. Remember that mania rarely resolves on its own in a short period. Untreated mania can last months, by which time the patient may have been arrested or bankrupted or may have committed murder. And when the mania does finally go away, the patient often slips into a severe depression, which can result in suicide. No matter how wonderful manic patients think they feel, it is no favor to leave them alone.

The Euthymic Bipolar Patient

Euthymic means normal mood—neither depressed nor manic. A bipolar patient in this state appears completely normal. Studies have shown that even trained mental health professionals cannot tell a bipolar person in the euthymic state from a person with no psychiatric problems. A bipolar patient who presents at this point in the illness should be placed on lithium, Lamictal, or Depakote to prevent the onset of highs and lows. Although two of the atypical antipsychotic drugs discussed in more detail in Chapter 10 are also approved as mood stabilizers, Zyprexa and Abilify, the former causes very substantial weight gain and the latter is, in my opinion, not yet convincingly proved to work. Of all the medications that are approved as mood stabilizers, I believe the oldest, lithium, is still the best, and Lamictal comes in second, although with the latter breakthrough manias are possible.

Once a patient is stabilized on lithium, Lamictal, or Depakote, the question that always arises is, is it for life? This question is difficult to answer for two reasons. First, no one likes to hear that he or she will have to take medication forever. Second, there is so much variability in the course of bipolar disorder that it is difficult to know how long the condition will remain active in an individual patient.

Bipolar illness can be devastating and severe, but its treatment is generally well tolerated and safe. So it is best to be cautious about stopping a mood stabilizer. After a patient has had serious manic and depressive episodes, I usually recommend that he or she remain on preventative medication for five to ten years. Then, if the patient has been completely stabilized, he or she may attempt to stop the medication. I always make it clear that this is a risk: After about one month off the drug the patient could become seriously depressed or manic again. It is helpful if a spouse or relative is available to alert me at the first sign that something is wrong so that treatment can be resumed immediately. Rather than take this risk, some patients elect to continue taking medication indefinitely.

On the other hand, it does happen that a patient who has been successfully treated with lithium for many years is forced to stop taking the drug because of medical problems. A patient may develop kidney problems, for example, and be forced to stop lithium. In this case, it is not necessarily the case that lithium produces the kidney problem, although it sometimes does, but regardless of the cause, reduction in kidney function may necessitate stopping lithium. Will such a patient be doomed to a life of highs and lows? Although lithium is in my opinion the best drug for bipolar patients, fortunately alternative medications are available. Consequently, if a bipolar patient is forced to stop lithium at some point, the chance is good that an alternative drug can be safely and successfully substituted.

Even if a patient takes lithium or similar medication religiously and has a generally good response, there may be bumps in the road. Breakthrough depression is usually easy to spot because patients don't like it and call the doctor right away. As mentioned earlier, this may mean that lithium has lowered the thyroid hormone level and indicate the need for thyroid medication.

Or a short course of antidepressants may be required. If it happens often, Lamictal may be introduced. Breakthrough highs are less easily spotted because the patient may confuse this with merely feeling well. One good rule of thumb is that a night or two of sleeping fewer than five hours without feeling tired the next day means that the doctor should be notified. Breakthrough mania is sometimes treated by increasing the amount of lithium for a while or by administering a brief course of an antipsychotic drug (see Chapter 10).

Bipolar disorder is a medical illness requiring skilled medical management. It should never be ignored. Although I mentioned earlier that all patients with bipolar disorder require medication, that does not at all mean that psychotherapy has no role. Thanks largely to Dr. Ellen Frank and her team at the University of Pittsburgh, it is now clear that psychotherapy that aims to help the patient cope with the stress of having a chronic illness, develop a regular schedule to daily activities, and reduce thoughts and behaviors that trigger depression is very helpful when administered in addition to medication.

DRUGS USED TO TREAT BIPOLAR MOOD DISORDER

LITHIUM

Brand Names: Lithobid, Lithonate, Lithotabs, Eskalith, Eskalith CR.

Used For: Long-term treatment of bipolar mood disorder to prevent future highs and lows, to enhance the effectiveness of antidepressant drugs.

Do Not Use If: You have kidney disease, are taking diuretics (water pills) for high blood pressure, or use anti-inflammatory drugs like Motrin, Naprosyn, and Indocin. It is still possible to use lithium in these situations, but it will require special attention from your doctor.

Tests to Take First: Before the first lithium tablet goes into your mouth, you should have blood tests to measure kidney function and thyroid function. As lithium can affect kidney and thyroid function, it is important that a baseline be established against which later levels can be judged. The doctor should also record your pulse, and, if you are over age fifty and on lithium for the first time, you may need to have an electrocardiogram.

Tests to Take While You Are on It: Blood tests are required frequently, especially after initiation of lithium treatment, because the only way to determine the correct dose for an individual is by monitoring the lithium blood level, which is obtained through a simple blood test. Levels are usually maintained between 0.5 and 1 mEq/L, although different situations may justify higher or lower levels. The lithium level is never allowed to rise above 1.2 because serious side effects emerge. Below 0.5, lithium probably doesn't do much good. The first blood level is usually drawn after the first week of lithium treatment, and, if necessary, the dose is adjusted. One week after each change in dose, a new level is obtained. When the correct dose is reached, lithium levels can be obtained less frequently. Ultimately, for people under age sixty, levels can be determined four or five times a year. Patients over sixty should have tests at least every month because the body's ability to metabolize lithium starts declining at this point. In addition to these relatively frequent lithium levels, blood tests for kidney and thyroid function are usually obtained every six months. Some doctors also obtain urine tests for kidney function. Finally, and particularly in patients over sixty, the doctor should check the patient's pulse once a month; rarely, lithium can produce a dramatic decrease in heart rate.

Usual Dose: Most lithium tablets and capsules come in one strength: 300 mg. There is also a 450-mg preparation (Eskalith CR). A patient is usually started on two or three a day; elderly patients are often started on only one tablet or capsule a day. Once again, it must be emphasized that the final dose can be determined only by measuring the blood level. One patient may take 900 mg a day to reach a "good" level, whereas another patient of exactly the same sex, height, and weight may require 1,500 mg to have the same blood level. After the correct dose is determined, it is best that the entire dose be taken once a day, although it makes no difference what time of day it is taken. Many patients prefer to take lithium on a full stomach.

How Long Until It Works: Lithium is given to *prevent* future highs and lows, and once a good blood level is reached, it should start to do this. The only way to determine if lithium is working is to observe the patient over time for further mood swings.

Common Side Effects: Upset stomach and diarrhea, usually in the early phase of treatment. Metallic taste in mouth, also usually in early phase. Increased frequency of urination, but not enough to disrupt a patient's schedule. Weight gain, anywhere from five to twenty or more pounds; the average is about ten pounds, usually in the first year of treatment. Acne. Decrease in thyroid gland function, which occurs in about one-fourth of people taking lithium, more often in women than men; in only about 5 percent of lithium-treated patients does thyroid hormone decrease to the point that treatment with thyroid hormone is essential. Tiredness and difficulty concentrating are reported in about 10 percent of patients but may be due, in some cases, to depression. Fine hand tremor.

Less Common Side Effects: Diabetes insipidus—this has nothing to do with "sugar" diabetes, which is technically called diabetes mellitus. In diabetes insipidus, there is a massive increase in thirst and urination. Patients feel as if they must drink almost constantly, and as soon as they drink they have to urinate. There is a need to wake up almost hourly through the night to urinate. This condition can be treated by adding a special drug or reducing the dose of lithium, but it must be taken care of immediately. Decrease in kidney function—several years ago there were reports of patients developing kidney damage after taking lithium for more than ten years. None of these patients developed kidney failure; that is, dialysis or a kidney transplant was not required. Most experts now doubt that lithium really caused the problem, as those patients were taking many drugs for other medical problems. However, there is no question that some patients who take lithium for years experience a decline in kidney function that only in very occasional cases means that lithium must be discontinued. To be on the safe side, we insist that patients undergo simple blood tests, and sometimes urine tests, that measure kidney function every six months to one year while on lithium. Lithium toxicity—this very serious medical emergency is almost entirely preventable: Regularly check the lithium blood level and never become dehydrated. Lithium toxicity occurs when the blood level climbs above 1.5. The patient begins to shake and tremble, feels confused, vomits, and develops diarrhea. The lithium level can be greatly increased by severe dehydration, such as can occur after more than a day without anything to drink, after persistent vomiting and diarrhea, or when mountain climbing in the desert when the temperature is 105°. Elderly people are more prone to develop lithium toxicity than younger people. A lithium-treated patient should always drink the equivalent of six glasses of water a day and not start a salt-restricted diet while on lithium. Also, if food poisoning or a stomach virus develops with vomiting or diarrhea, the doctor should be called immediately; the patient will probably be told to stop taking lithium until his or her stomach settles down.

What to Do About Side Effects: Most of the common side effects go away on their own after a few weeks. Taking lithium on a full stomach usually takes care of the stomach upset. The acne sometimes caused by lithium responds to the same treatments that dermatologists prescribe for teenagers. Thyroid gland underactivity is usually picked up by the lab tests; sometimes, low thyroid function results in depression or enlargement of the thyroid, the condition called goiter. These are easily reversed by prescribing thyroid hormone replacement medication. Tiredness and decreased concentration usually go away in time, but occasionally reduction of the dose of lithium is required. The fine hand tremor is usually barely noticeable. If it becomes annoying, propranolol or atenolol can be added, and these usually eliminate the tremor completely. The weight gain is the biggest headache. Dieting can help remove some of this weight, but fluid and salt intake should not be restricted.

If It Doesn't Work: Minor highs and lows may still occur while on lithium, and these are usually treated briefly with appropriate additional medications, such as antidepressants and antipsychotics. If major mood swings continue to occur while on lithium, however, most psychiatrists move to the next level of treatment, which is the addition of an atypical antipsychotic such as Lamictal, Depakote, or Tegretol (described in Chapter 10). Studies show that most bipolar patients wind up taking more than one medication in order to remain stable.

If It Does Work: How long should one stay on lithium? Unfortunately, this question remains unanswered because how long the illness remains active in a given patient is not known. After several bouts of life-threatening mania and depression, most patients are grateful for the relief lithium offers. After ten years of dutifully taking the medication and remaining symptom free, however, many wonder if they might get away with stopping the drug. I usually recommend that a patient remain on lithium indefinitely, but after many years of stability, I will go along with a try at discontinuation. At the first sign that symptoms are reemerging, however, lithium treatment is resumed.

Cost: Generic lithium is inexpensive and there is rarely a need to use one of the more expensive brands.

Special Comments: Lithium has proved to be one of the true miracle drugs in psychiatry. Most bipolar patients respond and remain symptom free. Lithium is safe and effective when administered under proper supervision. Any person with a serious bipolar disorder deserves a trial of lithium and should, in no way, fear this drug.

DIVALPROEX SODIUM AND VALPROIC ACID

Brand Names: Depakote, Depakote CR. Valproic acid is available as Depakene (see below for the distinction).

Used For: Seizure disorders, acute mania, bipolar mood disorder, migraine headache.

Do Not Use If: You have serious liver disease.

Tests to Take First: You should undergo blood tests of liver and thyroid function and a complete blood count to establish a baseline.

Tests to Take While You Are on It: Liver function, which is determined by a simple blood test, and the complete blood count (CBC) must be monitored several times in the first few months of treatment, and once every few months thereafter. Thyroid function tests should also be repeated about once a year. A blood test for determining the level of Depakote is available and is useful in adjusting the dose. It is not used to prevent toxicity the way lithium levels are used.

Usual Dose: Depakote is available in 250-mg capsules. The final dose is calculated with a formula based on body weight. Theoretically, a 165-pound person requires a final daily dose of 4,500 mg. Psychiatric patients, however, seem to require lower doses, 2,000 mg or less. Starting treatment at one capsule two or three times daily and increasing the dose by one to two capsules a week constitutes the best strategy. The entire daily dose can be taken at one time, although it is usually divided into two equal doses, taken morning and evening. Depakote ER is an extended-release form that can be taken once daily. Claims that it has fewer adverse side effects have not been substantiated. Also, at the equivalent dose it gives lower blood levels than ordinary Depakote. Depakene (valproic acid) is dosed the same way as Depakote.

How Long Until It Works: When used to treat the acutely manic patient, Depakote should work in a few days. When Depakote is given to prevent future highs and lows, the only way to determine if it is working is to observe the patient over several months to see if mood swings have indeed stopped. It is often useful to keep a daily diary of moods (see Figure 1 on page 195) to help evaluate how well the drug is working. Although clinicians believe that Depakote works as a mood stabilizer to prevent future highs and lows, it has not worked out that way in research trials.

Common Side Effects: Nausea, vomiting, indigestion, and drowsiness sometimes occur. Weight gain can be substantial.

Less Common Side Effects: If you look up Depakote in the *PDR* and similar books, you will read some terrifying warnings. Depakote has been reported to produce fatal liver damage. What the books don't emphasize is that all of the fatalities were in infants with brain damage who had also been taking several other medications. For adults, the risk of serious liver side effects from Depakote is virtually nonexistent. To be on the safe side, liver function is measured several times after initiation of Depakote treatment and then less frequently after the first three to six months of treatment. The dose is lowered or the drug discontinued if any abnormalities are found. Patients should not fear taking Depakote because of concern that a very rare liver problem could develop. Depakote can also cause anemia, hence the need to check the CBC. This can be especially a problem in the elderly and may necessitate switching to a different drug.

What to Do About Side Effects: The common side effects usually go away by themselves, but weight gain is a major problem. Liver failure probably does not occur at all in adults but is prevented by careful monitoring of liver function. If anemia develops, the dose should be lowered.

If It Doesn't Work: Most bipolar patients respond to lithium alone. Many of the remaining respond to lithium plus another mood stabilizer.

Depakote is very frequently the mood stabilizer successfully added to lithium in these cases.

If It Does Work: Stay on it for a long time. When it is time to stop Depakote, taper slowly.

Cost: There is technically no generic form for Depakote or Depakote ER (the latter is the more expensive of the two and generally not worth it). However, many experts believe that Depakene, which is available as the generic valproic acid, is really identical to sodium valproate (Depakote) and a cheaper substitute. Although some patients complain that Depakene upsets their stomach more, a few studies have shown that this is not the case. I remain unconvinced that Depakene is really just as good and still prescribe Depakote.

Special Comments: Depakote is generally effective and well tolerated and, because of drug company marketing, more often prescribed to bipolar patients than lithium. In fact, a whole new generation of psychiatrists is growing up thinking that Depakote is better than lithium. This is definitely not true. At the very least, the two are equally effective, and in my opinion lithium is superior and should be tried first.

CARBAMAZEPINE

Brand Names: Tegretol, Tegretol XR, Carbatrol, Equetro.

Used For: Treatment of seizures (epilepsy), treatment of bipolar mood disorder in patients who fail to respond to lithium alone. Only the brand-name Equetro form of carbamazepine is officially approved by the FDA for the treatment of bipolar disorder.

Usual Dose: Generic carbamazepine comes in 100-mg chewable tablets and 200-mg tablets (and a liquid form that is 100 mg per teaspoon). Equetro comes in 100-, 200-, and 300-mg tablets. They are both usually started at 200 mg twice a day and then slowly increased every three to four days to a maximum of 600 mg twice daily. Despite its XR designation, Tegretol XR is also usually taken in two equally divided doses.

Do Not Use If: You have serious blood or liver disease, are taking birth control pills (they won't work as well). Grapefruit juice may affect blood levels of carbamazepine.

Tests to Take First: A complete blood count (CBC) is required, as are blood tests of liver, kidney, and thyroid function. These tests establish a baseline against which any changes produced by Tegretol can be measured.

Tests to Take While You Are on It: Complete blood counts are performed frequently while patients are on Tegretol. In most patients, there is a small, but insignificant, drop in blood cells. In extremely rare cases (less than one in fifty thousand patients), however, a very large drop may occur and Tegretol must be stopped immediately. This condition is called aplastic anemia. If it is going to occur, it almost always happens in the first year of treatment. To watch for this, the CBC is obtained once every two weeks during the first two months of treatment and then every three months afterward. Tegretol can also rarely interfere with liver, kidney, or thyroid function, and the appropriate blood tests are obtained every six months to one year. Finally, blood levels of Tegretol can aid in dose adjustment, although such tests are not necessary to avoid toxicity, as are lithium levels. A good Tegretol level ranges from 8 to 12.

How Long Until It Works: As with lithium, Tegretol is prescribed to prevent future problems, not to treat acute depression or mania. Once it reaches a blood level of about 8, Tegretol should start to have its preventative effect. Then it is a matter of waiting to see if mood swings are indeed blocked over the next several months.

Common Side Effects: Dizziness, drowsiness, unsteadiness, nausea, and vomiting usually occur early in treatment and sometimes, but not always, go away. Most patients tolerate Tegretol well.

Less Common Side Effects: Two problems with Tegretol treatment demand immediate medical attention. First, the very rare (one in fifty thousand cases) severe drop in the production of blood cells called aplastic anemia puts patients at great risk of developing serious anemia, infections, and bleeding problems. Warning signs include fever, sore throat, easy bruising, purple spots on the skin, and ulcers in the mouth. To avoid aplastic anemia, CBCs should be drawn frequently and Tegretol must be stopped immediately if the results indicate aplastic anemia. Second, and also extremely rarely, Tegretol can cause a variety of skin reactions that require stopping the drug immediately. Therefore, any new rash should be shown to the doctor right away.

What to Do About Side Effects: The common side effects usually go away on their own, but temporarily lowering the dose may be necessary. The less common side effects are prevented by undergoing the appropriate blood tests and promptly reporting all new symptoms to the doctor.

If It Doesn't Work: Mild highs and lows may still occur on Tegretol and are usually treated symptomatically with brief courses of antidepressants or antipsychotic drugs (for mania). If severe mood swings continue, however, most psychiatrists recommend either combining it with another mood stabilizer or discontinuing Tegretol and moving on to another treatment.

If It Does Work: Follow the same advice given for patients treated with lithium alone: Stay on the drug indefinitely. After a few months on Tegretol, the risk of serious side effects virtually disappears and most of the common side effects also subside. Discontinuation of the drug always involves the risk of developing a new, serious depression or mania. When it is time to stop taking Tegretol, it should be tapered slowly.

Cost: In most instances, I am an advocate of generic medications. In the case of carbamazepine, however, there have been controversies about whether generic formulations are as good as the brand-name versions. It is wise to start with generic carbamazepine because it is certainly as safe as Tegretol or Equetro, but consider switching if the effect is not sufficient. For patients already stabilized on a brand-name form, it is best not to switch to a generic drug.

Special Comments: Tegretol has been prescribed by neurologists to treat seizure disorders for many years. Dr. Robert Post of the National Institutes of Health was the first to show that it works for bipolar patients, but because it was already off patent, no drug company was willing to spend the money to get the FDA to formally approve it. Some patients tolerate Tegretol well, whereas others never get over the dizziness and nausea and hate it. It causes less weight gain than lithium or Depakote, but is still generally prescribed only as an add-on to those drugs if they are not sufficiently effective. It is important to note that Tegretol affects the liver's system of breaking down drugs, including itself, so that doses of a host of drugs, too numerous to mention here, often have to be increased to maintain effectiveness. One of those drugs is the birth control pill, and having it become less effective is problematic, to put it mildly. Only recently, the manufacturer of the brand-name version of carbamazepine (Equetro) did get FDA approval

---

Table 25.

Order in Which Drugs Are Prescribed for Maintenance Treatment of Bipolar Patients

1. Lithium alone, Lamictal alone, or Depakote alone
2. Lithium plus Depakote or Lamictal
3. Lithium plus Tegretol
4. Lithium plus an atypical antipsychotic drug (like Zyprexa or Abilify)
5. Clozapine
6. Treat each separate depression with antidepressant medication in addition to a mood stabilizer, or Lamictal, and each separate manic period with antipsychotic drugs plus a mood stabilizer.

for bipolar disorder; hence generic carbamazepine now has some increased status for bipolar patients.

LAMOTRIGINE

Brand Name: Lamictal.

Used For: Treatment of seizures (epilepsy), treatment of bipolar disorder, especially the depressed phase.

Usual Dose: Because of the risk for a very serious rash (see below), Lamictal must be started at a very low dose, which is then increased over many weeks. Although different doctors have slightly different versions of how this is done, the basic dosing is one 25-mg pill, taken morning or night, for the first two weeks, then two 25-mg pills, taken together morning or night, for two weeks, then 100 mg a day for two weeks, then 150 mg a day for two weeks, and finally 200 mg a day. If more is needed, the top dose is usually 200 mg taken twice daily.

Do Not Use If: There are no absolute reasons not to take Lamictal.

Tests to Take First: None.

Tests to Take While You Are on It: None.

How Long Until It Works: Because of the need to raise the dose so slowly, it can be many weeks before Lamictal has an effect.

Common Side Effects: There are very few common side effects. Some patients may experience dizziness, headache, nausea, or sleepiness, but these are usually mild and quickly resolve.

Less Common Side Effects: The big issue with Lamictal is the rash. About one in one thousand people on Lamictal develops a rash that quickly goes on to become the devastating conditions known as Stevens-Johnson syndrome or toxic epidermal necrolytis. These are often fatal, and the first signs require going to the emergency immediately for treatment. The problem is greatly reduced (some would say made close to nonexistent) if the dose is started very low and advanced very slowly, as described above, and the drug is stopped immediately if any rash appears. That means that the patient must report any rash as soon as it appears and must check for rashes while on Lamictal. Fortunately, this problem is almost entirely confined to the first few months and after that almost never occurs. Cases of mania have also occurred that have been blamed on Lamictal, although it is never clear if these would have happened anyway to the bipolar patient.

What to Do About Side Effects: The common side effects usually go away on their own, but temporarily lowering the dose may be necessary. Rashes call for stopping the medication and contacting the doctor immediately. He or she may have you see a dermatologist (not all rashes are actually the kind that go on to serious problems) or go to the emergency room. Do what the doctor says.

If It Doesn't Work: Mild highs and lows may still occur on Lamictal and are usually treated symptomatically with brief courses of antidepressants or antipsychotic drugs (for mania). If severe mood swings continue, however, most psychiatrists recommend either combining it with another mood stabilizer or discontinuing Lamictal and moving on to another treatment.

If It Does Work: Follow the same advice given for patients treated with lithium alone: Stay on the drug indefinitely. After a few months on Lamictal, the risk of serious side effects virtually disappears and most of the common side effects also subside. Discontinuation of the drug always involves the risk of developing a new, serious depression or mania. When it is time to stop taking Lamictal, it should be tapered slowly.

Cost: No generic form is available and therefore Lamictal is very expensive.

Special Comments: Compared to the other mood stabilizers, Lamictal has the fewest side effects (including almost no chance of weight gain). As long as the dosing requirements are adhered to strictly and rashes are reported immediately, it is a safe and well-tolerated drug. Its main drawback (besides expense) is that although the FDA approved it for the prevention of both highs and lows, it is much better at treating and preventing depression than mania. Consequently, it is often added to lithium when the patient frequently has breakthrough depressions or used for bipolar II patients who get only mild manias (hypomania).

OTHER DRUGS FOR BIPOLAR PATIENTS

Although lithium, Lamictal, Depakote, and Tegretol are very effective mood stabilizers, studies have frequently shown that most bipolar patients take combinations of drugs, usually a mood stabilizer plus an antidepressant or antipsychotic or more than one mood stabilizer at the same time. All of the atypical antipsychotic drugs are approved for the treatment of acute mania and two (Zyprexa and Abilify) are also approved as mood stabilizers. Seroquel has a specifically additional indication for treating depression in bipolar patients. (They are discussed in more detail in Chapter 10.) A drug related to Tegretol (carbamazepine), Trileptal (oxcarbazepine), is showing promise for bipolar disorder with fewer side effects; it has almost none of the problematic interactions with other drugs but does sometimes lower the sodium level so this needs to be monitored. Because so many of the effective treatments for bipolar disorder happen also to be anticonvulsants (that is, drugs used to treat epilepsy), including Depakote, Tegretol, and Lamictal, some believe that all anticonvulsants should work. However, drugs like Neurontin (gabapentin), Keppra (levetiracetam), Gabitril (tiagabine), and Topamax (topiramate) do not seem to work at all for bipolar patients. If nothing works, the ultimate treatment is probably the atypical antipsychotic clozapine (also discussed further in Chapter 10). Finally, specific bipolar disorder psychotherapy has been shown to be effective and should be implemented whenever possible along with medication.

Chapter 10

Drugs Used to Treat Schizophrenia

In the 1960s, several books and articles appeared claiming that schizophrenia was not really an illness at all. Some called it an alternative way of viewing the world, "marching to a different drummer," another version of normal. We were told to understand people with schizophrenia and even to try to learn from them.

I doubt many of these "experts" bothered to ask patients or their families for their opinion. More recently, an editorial in the prestigious British scientific journal *Nature* began, "Schizophrenia is arguably the worst disease affecting mankind."

Although that statement may be an exaggeration, there is no debate that schizophrenia is a horrible illness. It strikes people in late adolescence to early adulthood and often never goes away. Occasionally, patients with schizophrenia go into full, spontaneous remission, but this often occurs only after years of devastating illness. In the meantime, most patients with schizophrenia endure many hospitalizations, are unable to work, and have little social interaction. Schizophrenia devastates the early adult years of most patients.

The situation is almost equally grim for families of schizophrenia patients. Living with a schizophrenia patient is usually a full-time and harrowing job. The patient lives in his or her own world, entertaining bizarre ideas and listening to voices. He or she may talk without making sense, pace the floors all night, and occasionally become violent or threatening. Parents, acting as if they have toddlers, are afraid to leave their children with schizophrenia alone. They, like the patient, become prisoners of the illness.

So, although schizophrenia may seem romantic or interesting to philosophers, it is plainly awful to its victims. Hence, we want to do whatever we can to relieve the symptoms of schizophrenia.

The different forms of schizophrenia and the different ways it begins could be the subject of another book. Here I provide information important in guiding drug treatment. Several books listed under Suggestions for Further Reading provide a more detailed picture.

SYMPTOMS OF SCHIZOPHRENIA

The hallmarks of schizophrenia are hallucinations, delusions, thought disorder, and disorganized behavior. These are often called positive symptoms. There are also negative symptoms such as abnormal affect, loss of motivation, and social isolation.

Hallucinations occur when people hear and see things and, less commonly, smell or feel things that are not really there. In schizophrenia, auditory hallucinations—hearing voices—are common. This patient does not say, "My mind is playing tricks on me and it sounds like someone is talking." This patient really hears the voice. Often, the person with schizophrenia is surprised that no one else can hear what he or she hears. The voices often say bizarre things, tell the patient what to do (so-called command hallucinations), or make comments on what the patient is doing. Some patients with schizophrenia like the voices and sit alone in a corner listening; others are tortured by them and plead that someone make them go away.

Delusions are false ideas that the patient passionately insists and believes are true. Paranoid delusions are very common in certain forms of schizophrenia. Patients have the unshakable belief that others are actively planning to harm them. Delusional patients may believe that the FBI is tapping their phone, that people from Mars are communicating with them, that bugs are crawling around inside them, or that someone is poisoning their food. No amount of reasoning with delusional patients changes their mind; there are no "facts" that will shake the delusion.

Thought disorder involves a number of marked abnormalities in mental processes. Most commonly, patients talk without making any sense; they string words together seemingly at random in what is often called a word salad. They are not being "deep" or esoteric. Paying more careful attention will not reveal hidden meanings. What they say is senseless because their brain is simply firing out words that don't fit together. At other times, patients with schizophrenia may be talking sensibly and suddenly stop; the idea they had suddenly disappeared.

Disorganized behavior is seen in some patients with schizophrenia when they become involved in bizarre or socially inappropriate behaviors, including undressing in public, collecting garbage, or shadow boxing and screaming in a public park.

Abnormal affect in schizophrenia usually means the absence of normal moods. Patients talk about something sad and laugh, or talk about something pleasant without any expression on their face. This is sometimes called inappropriate or flat or blunted affect. Patients seem emotionless and zombielike or inappropriately silly and giggly. It is not that they are depressed or happy; instead, they do not express or feel emotions consistent with their speech or the events around them.

Hallucinations, delusions, thought disorder, and disorganized behavior, and the negative symptoms such as abnormal affect are called psychotic symptoms. Psychotic symptoms can occur in disorders other than schizophrenia. Manic and depressed patients both develop psychotic symptoms. Certain drugs used to treat medical illnesses, for example, steroids, can produce psychotic symptoms. Street drugs like cocaine and angel dust (PCP) also induce psychosis. When patients with dementia, such as Alzheimer's disease, develop psychotic symptoms, they often cannot be maintained at home and need to be moved to a nursing home. Making the diagnosis of schizophrenia therefore requires skill and experience.

Eventually, however, the diagnosis of schizophrenia usually becomes all too obvious. The reason is that most other psychoses eventually go away, even without treatment. If a psychotically depressed patient doesn't commit suicide, she will get better eventually. Likewise, if a person stops taking steroids or PCP, the psychotic symptoms disappear. The person with schizophrenia, however, suffers from a chronic illness that usually gets worse and worse. Even when the most florid psychotic symptoms go away, the patient feels unmotivated and isolated. He cannot function at work or in social situations. Casual observers find him odd. At one time, patients with schizophrenia used to live in the wards of state psychiatric hospitals; now they all too often live on the streets of big cities.

So the diagnosis of schizophrenia involves the recognition of two factors: acute psychotic symptoms and a deteriorating course of illness. It is difficult to make the diagnosis in someone who has had a single episode of psychosis, which may represent a manic episode or the effect of a drug. The psychosis may never return. But after two or three episodes, especially if the patient doesn't bounce back to normal in between, the diagnosis of schizophrenia can reliably be made.

Positive, Negative, and Cognitive Symptoms

Perhaps the most useful distinction among different symptoms of schizophrenia will turn out to be the positive-versus-negative dichotomy. Positive symptoms are all the things traditionally used to define schizophrenia—hallucinations, delusions, thought disorder, and disorganized behavior. These are the symptoms that seem most obvious, are easiest to observe, and call the person with schizophrenia to the attention of others. They usually do not become apparent until very late in adolescence or early adulthood and often precipitate the first treatment encounter or hospitalization.

We now realize, however, that there are a whole other set of symptoms that patients with schizophrenia have, which we call negative symptoms. These include loss of motivation, loss of drive, decreased ability to experience pleasure, memory problems, and decreased speech production. These may be present before positive symptoms begin, start with them, or occur only years after positive symptoms have appeared.

Many experts now think that a third set of symptoms, called cognitive symptoms, may be the most critical ones in defining schizophrenia. Although patients with schizophrenia seem at first to have normal memory and some may even have a very high IQ before the illness begins, in-depth psychological testing has shown that abnormalities in memory are present at the very earliest stages of schizophrenia—some data even indicate they are present in early childhood among those destined to develop schizophrenia—and either never go away or get worse.

The original drugs for schizophrenia, like Haldol and Thorazine, do not do much for negative or cognitive symptoms and in fact may even make them worse. This means the positive symptoms are controlled, but the patient is left in an unmotivated, withdrawn, and socially isolated state. The newer drugs for schizophrenia, like clozapine, risperidone, and olanzapine, are effective for both positive and negative symptoms, and may make a small improvement in cognitive symptoms. For this reason, some patients not only stop having positive symptoms but also gain motivation and improved intellectual abilities. This has led some to be able to socialize more and even get jobs.

CAUSES OF SCHIZOPHRENIA

There is mounting evidence that schizophrenia is at least in part a genetic disease that involves abnormal development of the brain and loss of brain cells.

Much effort at finding abnormal genes in schizophrenia is now under way and several genes have already been identified that are good candidates for increasing the risk to develop schizophrenia. Many studies using specialized brain-imaging techniques such as PET and MRI scans (see Chapter 19) have shown that patients with schizophrenia basically have less brain tissue than normal people. A research group led by Dr. Kenneth Davis at the Mount Sinai School of Medicine in New York City has shown that the sheaths that wrap axons in the brain, the "wires" that connect brain cells, appear to be worn away or may never have formed normally. This also seems to be the result of abnormal gene function. It is also possible that events occurring during pregnancy, such as viral infections and nutritional deprivation, may contribute to damaging the brain of people who later develop schizophrenia. Finally, severe social stress may play a role in causing schizophrenia, as recently shown by Dr. Robin Murray of the Institute of Psychiatry in London.

We also now know that schizophrenia is not one disease. There are so many different forms, presentations, outcomes, and symptoms that it is likely to be a collection of several different diseases. In this respect, schizophrenia is similar to pneumonia, which can be caused by a number of different bacteria, viruses, and parasites yet almost always manifests as cough, fever, and chest pain. So too, there are probably many different causes of the hallucinations, delusions, thought disorder, and abnormal affect of schizophrenia. It is encouraging that more research money is now being spent to find the causes of schizophrenia, but the answers probably will require many more years of research.

One thing that clearly does not cause schizophrenia is bad parenting. This does not mean that I am endorsing parental neglect! Psychiatrists' offices are full of people whose parents were too busy or self-involved to take proper care of their children. Schizophrenia, however, is not an outcome of an unhappy childhood. We see patients with schizophrenia who had terrible parents and patients with schizophrenia who had good parents. Some patients with schizophrenia are the children of patients with schizophrenia; others are the children of completely normal people. Schizophrenia must be regarded as a tragic disease of uncertain cause that strikes one out of a hundred people in the United States. It can strike anybody.

The news that schizophrenia is not caused by bad parents has helped many family members of patients with schizophrenia shed their guilt and join forces to urge better treatment and more research. Such organizations as the National Alliance for the Mentally Ill have as members many parents of patients with schizophrenia who courageously come forward to make their stories known. Another extremely important organization in the fight against schizophrenia is the National Association for Research of Schizophrenia and Depression. Founded by Connie and Steve Lieber, NARSAD is the largest private philanthropic organization to fund psychiatric research in the world. As federal funds for biomedical research shrank tragically under the Bush administration in the twenty-first century, NARSAD has tried to step in to fill some of the gaps and keep the laboratories going.

The relatives of patients with schizophrenia, who are often charged with their care, need to know as much as possible about the drug treatment of schizophrenia so they can help guide the treatment. Usually, asking a schizophrenia patient in the middle of a psychotic episode to make a rational decision about taking drugs is not sensible. This does not mean that patients with schizophrenia should routinely be given medication against their will or that information should be withheld from them. It is often surprising to find out how much the psychotic patient actually understands if doctors take the time to explain things. And patients with schizophrenia clearly have the right to participate in all treatment decisions. The courts have also insisted that patients with schizophrenia have the right to refuse treatment and stay psychotic, even if it means they must remain hospitalized for years.

Informed family members are a great asset to both patient and doctor. The drugs used to treat schizophrenia are serious medications with many side effects. Family members must serve as advocates for their schizophrenia relatives, as well as assistants to the doctor in identifying side effects.

The drugs used to treat schizophrenia are often referred to as *neuroleptics*. I prefer the term *antipsychotic* because these medicines are effective against all psychoses, including those caused by schizophrenia, depression, mania, dementia, and drug abuse. The term *neuroleptic* is based on the incorrect idea that these drugs work because of certain side effects they sometimes produce.

WHEN SHOULD ANTIPSYCHOTIC DRUGS BE PRESCRIBED?

It is important to have some understanding of the antipsychotic drugs. These drugs are sometimes prescribed when they shouldn't be. At one point they were called major tranquilizers and were administered indiscriminately to people who were very anxious, agitated, or even annoying. This is almost never justified; antipsychotic drugs are not the first to consider for patients with anxiety disorders or depression. Other drugs work better. However, there are many cases in which patients with anxiety disorders, depression, or severe personality disorders (such as schizotypal disorder or borderline personality disorder) do not respond to medications and psychotherapies designed for these illnesses and the addition of one of the newer antipsychotic drugs is warranted. This should, however, be done carefully because antipsychotic drugs have serious side effects, as explained below.

Schizophrenia is not the only illness, however, for which antipsychotic drugs are correctly prescribed as the first-line agents. Four other conditions are so treated:

1. **Mania, with or without psychotic symptoms.** As I explained in Chapter 9, patients with bipolar disorder who are in the manic phase are sometimes first treated with antipsychotic drugs because lithium takes too long to work. Sometimes, manic patients also have psychotic symptoms, for example, hallucinations and delusions. It is sometimes necessary to treat acute mania with antipsychotic drugs, but these drugs should usually be discontinued in favor of long-term lithium treatment once the acute situation resolves. Two antipsychotic drugs, Zyprexa and Abilify, are approved by the FDA for the long-term treatment of patients with bipolar disorder, although I still prefer lithium or Lamictal, as explained in Chapter 9. An exception is when the antipsychotic drug clozapine is used to treat bipolar patients who fail to respond to all other treatments.

2. **Depression with psychotic symptoms.** Most depressed patients do not become psychotic, but occasionally a depressed patient hears voices telling him he is a horrible person or he is responsible for terrible crimes or he should kill himself. Or the depressed patient may develop delusions; for example, she may believe that she has caused someone else's death or is herself dying or that she has lost all of her money. In this case, antipsychotic drugs are usually combined with an antidepressant drug until the psychotic symptoms are eliminated. The antidepressant is then usually continued but the antipsychotic discontinued.

3. **Dementia with extreme agitation or psychotic symptoms.** Patients with dementias such as occur with Alzheimer's disease (formerly called senile dementia), Huntington's disease, or late-stage Parkinson's disease sometimes become agitated to the point that they cannot sleep or sit still longer than a minute. They may also develop psychotic symptoms including delusions and hallucinations. Low doses of antipsychotic medications are very effective in calming these patients and eliminating psychotic symptoms. Demented and elderly patients should not simply be placed on these medications and forgotten about as occurs tragically in too many American nursing homes; there is a constant need for medical supervision and reevaluation. Furthermore, some research studies recently demonstrated an increased risk for death, either from cardiac problems or infections, among patients with dementia given antipsychotic drugs. Although the risk is small, it has discouraged some doctors from

prescribing antipsychotic drugs to patients with dementia. On the other hand, behavioral disturbances in patients with dementia are extremely disruptive and are the leading cause of hospitalization and nursing home confinement for people with Alzheimer's disease. With few other choices that work, sometimes there is no other option.

4. **Certain tics and abnormal movements.** Antipsychotic medications are used for disorders such as Tourette's syndrome.

TREATMENT OF SCHIZOPHRENIA

Here are some examples of patients who should be placed on antipsychotic medications. All three patients have schizophrenia.

Patti was not a particularly remarkable child. She was neither exceptionally bright nor troublesome. Her teachers liked her, she earned good but not outstanding grades, and she always had plenty of friends without being the most popular girl in school. She got along very well with her older brother. Her parents, hardworking people who made a modest but sufficient income, were justifiably proud of her. After graduation from high school, Patti decided to attend a local community college to try and improve her grades and her chances of getting into a good university.

Things went badly at the college. Patti seemed to lose interest in classes after the first few months and then began having trouble getting up in the morning. She also seemed listless and preoccupied. Her parents first wondered if perhaps she was in love, then worried if she might be pregnant or taking drugs or sick. She lost weight and missed meals. One evening, for no apparent reason, she flung a plate of food across the room, yelled out an obscenity, and ran out of the house. She returned several hours later, and when her parents questioned her about her behavior, she screamed, "You will never take me alive."

After that, her behavior became more and more strange. She stopped going to college and remained in her room all day. She spoke to almost no one, refused to come to the telephone when somebody called, and picked at her food. Her parents asked her to see the family doctor, but she angrily refused.

The final crisis occurred when Patti barricaded herself in her room and refused to let anyone in. She screamed incoherently for hours. Her father finally broke down the door and found Patti sitting in the middle of the floor, rocking back and forth and lighting matches. She was taken to the hospital emergency room.

In the emergency room, Patti was first seen by a medical doctor who did her best to conduct a physical examination and obtain blood tests, but Patti thrashed about, insisting she was being persecuted for her "secret knowledge." The blood tests were all normal, including a screen for drugs such as marijuana, cocaine, amphetamines, and angel dust—all drugs that can cause psychotic behavior. Next, a psychiatrist was called in. The psychiatrist asked questions and attempted to gain Patti's confidence. Patti told him that she was being watched closely by "secret forces" and that these "forces" were putting new "thoughts in my head." Patti was hostile and suspicious but agreed with the psychiatrist that the voices and thoughts she was experiencing were unpleasant. She agreed to drink a solution containing 1 mg of the antipsychotic drug risperidone (Risperdal). An hour later she was calmer and cooperated with the complete physical examination.

Patti was then admitted to the psychiatric ward of the hospital, where she was placed on 1 mg of risperidone two times daily. She also underwent extensive medical tests including an electroencephalogram (EEG) and an MRI scan of the brain. The tests were normal, and over a two-week period, with the dose of her medication increased to 4 mg daily, Patti became calm, started eating, and decided the "secret forces" were only her imagination. She was kept on risperidone several more months, during which time she returned to college. The drug was then discontinued.

Patti's case represents an acute paranoid psychosis—"acute" because it came on relatively quickly and involved many active symptoms; "paranoid" because Patti had delusions that people were persecuting her, beliefs that were obviously false but unshakable; and "psychosis" because of the presence of hallucinations and delusions. She was treated with one of the newer, or "ayptical" antipsychotic drugs after medical problems and drug use were ruled out as the cause of her psychotic behavior.

At this point, we do not know whether Patti will go on to meet the diagnostic criteria for schizophrenia. Some patients, for reasons we do not understand, have a single psychotic episode and never become seriously psychiatrically ill again. If Patti has several similar episodes, she would be diagnosed as having chronic paranoid schizophrenia. Long-term prescription of antipsychotic drugs would then become necessary to control her symptoms.

The next case is quite different. Looking back, Mark's mother remembers that he was always a shy and lonely child. He had few friends in school and was often scapegoated by the other children. He was physically awkward and clumsy. His grades were poor and he seemed to get interested in unusual subjects, like staring at pictures in a book of houseplants, for hours on end.

By the time he was fourteen, Mark's teachers were already commenting that he was disruptive in school. He would burst out laughing for no good reason or suddenly push another child without provocation. His parents had a hard time getting him to wash or brush his teeth. Most disturbing, he seemed to talk to himself, and often, when talking to others, he made little sense. By age sixteen, Mark dropped out of school because his grades were terrible and he was unable to concentrate. He talked about his "friends," who were actually imaginary people with whom he carried on conversations all day long. He watched television most of the time and described in great detail the shows he watched as if they were real-life events. Many times his speech was slurred and difficult to understand.

Mark is now thirty years old and a patient in the research psychiatric ward of a university medical center hospital. His doctors are studying the causes and treatment of serious mental illnesses. Since age sixteen, Mark has seen many psychiatrists and undergone many diagnostic tests. He has also been admitted to hospitals from time to time for short periods, usually after he had paced through the night, laughing and talking to himself so loudly that people became frightened. He has been treated with many different antipsychotic drugs, first the "typical" drugs, including Thorazine, Mellaril, and Stelazine, and then in the 1990s the "atypical" drugs, including Zyprexa, Risperdal, and Geodon. He usually forgets to take his medication, so he now receives injections once every month of the very long-acting antipsychotic drug Haldol Decanoate. The doctors in the research hospital are planning to place him on clozapine, the most effective antipsychotic drug but also the one most fraught with side effects, and stop the monthly injections once it begins to work.

Mark is fortunate in some respects. Despite his odd and often frightening behavior, his family has stuck by him, allowing him to live at home and encouraging him to take his medication and see his doctor regularly. After hearing about experimental approaches to treatment of his illness, they arranged for admission to the medical center but understand that even top experts usually do not produce "cures." Clozapine, which is not experimental and has been available since 1990, sometimes works when nothing else has, so there is definitely hope for Mark.

Mark clearly suffers from chronic schizophrenia, "chronic" because the illness has been apparent for many years. Unlike Patti, Mark showed some symptoms of abnormal behavior from a very early age. This is referred to as prodromal schizophrenia. In hindsight, the diagnosis of schizophrenia might have been made when he was fourteen or fifteen years old, but the vast majority of shy and odd teenagers do not grow up to have schizophrenia. Also, recent studies have not made it clear whether offering antipsychotic treatment to people in prodromal phrases works. Mark never had an abrupt "psychotic" break but moved slowly into schizophrenia with delusions, hallucinations, abnormal affect, and thought disorder. Antipsychotic drugs may reduce the severity of some symptoms, like hallucinations and delusions, but do not cure the illness. Mark has never held a job and never had a date. Neuropsychological tests done in the research hospital showed that his memory is poor. When his parents die he may have to be institutionalized permanently because he never developed the capacity to support himself. He is not retarded: IQ tests are normal. He is, however, severely mentally disabled for life.

Now the last case of schizophrenia. Marty is fifty years old. He had his first psychotic break when he was in the army at age twenty. Since then he has had fifteen psychiatric hospitalizations. He has worked intermittently as a messenger and as a floor sweeper in an office. Now Marty lives in a group home for chronic patients with schizophrenia maintained by a community-based mental health organization.

Marty never laughs and he never cries. He does not look happy and he does not look sad. His face is expressionless. He moves slowly and talks as little as possible. When asked a question, he responds in short but appropriate answers. He does not hear voices or see things or have delusions, but he remembers that he did have these symptoms until about ten years ago. Marty makes uncontrollable chewing movements with his mouth and often grimaces involuntarily, a syndrome called tardive dyskinesia. These are permanent neurological side effects of the first-generation or typical antipsychotic drugs (like Haldol and Stelazine) that he took almost continuously from the time his illness began until the 1990s when the new or atypical drugs became available. He now takes a low dose of the antipsychotic drug Seroquel (quetiapine), which mostly helps control his anxiety and helps him sleep through the night. He has gained forty pounds as a result of taking higher doses of Seroquel and Zyprexa in the past.

After many years of psychotic symptoms (hallucinations, delusions, thought disorder), some patients with schizophrenia have a burnt-out appearance. They no longer exhibit formal psychotic symptoms, but they look and act like zombies. These negative and cognitive symptoms do not respond to antipsychotic drugs as well as do the positive symptoms of hallucinations, delusions, and thought disorder, although the newer drugs like clozapine, risperidone (Risperdal), olanzapine (Zyprexa), and aripiprazole (Abilify) may be effective for negative symptoms.

The three schizophrenia cases I have presented represent three different aspects of antipsychotic drug use. Patti is an acutely psychotic patient; antipsychotic drugs work very well in this situation. Mark has chronic schizophrenia but still has psychotic symptoms; antipsychotic drugs may reduce the severity of or even eliminate psychotic symptoms but do not usually return the patient to normal functioning permanently. Marty also has chronic schizophrenia, but most of his psychotic symptoms have subsided with the use of medication. He has mostly negative and cognitive symptoms that do not respond well to antipsychotic drugs. He also has side effects from taking antipsychotic drugs for many years. The next step will be to try him on clozapine.

Remember, these are only examples. There are rare cases in which even acute psychosis does not respond to antipsychotic drugs. Sometimes, negative symptoms do improve with drug treatment. Patients who became ill after the introduction in the 1990s of the atypical antipsychotic drugs have relatively little chance of developing tardive dyskinesia (none if they are on clozapine). Weight gain from the newer drugs, however, has become the big headache, often leading to diabetes and heart disease.

Three important messages should be learned from these cases:

1. Antipsychotic drugs work.

2. Antipsychotic drugs do not "cure" schizophrenia.

3. Antipsychotic drugs can cause serious side effects.

OTHER PSYCHIATRIC ILLNESSES

Now I present two cases in which antipsychotic drugs are appropriately prescribed to patients who do not have schizophrenia.

John is a forty-two-year-old actor. He was diagnosed with bipolar disorder at age twenty-five after a series of manic and depressive episodes. (This illness is described in more detail in Chapter 9.) For more than ten years John has taken lithium every night and, except for occasional mild depression, has been free of manic highs and depression.

Several months ago, however, he decided he had taken lithium long enough and, without telling his wife or friends or doctor, stopped taking it. He was fine for a month and this convinced him he was completely over the illness. After about six weeks off lithium, friends noticed that he was talking fast, seemed restless, and frequently argued with coworkers. He started writing a play, working far into the night, and waking up at the crack of dawn. He felt productive, but his wife read the play and found it to be mostly an endless collection of random ideas and speeches. She mentioned this to John, and he accused her of being envious and not deep enough to understand his talent. He started calling producers in Hollywood and running up enormous phone bills. His wife became alarmed when John told her he had invested most of their savings in an experimental off-Broadway play without consulting her or even checking out the investment.

Finally, John's wife called his psychiatrist and reported his odd and impulsive behavior. The psychiatrist diagnosed acute mania and prescribed the antipsychotic medication Risperdal (risperidone). John agreed to take it only because he wanted to get some sleep. After several days he began to calm down; the psychiatrist strongly recommended that he resume taking lithium along with the antipsychotic drug. After three weeks, John was back to normal. The antipsychotic drug was discontinued and he remained on lithium another ten years.

As I explained in Chapter 9, during an acute mania in a patient with bipolar disorder, it is often necessary to prescribe antipsychotic drugs to control the symptoms rapidly. Lithium alone takes too long once the manic episode is in full force. As soon as the episode is under control, the antipsychotic drug is usually stopped. The patient remains on lithium to prevent another manic episode.

Vivian is seventy-five years old and suffers from the degenerative illness Alzheimer's disease. Alzheimer's is the most common form of dementia. Patients with Alzheimer's gradually lose their memory and ability to perform many intellectual activities. This is not the mild memory loss that sometimes accompanies normal aging but a progressive loss of mental capacity that usually renders the patient incapacitated before death.

Vivan lives in a nursing home. She reads the newspaper every day, but a few minutes after reading an article cannot explain what it is about. She remembers what she wore to her sweet sixteen party almost sixty years ago but cannot recall what she had for breakfast an hour after the meal is over. She has difficulty remembering faces and is often confused about whether it is day or night.

Vivian's children and grandchildren visit her frequently. One day her son came to see her and she began yelling at him, accusing him of being an attendant who she insisted had stolen her glasses. It took an aide almost an hour to calm her down and convince her the man was her son. The next day she called her daughter and told her that the attendants were stealing money from her purse and giving her secret injections in the middle of the night. Given the horror stories sometimes heard about nursing homes, her daughter was understandably worried. When she went to check things out, her mother yelled at her also and accused her of stealing money. Vivian's children then heard the sad news from the nursing home director: Vivian had been making up stories about people stealing things from her for about two weeks. She had reached the point where an aide had to stay with her at all times, because she threatened to walk out of the nursing home in the middle of the night. The nursing home staff considered transferring her to a hospital with a specialized geriatric unit.

A psychiatrist was called in to evaluate Vivian. She ordered the doctor out of the room and accused him of being sent to kill her. Vivian then threw her food tray in the garbage, insisting the food was poisoned. The psychiatrist first ordered medical tests to ensure that a new medical problem was not causing her psychotic symptoms. The tests showed no change from her checkup six months earlier, so he prescribed a very low dose of an antipsychotic drug. Three days later, Vivian's psychotic symptoms had disappeared, she recognized her son, and she ate her meals. Her memory, however, was unimproved.

In Chapter 17, I discuss special considerations in prescribing psychiatric drugs for elderly patients. The case of Vivian illustrates several important points. First, psychotic symptoms like Vivian's paranoid delusions often complicate Alzheimer's disease. These symptoms sometimes jeopardize a patient's well-being to the point that there is no choice but to treat. It is crucial that a physician evaluate a patient in this situation because many new medical problems on top of the Alzheimer's disease, for example, strokes, uncontrolled diabetes, and dehydration, can cause psychotic symptoms in elderly people. After a medical doctor has excluded a physical medical cause, it may be necessary to prescribe antipsychotic drugs. These should be administered in very low doses, because elderly patients—especially demented elderly patients—are very susceptible to side effects. Also, very recently some puzzling research suggests that there is a small risk for increased death when elderly patients with dementia are given antipsycohotic drugs. However, there are few viable alternatives and Vivian obviously could not be left in the state she was in for much longer. The drugs usually work quickly. They should be stopped and resumed only if the symptoms return. Elderly people should be seen regularly by a doctor once an antipsychotic drug is prescribed. They should never be left on the drugs indefinitely without medical supervision.

IMPROPER USE OF ANTIPSYCHOTIC DRUGS

Having presented these five cases—three patients with schizophrenia, one with mania, and one with psychosis resulting from Alzheimer's disease—for whom antipsychotic medications were properly prescribed, I now present a case in which drugs were *improperly prescribed*.

Janice is a commercial photographer trying to start her own business after years of taking pictures at weddings. Although she is a very talented photographer, she has little skill for business. Characteristically, she impulsively quit her job and rented studio space that was much too expensive. She got very little advice on the proper way to set up a new business and did not take into consideration the competition she would have.

Consequently, Janice began having serious financial problems. With these, she felt extremely anxious, had trouble falling asleep, and lost weight.

Her friends grew tired of listening to her constant preoccupation with the business and her financial problems, and many avoided seeing her. This made Janice feel abandoned, and she angrily thought that the world was simply against a young woman trying to make a go of it on her own.

Janice's worried parents agreed to lend her some money and also to pay for her to see a psychotherapist. The psychotherapist believed Janice needed to work on two problems: the short-range problem of getting herself out of a tight practical situation and the long-range problem of her continuous refusal to deal with the world in a realistic, adult way. In essence, the therapist explained, Janice maintained a childlike vision of the world in which good intentions and talent alone are enough to win praise and reward. Whenever things contradicted that view, Janice quickly became bitter, accusatory, and angry.

Despite this sound advice, Janice believed she should take some kind of medication. She refused to accept the possibility that she had psychological problems; her main problems, she believed, were anxiety and lack of sleep.

Reluctantly, the therapist referred her to a psychiatrist who put Janice on a medication for anxiety, Xanax (alprazolam). This helped calm her down and improved her sleep; however, Janice remained angry, frantic, and bent on a course of professional and financial disaster. A month later she returned to the psychiatrist and complained that the medication was not strong enough. She cried a bit and blamed the doctor for not understanding her problems or taking her seriously enough. The doctor explained that the drug he placed her on was a minor tranquilizer. Since it obviously was not strong enough for Janice's problems, he now gave her a major tranquilizer. And so Janice was placed on the atypical antipsychotic drug Seroquel (quetiapine). This made her very sleepy and she also felt "drugged." She gained more than five pounds. After two weeks on Seroquel, she accepted her therapist's recommendation that she get a second opinion from another psychiatrist.

Janice's story illustrates a common mistake made with antipsychotic drugs. Because they do calm very psychotic patients, some people, including a few physicians, think they are simply very powerful tranquilizers. If an anxious patient doesn't respond to one of the antianxiety drugs described in Chapter 8, why not try one of these more powerful drugs?

The answer to this question is simple: Antipsychotic drugs are not powerful tranquilizers; they are medications designed to treat specific sets of psychotic symptoms found in patients with specific diagnoses. Psychosis may occur in a variety of settings, including mania, schizophrenia, psychotic depression, and dementia. In those cases, antipsychotic drugs are warranted. Medications like Seroquel are sometimes helpful for patients with severe anxiety disorders or depression when more standard drugs don't work sufficiently and the patients still suffer from substantial agitation and insomnia.

A severe form of personality disorder, borderline personality disorder, is sometimes best treated with antipsychotic drugs for short periods. However, they are not well used as initial treatments or as backups to antianxiety drugs for patients who are not suffering from a properly diagnosed psychiatric disorder.

Janice probably should not be treated with any medication. A short course of Xanax is not a terrible idea if it temporarily helps her sleep and feel calm enough to deal rationally with her problems. However, given her penchant for irresponsible behavior, she is at risk for wanting to keep taking it and not agree to a "short course." Her therapist had been correct in explaining to Janice that what she needed was counseling and therapy. I do not mean to imply that use of an antipsychotic drug in any patient who is not psychotic or manic is automatically wrong. I do mean to warn against the use of antipsychotic drugs for the routine treatment of anxiety and depression. By no means should anybody take these drugs without regular visits to a psychiatrist who understands how to prescribe them.

WHAT ARE THE SERIOUS SIDE EFFECTS OF ANTIPSYCHOTIC DRUGS?

Given the beneficial effects of antipsychotic drugs on some patients, why is there so much fuss? How dangerous can these drugs be?

Let me start by stating again one of the guiding principles behind the recommendations in this book and the use of medication to treat any medical problem: *The benefit must always clearly outweigh the risk.*

Schizophrenia is a devastating disease. We are willing to accept more risk in treating very serious diseases than in treating less serious diseases. The drugs used to treat cancer, for example, can themselves threaten the lives of patients. But to save a life we often take the risk—with the patient's full consent and understanding—of administering potentially very toxic treatments.

The antipsychotic drugs produce powerful changes in brain chemistry. Many of these changes involve blocking the action of the brain chemical dopamine (this is described more fully in Chapter 21). We do not yet know if blocking dopamine is the way antipsychotic drugs work to treat psychosis— indeed, the newer antipsychotic drugs are not particularly strong dopamine blockers—but we do know that blocking dopamine produces a number of adverse side effects in patients who take the older antipsychotic drugs. These side effects have technical names and are often confusing to patients and families. Therefore, before proceeding to describe the individual drugs, I want to detail this particular group of side effects, bearing in mind that they are most problematic with the older or "typical" antipsychotic drugs like Thorazine and Haldol, which are infrequently used today.

Acute dystonic reaction. Within hours or a few days of starting one of the older antipsychotic drugs, some patients, particularly young men, may suddenly experience painful, tightening spasms of the muscles, particularly in the head and neck. The tongue may protrude and the patient may drool. Sometimes the eyes appear locked in place. Rarely, muscles of the larynx (windpipe) also begin to spasm and the patient has difficulty breathing. This effect is called dystonia and occurs in between 1 percent and 8 percent of patients who take the older antipsychotic drugs. Acute dystonia can be reversed in a matter of seconds by injection of the proper antidote (Benadryl or Cogentin). Of the newer "atypical" antipsychotic drugs, it is most likely to occur with Risperdal (risperidone), less likely with Zyprexa (olanzapine), Seroquel (quetiapine), Geodon (ziprasidone), and Abilify (aripiprazole), and never occurs with Clozaril (clozapine).

To prevent acute dystonia, many clinicians place patients on one of these antidotes, which are taken by mouth, at the same time the older antipsychotic drug is started. Several categories of antidotes are available. Some brand names are Cogentin, Artane, Akineton, and Benadryl (see Table 26).

Parkinsonian syndrome. After a few weeks of taking one of the older antipsychotic medications, some patients develop a neurological syndrome that is very similar to Parkinson's disease. The most obvious sign of this is tremor, especially of the hands. But patients with drug-induced Parkinsonian syndrome may also have a loss of facial expression, slowed movements, rigidity in the arms and legs, drooling, and shuffling gait. It occurs in as many as one-third of patients who take the older antipsychotic drugs. The same order of risk as mentioned above for dystonia holds for the newer drugs (Risperdal > Zyprexa, Seroquel, Geodon, Abilify > Clozaril). Drugs that treat acute dystonia are also effective in reversing Parkinsonian syndrome. These include Cogentin, Artane, Akineton, and Symmetrel (see Table 26).

Akathisia. Perhaps as many as 75 percent of patients treated with the older antipsychotic drugs develop some degree of akathisia, although it is usually problematic in only about 10 percent to 20 percent. Patients with akathisia feel restless and are unable to sit still. They may appear agitated and jumpy, but the problem is not psychological. The restlessness is a direct side effect of the medication. It occurs with the newer antipsychotic drugs as well (but not with clozapine), although less frequently than with the older drugs. Akathisia is a leading cause of patient refusal to continue taking antipsychotic drugs. Akathisia is also difficult to treat, but some medications may be helpful. These include propranolol (Inderal), clonidine (Catapres), and benzodiazepines like diazepam (Valium). It is extremely important to treat akathisia vigorously if it is necessary to keep the patient on the antipsychotic drug.

Akinesia. Usually occurring many weeks after initiation of the older antipsychotic drugs, akinesia involves a decrease in spontaneous movements and apathy. It resembles depression or negative symptom schizophrenia but is actually a drug side effect. It is rare with the newer antipsychotic drugs. It can usually be reversed with the same drugs that reverse acute dystonia and Parkinsonian syndrome (for example, Cogentin, Akineton, Artane, and Benadryl).

Tardive dyskinesia. Tardive dyskinesia, or TD, is one of the dreaded, but often unavoidable, outcomes of treatment with the older antipsychotic drugs and possibly also the antidepressant drug Asendin. Usually developing after a year or more of continuous use of the older antipsychotic drugs, TD is characterized by involuntary and purposeless movements of the head, neck, trunk, and extremities. TD often begins with wormlike movements of the tongue, grimacing, chewing, and lip smacking. There may also be a variety of sudden or writhing movements of the hands, arms, and legs. The patient cannot control the movements, which may be made worse by stress. TD is especially likely to occur in older people and in people with brain damage who are treated with antipsychotic drugs. The longer the patient is kept on the medication, the more likely TD is to occur.

Most patients do not begin to show signs of TD until they have taken antipsychotic drugs for many years, but signs can emerge more quickly, particularly in the elderly. The risk of developing severe TD from the older, typical antipsychotic drugs probably lies between 20 percent and 40 percent, but mild signs may appear in up to 70 percent of patients. Studies have shown that the newer atypical drugs have a much lower risk of causing TD, perhaps a 25 percent lower risk. Furthermore, clozapine (Clozaril) seems to have no risk of TD at all. Patients on any antipsychotic drug, except clozapine, should be examined carefully by the doctor at least every six months for signs of TD. Many psychiatrists use the guidelines for examination found in the Abnormal Involuntary Movements Scale (AIMS) of the National Institutes of Health. When signs of TD are first observed, an attempt is made to lower the dose of the drug and even to taper the patient off the medication. In some cases, the movements worsen after the medication is stopped; this is usually temporary and in most instances, especially if caught early, TD goes away after the drug is stopped. There are, however, cases in which stopping the medication results in no decrease, and even a permanent increase, in TD. This difficult-to-treat situation often requires the expertise of neurological specialists in movement disorders. Some drugs may help reverse TD, for example, tetrabenazine.

However, the only reliable treatment for reducing or even eliminating TD is to switch the patient to clozapine.

It is impossible to predict which patients will develop TD. Studies give different estimates, but probably about one in four patients on the older drugs and far fewer on the newer ones experience some degree of full-blown TD. It is also impossible to determine how long a given person will be on medication before TD develops. Therefore, it is often hard for psychiatrists to decide how much information to give acutely psychotic patients before starting an antipsychotic drug. On the one hand, we want well-informed patients who make important decisions about their medical care. On the other hand, telling a paranoid patient who hears voices that a drug may cause abnormal movements in a few years is obviously risky. The patient usually does not understand what he or she is being told and is therefore unable to make an informed decision. The following recommendation seems to me the best compromise. Before giving the antipsychotic drug, the family should be fully informed about all side effects but should also be made to understand that TD virtually never develops after only a few weeks or months of taking the antipsychotic drugs. As soon as possible, when the patient is calm, an explanation should be given of the long-term risks of taking the medication. Some state laws may apply in this situation. Although the risk of TD is frightening and serious, so is the risk of allowing acute psychosis to remain uncorrected.

Neuroleptic malignant syndrome. Neuroleptic malignant syndrome (NMS) is an unusual but potentially life-threatening side effect of all antipsychotic drugs, including the newer drugs and even clozapine. The patient becomes severely rigid, to the point of not moving at all. Other characteristics are high fever, rapid heart rate, labored breathing, sweating, and abnormalities on blood tests. This syndrome is a medical emergency. Patients with neuroleptic malignant syndrome are usually admitted to the hospital, where the antipsychotic drug is immediately stopped. Two medications are recommended to treat this condition, dantrolene and bromocriptine. However, supportive care (cooling the patient and monitoring heart and breathing functions) is the most important intervention.

These six adverse reactions—acute dystonia, Parkinsonian syndrome, akathisia, akinesia, tardive dyskinesia, and neuroleptic malignant syndrome— are not the only side effects of antipsychotic drugs. Different drugs in this class may cause different side effects, all of which are described in the pages that follow. These six, however, are complex and specific to antipsychotic drugs. Dystonia, Parkinsonian syndrome, akathisia, and akinesia are often referred to as "extrapyramidal symptoms" (EPS). All of the older antipsychotic drugs have the potential to produce any one of them and, except for clozapine (which can cause NMS), so do the newer ones although at much reduced frequency.

Table 26.

Drugs Used to Counteract the Side Effects of Antipsychotics

GENERIC NAME	BRAND NAME	USED FOR	DAILY DOSE
Benztropine	Cogentin	Acute dystonia Parkinsonian syndrome Akinesia Akathisia	2–8 mg
Trihexyphenidyl	Artane	Acute dystonia Parkinsonian syndrome Akinesia Akathisia	1–15 mg
Diphenhydramine	Benadryl	Acute dystonia	25 mg (injection)
Biperiden	Akineton	Acute dystonia	2–6 mg
Amantadine	Symmetrel	Parkinsonian syndrome	100–300 mg
Diazepam	Valium	Akathisia	2–20 mg
Lorazepam	Ativan	Akathisia	0.5–6 mg
Propranolol	Inderal	Akathisia	20–60 mg
Bromocriptine	Parlodel	Neuroleptic malignant syndrome	Given by injection
Dantrolene	Dantrium	Neuroleptic malignant syndrome	Given by injection
Levodopa	Many	Tardive dyskinesia	Varies

Given the fact that the ayptical antipsychotic drugs are so much less likely to cause EPS and TD, they were at first heralded as miracles. However, it quickly became apparent that clozapine (Clozaril), Zyprexa (olanzapine), Risperdal (risperidone), and Seroquel (quetiapine) have a very different side effect—weight gain. The risk is as follows: clozapine and Zyprexa > Seroquel > risperidone. Geodon (ziprasidone) and Abilify (aripiprazole) seem to have a smaller risk, but most psychiatrists question whether they are as effective as the first four. This is not the level of weight gain seen with Depakote or Paxil (although it can be pretty bad with those drugs) but rather often massive weight gain of twenty to fifty pounds. Patients who sustain that much weight gain are at very high risk for diabetes, heart disease, and other medical complications of obesity. It is unclear why these drugs cause so much weight gain. Many medication strategies have been tried, and some, like metformin (Glucophage), used to treat diabetes, may help a bit, but it is very hard to prevent or reverse. Some people say that the weight gain from the newer drugs is harder to live with than the side effects of the older drugs, which were cosmetically annoying but generally not medically serious. That is, shaking with Parkinson's syndrome or TD from Trilafon (perphenazine) might seem better to some patients than getting diabetes from Zyprexa. It is very clear that doctors prescribing antipsychotic medications must weigh their patients frequently, check blood glucose and lipid levels on a regular basis, and design diet and exercise programs for them. The latter is something psychiatrists have traditionally not gotten involved with; one psychiatrist I know had to see a nutritionist when he himself developed a problem with obesity because he knew so little about how to be on a diet and lose weight. Hence there is going to have to be a lot of education for doctors, patients, and families about how to reduce the weight gain impact of antipsychotic drugs. In terms of side effects in addition to weight gain—clozapine (Clozaril) is in a class of its own—these will be described below.

THE TWO TYPES OF ANTIPSYCHOTIC DRUGS

By now you have noticed my use of the terms *older, typical, newer,* and *atypical* antipsychotic drugs. As is the case with the antidepressants discussed in Chapter 7, with which we now have "older" and "newer" medications, so with antipsychotics we are currently in the midst of a treatment revolution. This began in 1990 when clozapine (Clozaril) was first introduced to the United States and has continued through the decade with the introduction of risperidone (Risperdal), olanzapine (Zyprexa), Seroquel (quetiapine), Geodon (ziprasidone), and Abilify (aripiprazole).

At first, clozapine was called an atypical antidepressant. This is because it has features that are distinct from the older drugs that had been introduced between the 1950s and 1970s for the treatment of schizophrenia. Unlike those drugs, which include Haldol, Thorazine, Trilafon, and Mellaril, clozapine has virtually no ability to produce the extrapyramidal side effects of dystonia,

234. PSYCHIATRIC DRUG REFERENCE GUIDE

Table 27.

Atypical Antipsychotic Drugs

DRUG	DOSE	AGRANULO-CYSTOSIS?	EPS[a]	SIDE EFFECTS
Clozaril (clozapine)	300–900 mg	About 1%	No	Sedation, seizures, weight gain, salivation
Risperdal (risperidone)	1–6 mg	No	Some at doses over 6 mg	Sedation
Zyprexa (olanzapine)	5–20 mg	No	Little	Sedation, weight gain
Seroquel (quetiapine)	50–60 mg	No	No	Sedation, weight gain
Geodon (ziprasidone)	20–160 mg	No	No	Dry mouth, constipation, agitation
Abilify (aripiprazole)	10–15 mg	No	No	Headache, insomnia, tremors
Invega (paliperidone)	6–12 mg	No	Yes	Sedation, weight gain

[a]Loss of blood cells needed for immune response
[b]Extrapyramidal side effects (e.g., dystonia, Parkinsonian syndrome)

akathisia, or Parkinsonian syndrome. It does not even produce tardive dyskinesia. So clozapine does not have any of the serious neurological side effects associated with the traditional antipsychotic drugs. Furthermore, clozapine works in at least one-third of patients with schizophrenia who fail to respond to other antipsychotic drugs, and it appears to be helpful for reversing negative symptoms. From a chemical point of view, clozapine has less dopamine-blocking and more serotonin-blocking properties than the older drugs.

Clozapine clearly has major advantages over Prolixin and Haldol. But of course, nothing is perfect. Clozapine produces some sedation and a lot of weight gain, causes seizures in about 4 percent of people who take it (most of the older drugs do this in only 1 percent of patients), and can make someone who takes it salivate uncontrollably. Rarely, it can have potentially serious effects on the heart, liver, and pancreas. Although clozapine was actually discovered in the 1950s along with the older drugs like Thorazine, its introduction in the United States was delayed because less than 1 percent of people who take it develop a serious and potentially life-threatening side effect called agranulocytosis in which the bone marrow stops producing a type of blood cell that is crucial for the immune system to fight infection. To protect against this side effect, patients taking clozapine must have their blood drawn every week during the first six months, then every other week for the rest of the time they take clozapine and must stop the medication if the granulocyte count starts to drop. With this weekly and every other week blood monitoring, there is almost no chance that a patient will die from agranulosytosis by taking clozapine. On the other hand, weekly blood tests are inconvenient and expensive. And so the search was on to find a drug that would have properties similar to clozapine's without the risk of agranulocytosis. This new class of antipsychotic drugs, shown in Table 27, is called the atypical antipsychotics, although they have totally replaced the "typical" drugs as the most often prescribed.

Risperdal (risperidone) was the next drug after clozapine. Although it is not as potent as clozapine, it works at least as well as the older drugs, is better for negative symptoms, produces fewer neurological side effects at doses under 6 mg a day, and does not cause agranulocytosis. Risperdal is the only atypical drug available in a depot formulation, called Risperdal Consta, which is injected and lasts two weeks. This is important for patients with schizophrenia who don't remember to take their pills on a regular basis, but is also expensive. In 1996, the third atypical antipsychotic, olanzapine (Zyprexa), was introduced. Zyprexa may be the most effective of the atypical drugs after clozapine (although in studies it runs neck and neck with Risperdal), and it definitely produces fewer neurological side effects than the older drugs. It also does not cause agranulocytosis. However, except for clozapine, it causes the most weight gain (perhaps of any drug in psychiatry) and has been linked to diabetes and increased cholesterol levels. After Zyprexa came Seroquel (quetiapine). Quetiapine is virtually devoid of neurological side effects and does not cause agranulocytosis but is quite sedating and is midway between Risperdal and Zyprexa in terms of weight gain. Also, in order to treat psychosis, very high doses are needed (at least 600 mg) and the drug must be given twice a day, unlike Zyprexa and Risperdal, which can both be given once a day. Seroquel has gained an important niche at low doses (less than 200 mg a day, often given in one dose at bedtime) as a drug that is added to other drugs, like antidepressants, to calm agitation and anxiety and treat insomnia.

Geodon (ziprasidone), the fifth atypical antipsychotic drug, has an interesting history. Early studies suggested that it might have a side effect involving the heart called QT interval prolongation. In the worst-case scenario, QT prolongation, seen on an electrocardiogram, can result in sudden death. The FDA ordered more studies and a competitor drug company went all-out to "warn" doctors that Geodon might be dangerous. It turns out that QT prolongation is not a side effect of consequence for Geodon, but the initial scare made psychiatrists reluctant to prescribe it. Geodon does not cause EPS, weight gain, or agranulocytosis. However, some psychiatrists complain that Geodon does not work as well as Risperdal or Zyprexa, at least unless the dose is raised to 160 mg a day, and not infrequently causes agitation. It is available in an injectable form that is sometimes used in emergency rooms to treat very agitated patients quickly but is more expensive than the generic forms of the typical drugs, like Haldol (haloperidol), or the benzodiazepine Ativan (lorazepam), which can also be injected for this purpose. It remains to be seen how much use Geodon gets for schizophrenia.

The most recently introduced atypical antipsychotic drug is Abilify (aripiprazole). Unlike all of the other antipsychotic drugs, both typical and atypical, it does not block the dopamine receptor in the brain but actually stimulates it. This would seem to be the best way to make schizophrenia worse, but animal studies suggested that Abilify does in fact block the dopamine receptor when there is too much dopamine (which is directly related to positive symptoms of schizophrenia) but stimulates it when there isn't enough (which may be related to negative and cognitive side effects). Other attractive features of Abilify are a lack of weight gain, no agranulocytosis, no EPS, and no sedation. Some psychiatrists have tried to add it to antipsychotic drugs that do cause weight gain, like clozapine, Zyprexa, and Seroquel, in order to get some weight loss, but only to mixed success. Abilify is one of those drugs that sometimes seem to work for schizophrenia, sometimes don't, and sometimes make the patient worse.

Released too recently to allow a full description in this book is Invega (paliperidone), an antipsychotic drug related to Risperdal.

All of the atypical antipsychotic drugs, except clozapine, are officially approved by the FDA for the treatment of acute mania in bipolar patients. Zyprexa and Abilify are also indicated as mood stabilizers, which means the FDA thinks they work to prevent highs and lows in bipolar patients.

It is a sad irony that the better the atypical drugs work, the more side effects they have. Clozapine and Zyprexa, the two most potent for schizophrenia, cause the most weight gain. Risperidone is also very potent, but if the dose is raised to 6 mg or more it starts causing the same neurological side effects (EPS) as the typical drugs, and some people call it "expensive Haldol." Geodon and Abilify have the best side effect profiles, but there are questions about effectiveness. Thus, picking the right drug for any given patient is tricky. My own recommendation for patients with schizophrenia, psychosis secondary to dementia, and psychosis secondary to mania in bipolar patients, is to try Risperdal first to see if relatively low doses (3–4 mg a day) work. That strategy is associated with relatively little weight gain or EPS. Another plus about Risperdal is that generic risperidone, the cheaper version, will be available in a year or two. It is attractive to start with Zyprexa, however, because it calms psychotic patients quickly.

Although the typical antipsychotic drugs are rarely used these days, one of them, Trilafon (perphenazine), was included in a huge National Institute of Mental Health study led by Jeffrey Lieberman of Columbia University called CATIE that compared all of the atypical drugs (except Abilify, which was not available when the study began) and Trilafon. In that study, Zyprexa did slightly better than Risperdal, Seroquel, Geodon, or Trilafon, but caused the most weight gain. Surprisingly, Trilafon did as well as those three atypical drugs, although it did cause more EPS. Because Trilafon is so much less expensive than the atypicals, and causes very little weight gain, the CATIE study has stimulated debate about whether the atypical drugs are really that much better than the typical drugs. Thus it is still important to know about the typical drugs. They are divided into two types: high potency and low potency. They work equally well against psychosis. Low-potency typical antipsychotic drugs tend to lower blood pressure and cause sedation as their main side effects—examples are Thorazine and Mellaril. High-potency typical antipsychotic drugs do not affect blood pressure or produce sleepiness as much, but they produce more dystonias and Parkinsonian syndrome—examples are Haldol and Stelazine. Trilafon falls in between high- and low-potency typical antipsychotic drugs and before Risperdal was my antipsychotic drug of first choice. It may make a small comeback since the CATIE study, but to my mind the risk of tardive dyskinesia outweighs the benefits. Haldol, like Risperdal, is available in a depot injectable form called Haldol Decanoate. It has an advantage over Risperal Consta in that it needs to be injected only once a month instead of every two weeks, but patients say injections of Haldol Decanoate hurt more than Risperdal Consta. Haldol Decanoate is, of course, cheaper.

HOW LONG SHOULD TREATMENT LAST?

How long should patients be treated with antipsychotic drugs? For patients with mania, psychotic depression, or dementia who also have psychosis, the answer is easy: the shortest time possible. The antipsychotic drug is usually stopped as soon as the symptoms subside. Manic patients are then kept on lithium, Lamictal, or Depakote and depressed patients on antidepressants. Elderly patients should be kept off medication whenever possible.

The length of treatment for patients with schizophrenia is more difficult to determine. After the first psychotic break, many psychiatrists recommend at least one year of treatment, then discontinuation of the medication and careful observation. After the second psychotic break, patients should be treated for several years. Study after study has shown that patients with schizophrenia who discontinue their medication stand a good chance of returning to the hospital. During treatment with an antipsychotic medication, however, patients should be kept on the lowest possible dose that keeps the symptoms of psychosis in check. Patients should also be observed and examined frequently for any signs of tardive dyskinesia, weight gain, or diabetes.

GUIDELINES FOR THE PATIENT WITH SCHIZOPHRENIA

Treatment of patients with schizophrenia is summarized by the following list.

1. Risperidone or olanzapine should be started. If the former, watch for EPS; if the latter, remember that weight gain will inevitably occur.

2. The dose of the antipsychotic drug should be increased as neded to get the desired result—resolution of positive symptoms. Doses of Zyprexa above 30 mg rarely offer much more benefit than lower doses, and doses of Risperdal of 6 mg or greater will start to cause EPS.

3. The dose should be kept as low as possible to control symptoms.

4. A different antipsychotic drug should be prescribed only if the patient does not respond to the first drug after four weeks. Many psychiatrists add antipsychotic drugs with fewer side effects than Zyprexa and Risperdal (like Seroquel, Geodon, and Abilify) and then try to lower the dose of the first drug. This sometimes works. Others slowly lower the dose of and then discontinue Zyprexa or Risperdal once the patient is better at the same time that they add and slowly increase the dose of Seroquel, Geodon, or Abilify, again hoping to minimize side effects.

5. Propranolol (Inderal), diazepam (Valium), or lorazepam (Ativan) should be given if the patient develops akathisia (restlessness caused by the antipsychotic drug).

6. A patient who has had only one psychotic episode should be kept on the drug for about one year.

7. A patient who has had two or more episodes should be kept on the drug for several years.

8. Patients should see a psychiatrist at least once a month and also be examined regularly for signs of tardive dyskinesia, weight gain, and diabetes.

9. Patients who persistently forget to take their medication may be switched to long-acting, injectable forms of antipsychotic medications (Haldol Decanoate or Risperdal Consta).

10. Patients who fail to respond to any of the atypical antipsychotic medications should always be offered a trial of clozapine. Far too few patients with schizophrenia are placed on clozapine.

Although all patients with schizophrenia need to take antipsychotic medication, this does not mean that various forms of talk and rehabilitation therapies are unimportant. In fact, studies persistently have shown that interventions like family therapy, vocational rehabilitation, and social skills training are extremely beneficial. For patients who repeatedly relapse and require hospitalization, assertive community therapy (ACT) is extremely helpful. ACT involves teams of mental health professionals who work in the community with patients to ensure that they not only make it to their appointments with psychiatrists and take their medication but also have sufficient money for basic needs and a place to live. Robert Drake of Dartmouth University has been a pioneer in developing "psychosocial" therapy programs that address more than just the medication needs of patients with schizophrenia. States vary tremendously in how well they fund programs like ACT and family intervention. The National Alliance for the Mentally Ill has been a vital advocate for these services.

Above all, remember that no matter how distant, volatile, or antisocial the person with schizophrenia seems, he or she is a suffering human being. It is not the patient's fault that the causes of schizophrenia and its cure have not been found. Although I do not believe that love and kindness can cure schizophrenia any more than I believe abuse and neglect cause the illness, it is clear that mistreatment of the patient with schizophrenia can worsen the condition. By the same token, understanding, acceptance, and kindness may make it easier to live with "the worst illness in the world."

DRUGS USED TO TREAT PSYCHOSIS

Many medications are used to treat psychosis. The following descriptions include only those available in the United States.

HALOPERIDOL

Brand Names: Haldol, Haldol Decanoate (long-acting depot formulation).

Used For: Psychosis associated with schizophrenia, mania, or depression; psychosis in elderly people with dementia; severe tics in patients with the neurological disease Tourette's syndrome.

Do Not Use If: You do not have psychotic symptoms. However, there are rare circumstances in which Haldol is prescribed for nonpsychotic patients. Some psychiatrists believe that Haldol should not be combined with lithium; this topic is controversial, but so many other antipsychotic drugs are available that it is easy to substitute a different one if you are also on lithium. People with a history of epilepsy (convulsions) should use these drugs with caution.

Tests to Take First: None required.

Tests to Take While You Are on It: A physical examination called the AIMS test should be performed by the psychiatrist or nurse practitioner at least every six months to detect early signs of tardive dyskinesia. Weight should be monitored monthly.

Usual Dose: In very acute emergency situations, Haldol can be given by injection, usually 5 mg every hour up to six doses. Sometimes, a higher dose is given over a shorter time to control dangerously psychotic behavior. In less serious situations, a patient is usually started at 5 mg two or three times daily and watched for about two weeks. If the response is still not good enough, the dose can be raised as high as 60 mg daily. It is best to keep the dose at 10–15 mg daily whenever possible. Elderly patients should be started at 0.5–1 mg once or twice a day. Haldol Decanoate is given in 50- to 100-mg injections once a month.

How Long Until It Works: Very psychotic patients may show signs of improvement after a few doses of Haldol, but full relief of symptoms usually takes two to four weeks.

Common Side Effects: Acute dystonia (sudden muscle stiffness), Parkinsonian syndrome (tremors and muscle stiffness), akathisia (jumpiness), akinesia (loss of interest and decreased movements)—all defined more fully earlier in this chapter; weight gain.

Less Common Side Effects: Neuroleptic malignant syndrome (serious increase in temperature and muscle rigidity—rare), tardive dyskinesia (involuntary movements after prolonged use), production of breast milk in men and women, seizures in people who already have epilepsy, loss of menstrual period and sex drive.

What to Do About Side Effects: At the same time Haldol is started, patients under age forty should also be placed on one of the drugs listed in Table 26 to prevent dystonia, Parkinsonian syndrome, and akinesia. Patients over forty should be given these drugs only if the side effects actually occur. Akathisia is treated with Inderal, Valium, or Ativan. The only treatment for weight gain is a diet, which sometimes helps. Neuroleptic malignant syndrome is an emergency that requires immediate medical care. Tardive dyskinesia usually occurs only after years of taking these drugs; in most cases it can be controlled by stopping the drug when the first signs occur. Clozapine is the only effective treatment for tardive dyskinesia. Production of breast milk is very rare and can be treated with special medication.

If It Doesn't Work: After four weeks at high enough doses, the best move is to switch to another antipsychotic drug.

If It Does Work: Except for patients with schizophrenia, Haldol should be discontinued shortly after the psychotic symptoms are under control. Patients with schizophrenia must remain on the drug indefinitely, but attempts to lower the dose should be made frequently and the patient should be watched for signs of tardive dyskinesia.

Cost: Generic haloperidol is as safe and effective as brand-name Haldol and much less expensive. Haldol Decanoate is cheaper than Risperdal Consta.

Special Comments: Haldol was once the most widely prescribed antipsychotic drug, but it is rarely used any longer. It is medically safe and very effective but can cause many uncomfortable and occasionally dangerous nervous system side effects. Therefore, a patient on Haldol must see a physician on a regular basis. Haldol Decanoate, the long-acting form of Haldol that can be injected once every four weeks, is prescribed mainly for patients who do not remember to take their medicine every day. Unfortunately, the American health care system does not seem capable of figuring out how to deliver depot medications to patients with schizophrenia.

CHLORPROMAZINE

Brand Name: Thorazine. (Brand-name Thorazine is no longer available in the United States.)

Used For: Psychosis associated with schizophrenia, mania, or depression; occasionally, in low doses, to control severe nausea or vomiting.

Do Not Use If: You have low blood pressure, an enlarged prostate, narrow-angle glaucoma, or epilepsy, unless your doctor knows about this.

Tests to Take First: None required.

Tests to Take While You Are on It: A physical examination called the AIMS test should be performed by the psychiatrist or nurse practitioner at least every six months to detect early signs of tardive dyskinesia. Weight should be monitored monthly.

Usual Dose: In very severe cases, Thorazine can be given by injection, usually 25 or 50 mg at a time. Less severely ill patients are started on 100 mg once or twice a day and are then observed for a few days. The dose can be raised to 600 mg a day, sometimes even higher. More and more evidence is now accumulating that for maintenance treatment of patients with schizophrenia, between 300 and 600 mg a day is probably the best dose.

How Long Until It Works: The patient may show some reduction in symptoms, especially violent agitation, after a few doses, but complete relief from psychosis may take up to four weeks.

Common Side Effects: Sedation, low blood pressure and dizziness, dry mouth, constipation, difficulty urinating, blurry vision, akathisia (jumpiness), Parkinsonian syndrome (tremors and muscle stiffness), akinesia (loss of motivation and decreased movement), weight gain, increased sensitivity to the sun.

Less Common Side Effects: Acute dystonia (sudden muscle stiffness), tardive dyskinesia (involuntary movements after prolonged use), neuroleptic malignant syndrome (serious muscle rigidity and fever—rare), production of breast milk in men and women, seizures in patients with a history of epilepsy, loss of menstrual period and sex drive.

What to Do About Side Effects: Thorazine makes patients sleepy and lowers blood pressure. There is no way to counteract these effects except by lowering the dose. The sedation is sometimes an advantage in quieting violent patients and helping agitated patients sleep better. Reduction of blood pressure produces dizziness, especially after rising from a lying or sitting position. It can cause an elderly person to black out and fall, making Thorazine a risky choice in older people.

The neurological side effects of Parkinsonian syndrome and akinesia are seen less often with Thorazine than with Haldol but still occur and are treated with counteracting drugs (Cogentin or Artane). Akathisia, described in more detail earlier in this chapter, is treated with counteracting medications (Inderal, Valium, or Ativan). It can be very disturbing and sometimes requires reduction of the dose. The quartet of side effects—dry mouth, constipation, difficulty urinating, and blurry vision—is known collectively as anticholinergic side effects. They are annoying but not dangerous; the one exception is difficulty urinating, which can be serious in a man with an enlarged prostate. These side effects are usually treated conservatively with laxatives and bran for constipation, sugarless hard candies and mouthwash for dry mouth, bethanechol (Urecholine) for difficulty urinating, and occasionally new glasses for blurry vision. Because of increased sensitivity to the sun, it is important that people on Thorazine use a sunblock with an SPF of at least 30 when exposed to the sun. Drinking plenty of fluids on hot days is also desirable. Weight gain, which can be up to twenty pounds in some people, can sometimes be controlled by calorie reduction.

Of the less common side effects, acute dystonia is treated with counteracting medications (Cogentin, Artane, or Benadryl). This effect occurs less often with Thorazine than with Haldol. Tardive dyskinesia, the involuntary movements caused by prolonged use of antipsychotic medications, is described more fully earlier in this chapter. TD usually goes away if the medication is stopped as soon as the first signs appear. Therefore, a patient on Thorazine should be examined by a doctor regularly. Neuroleptic malignant syndrome is rare and requires emergency medical care. Production of breast milk is also rare and can be treated. Thorazine increases the chance of having a seizure in patients who have or have had a seizure problem, so the doctor must be informed if the patient has ever had a convulsion or is taking anticonvulsants.

If It Doesn't Work: First be sure that the patient is taking the medication. Many psychotic patients do not take prescribed medication regularly. If the problem is not lack of adherence and the patient has been taking Thorazine for four weeks at a dose of at least 600 mg with no response, then it is usually best to switch to a different drug.

If It Does Work: Manic and depressed patients with psychosis who are given Thorazine should remain on it only until the psychotic symptoms resolve. Patients with schizophrenia may have to remain on the drug indefinitely, but attempts should always be made to reduce the dose to the lowest possible amount that still controls psychotic symptoms.

Cost: In psychiatry, and even in popular culture, the word *Thorazine* was once nearly a household word. Today, it is so uncommonly used that the brand-name drug Thorazine is actually no longer produced. Generic chlorpromazine is just as good and very inexpensive.

Special Comments: Thorazine was one of the first medications for psychosis introduced into clinical practice, in the early 1950s. It is medically safe and very effective but also makes the patient feel very sleepy and sluggish. Patients on Thorazine often appear drugged. Therefore, it is now given mostly to patients in whom some amount of sedation is specifically called for, for example, very agitated or violent patients. It should never be used as a sleeping pill for nonpsychotic patients.

THIORIDAZINE

Brand Name: Mellaril. (Brand-name Mellaril is no longer available in the United States.)

Used For: Psychosis associated with schizophrenia, mania, or depression.

Do Not Use If: You have low blood pressure, an enlarged prostate, narrow-angle glaucoma, epilepsy, or a heart condition, unless your doctor knows about this.

Tests to Take First: An electrocardiogram should be performed.

Tests to Take While You Are on It: A physical examination called the AIMS test should be performed by the psychiatrist or nurse practitioner at least every six months to detect early signs of tardive dyskinesia. Weight should be monitored monthly.

Because Mellaril can rarely produce changes in the retina, patients should be examined by an ophthalmologist every six months to a year while on the drug. An electrocardiogram should be performed about one week after starting, one month later, and then any time pulse rate drops.

Usual Dose: The patient is usually started at 100 mg once or twice daily, and the dose is raised as high as 600 mg over subsequent weeks until psychotic symptoms are resolved. Most patients respond to doses between 300 and 600 mg. More than 800 mg a day should never be given because of the risk of damaging the retina.

How Long Until It Works: The patient will probably become calmer and somewhat less violent after a few doses, but complete relief of psychotic symptoms may take up to four weeks.

Common Side Effects: Sedation, low blood pressure and dizziness, dry mouth, constipation, difficulty urinating, blurry vision, akathisia (jumpiness), Parkinsonian syndrome (tremors and muscle stiffness), akinesia (loss of motivation and decreased movement), weight gain, increased sensitivity to the sun.

Less Common Side Effects: Acute dystonia (sudden muscle stiffness), tardive dyskinesia (involuntary movements after prolonged use), neuroleptic malignant syndrome (serious muscle rigidity and fever), production of breast milk in men and women, seizures in patients with a history of epilepsy, loss of menstrual period and sex drive, damage to the retina (usually only if the dose exceeds 800 mg per day), changes on the electrocardiogram, known as QT or QTc prolongation (rare but potentially life threatening).

What to Do About Side Effects: Mellaril makes patients sleepy and lowers blood pressure. There is no way to counteract these effects except by reducing the dose. The sedation is sometimes an advantage in quieting violent patients and helping agitated patients sleep better. Lowering of blood pressure produces dizziness, especially after rising from a lying or sitting position. It can cause an elderly person to black out and fall, making Mellaril a risky choice in elderly people.

The neurological side effects of Parkinsonian syndrome and akinesia are seen less often with Mellaril than with Haldol but still occur and are treated with counteracting drugs (Cogentin or Artane). Akathisia, described in more detail earlier in this chapter, is treated with counteracting medications (Inderal, Valium, or Ativan). It can be very disturbing and sometimes requires reduction of the dose. The quartet of side effects—dry mouth, constipation, difficulty urinating, and blurry vision—is known collectively as anticholinergic side effects. They are annoying but not dangerous; the one exception is difficulty urinating, which can be serious in a man with an enlarged prostate. These side effects are usually treated conservatively with laxatives and bran for constipation, sugarless hard candies and mouthwash for dry mouth, bethanechol (Urecholine) for difficulty urinating, and occasionally new glasses for blurry vision. Because of increased sensitivity to the sun, it is important that people on Mellaril use a sunblock with an SPF of at least 30 when exposed to the sun. Drinking plenty of fluids on hot days is also desirable. Weight gain, which can be up to twenty pounds in some people, can sometimes be controlled by calorie reduction.

Of the less common side effects, acute dystonia is treated with counteracting medications (Cogentin, Artane, or Benadryl). This effect occurs less often with Mellaril than with Haldol. Tardive dyskinesia, the involuntary movements caused by prolonged use of antipsychotic medications, is described more fully earlier in this chapter. It usually goes away if the medication is stopped as soon as the first signs appear. Therefore, a patient on Mellaril should be examined by a doctor regularly. Neuroleptic malignant syndrome is rare and requires emergency medical care. Production of breast milk is also rare and can be treated. Mellaril increases the chance of having a seizure in patients who have or have had a seizure problem, so the doctor must be informed if the patient has ever had a convulsion or is taking anticonvulsants. The patient should see an ophthalmologist about once a year to check for any changes in the retina. The heart problem known as QT prolongation was always known but only recently did a study reveal that it can potentially be life threatening. Although getting an electrocardiogram before starting Mellaril is a good idea, it doesn't necessarily help predict who is going to get QT prolongation. Certain other medications, too numerous to mention here, increase the risk. The doctor should take the patient's pulse regularly and if it drops stop Mellaril and get an electrocardiogram right away.

If It Doesn't Work: Assuming that the patient has been taking the medication (nonadherence is often a problem with psychotic patients), if there is no response after four weeks at a dose of at least 600 mg a day, a different antipsychotic drug should be tried.

If It Does Work: Patients treated with Mellaril because of psychotic symptoms associated with depression or mania should take the medication only until the psychosis is resolved. Schizophrenia patients may have to remain on Mellaril indefinitely, but attempts should always be made to keep the dose as low as necessary to control psychotic symptoms.

Cost: Although once a frequently prescribed drug, Mellaril is so rarely prescribed today that brand-name Mellaril is no longer produced. Generic thioridazine is just as good. *Special Comments:* Mellaril is almost identical to Thorazine. It tends to produce fewer nervous system side effects, like dystonia and akathisia, than Haldol but more sleepiness and greater reduction of blood pressue. It used to be prescribed to psychotic patients who are very agitated or violent because in these cases sedation is often desirable. It has been claimed that Mellaril is less likely than other antipsychotic drugs to cause tardive dyskinesia, but this is doubtful. Furthermore, the side effects involving the heart and the eyes make it a risky choice and most doctors refuse to prescribe it any longer given the wide range of alternative choices.

TRIFLUOPERAZINE

Brand Name: Stelazine. (Brand-name Stelazine is no longer available in the United States.)

Used For: Psychosis associated with mania, depression, or schizophrenia; control of psychotic symptoms in the elderly.

Do Not Use If: You do not have psychotic symptoms, except in rare circumstances. Stelazine increases the chance of having a seizure in patients with a history of epilepsy.

Tests to Take First: None required.

Tests to Take While You Are on It: A physical examination called the AIMS test should be performed by the psychiatrist or nurse practitioner at least every six months to detect early signs of tardive dyskinesia. Weight should be monitored monthly.

Usual Dose: Patients are usually started at 5 mg two or three times daily and observed for several weeks. If there is no response, the dose can be raised to as high as 60 mg, but a dose between 15 and 40 mg a day is probably optimal for treating schizophrenia.

How Long Until It Works: A severely psychotic patient may feel calmer and be less agitated after a few doses, but full relief of psychotic symptoms usually takes up to four weeks.

Common Side Effects: Acute dystonia (sudden muscle stiffness), Parkinsonian syndrome (tremors and muscle stiffness), akathisia (jumpiness), akinesia (loss of interest and decreased movements)—all defined more fully earlier in this chapter; weight gain.

Less Common Side Effects: Neuroleptic malignant syndrome (serious increase in temperature and muscle rigidity—rare), tardive dyskinesia (involuntary movements after prolonged use), production of breast milk in men and women, seizures in people who already have epilepsy, loss of menstrual period and sex drive.

What to Do About Side Effects: At the same time Stelazine is started, patients under age forty should also be placed on one of the drugs listed in Table 26 to prevent dystonia, Parkinsonian syndrome, and akinesia. Patients over forty should be given these drugs only if the side effects actually occur. Akathisia is treated with Inderal, Valium, or Ativan. The only treatment for weight gain is a diet, which sometimes helps. Neuroleptic malignant syndrome is an emergency that requires immediate medical care. Tardive dyskinesia usually occurs only after years of taking these drugs; in most cases, it can be controlled by stopping the drug when the first signs occur. Production of breast milk is very rare and can be treated with special medication.

If It Doesn't Work: Assuming the patient has been taking the medication as prescribed, if there is no response after four weeks, it is best to switch to a different drug.

If It Does Work: Manic or depressed or elderly patients who have been given Stelazine to treat their psychotic symptoms should take it only until those psychotic symptoms go away. Patients with schizophrenia may have to stay on Stelazine indefinitely, but frequent attempts should be made to lower the dose to the minimum required to control psychotic symptoms.

Cost: Brand-name Stelazine is no longer manufactured in the United States, but trifluoperazine is just as good.

Special Comments: Stelazine is almost identical in action and side effects to Haldol. Like Haldol, it is well suited for patients for whom sedation is not desirable. It has been said that Stelazine is also useful for nonpsychotic anxiety, but I feel this is almost always a mistake. Patients with anxiety who are not psychotic and need medication should almost always be given an antidepressant, buspirone (BuSpar), or a benzodiazepine (for example, Valium or Xanax) instead of Stelazine. Stelazine is rarely prescribed any longer in favor of the atypical antipsychotics.

FLUPHENAZINE

Brand Names: Prolixin, Permitil.

Used For: Psychosis associated with schizophrenia, mania, or depression; psychosis in elderly patients with dementia.

Do Not Use If: You do not have a psychotic illness.

Tests to Take First: None required.

Tests to Take While You Are on It: None required.

Usual Dose: For severely psychotic patients requiring emergency treatment, Prolixin can be given by injection. Usually, an injection of 5 mg is given first; this can be repeated every fifteen minutes to an hour until a total of six doses have been given. In less urgent situations, the patient is usually given 5 mg two or three times daily and observed for about two weeks. The dose can then be increased to as much as 60 mg a day, but doses of 10–15 mg daily are best. Elderly patients should be started at very small doses, sometimes as low as 0.5 mg. It is also available in liquid form of 2.5 mg per teaspoon.

How Long Until It Works: Some decrease in agitation, violent behavior, and psychotic symptoms may be seen after the first few doses, but full control of psychosis usually takes up to four weeks.

Common Side Effects: Acute dystonia (sudden muscle stiffness), Parkinsonian syndrome (tremors and muscle stiffness), akathisia (jumpiness), akinesia (loss of interest and decreased movements)—all defined more fully earlier in this chapter; weight gain.

Less Common Side Effects: Neuroleptic malignant syndrome (serious increase in temperature and muscle rigidity—rare), tardive dyskinesia (involuntary movements after prolonged use), production of breast milk in men and women, loss of menstrual period and sex drive.

What to Do About Side Effects: At the same time Prolixin is started, patients under age forty should also be placed on one of the drugs listed in Table 26 to prevent dystonia, Parkinsonian syndrome, and akinesia. Patients over forty should be given these drugs only if the side effects actually occur. Akathisia is treated with Inderal, Valium, or Ativan. The only treatment for weight gain is a diet, which sometimes helps. Neuroleptic malignant syndrome is an emergency that requires immediate medical care. Tardive dyskinesia usually occurs only after years of taking these drugs; in most cases it can be controlled by stopping the drug when the first signs occur. Production of breast milk is very rare and can be treated with special medication.

If It Doesn't Work: If Prolixin has not worked after four weeks and non-adherence is not the problem, it is best to try a different antipsychotic drug.

If It Does Work: Patients with mania, depression, or dementia who are given Prolixin should remain on it only until the psychotic symptoms resolve. Patients with schizophrenia may have to take Prolixin for a long time, but attempts to lower the dose to the minimum required to control psychotic symptoms should be made frequently.

Cost: Generic fluphenazine is not available, so expensive Prolixin must be prescribed.

Special Comments: Prolixin is very similar to Haldol and Stelazine and therefore was once commonly used to treat psychotic patients who do not want to be sedated. Prolixin may be less likely than the other antipsychotic drug to cause seizures in patients who also have epilepsy. It is rarely prescribed today in favor of the atypical antipsychotic drugs.

PERPHENAZINE

Brand Name: Trilafon.

Used For: Psychosis associated with mania, depression, or schizophrenia.

Do Not Use If: You do not have psychotic symptoms, have epilepsy and your doctor doesn't know it, have an enlarged prostate, or have narrow-angle glaucoma.

Tests to Take First: None required.

Tests to Take While You Are on It: A physical examination called the AIMS test should be performed by the psychiatrist or nurse practitioner at least every six months to detect early signs of tardive dyskinesia. Weight should be monitored monthly.

Usual Dose: The patient is usually started on 8 mg once or twice a day. This can be increased up to 64 mg a day until symptoms are relieved.

How Long Until It Works: Some relief from agitation and psychotic symptoms may be obtained after the first few doses, but full remission from psychosis usually takes up to four weeks.

Common Side Effects: Mild sedation, mild dizziness from lowered blood pressure, dry mouth, constipation, difficulty urinating, blurry vision, akathisia (jumpiness), Parkinsonian syndrome (tremors and stiffness), akinesia (loss of motivation and decreased movements), weight gain, increased sensitivity to the sun.

Less Common Side Effects: Acute dystonia (sudden tightening of muscles), tardive dyskinesia (involuntary movements after prolonged use), neuroleptic malignant syndrome (severe muscle rigidity and fever—rare), loss of menstrual period and sex drive, breast milk production in men and women, seizures in people with a history of epilepsy.

What to Do About Side Effects: The only remedy for sedation and dizziness is reduction of the dose, although drinking a lot of fluids and taking extra salt may also help the latter problem. The four anticholinergic side effects—dry mouth, constipation, difficulty urinating, and blurry vision—are usually annoying but not dangerous. Dry mouth is best relieved by mouthwash and sugarless hard candies, constipation by eating bran and using laxatives, difficulty urinating by bethanechol (Urecholine), and blurry vision by new glasses.

The best way to treat the neurological side effects of Parkinsonian syndrome, acute dystonia, and akinesia is with one of the counteracting medications listed in Table 26, for example, Cogentin and Benadryl. Some psychiatrists place the patient on these counteracting drugs as soon as Trilafon is started. Weight gain is controlled by diet and sensitivity to the sun by using sunblock of at least an SPF 30 and drinking plenty of fluids. Tardive dyskinesia, the development of involuntary movements in some patients treated with Trilafon for prolonged periods, usually goes away if the drug is stopped after the first signs appear. Therefore, the patient should be checked by the doctor at least every six months. Neuroleptic malignant syndrome is very rare and usually requires emergency treatment in the hospital. Breast milk production is similarly very rare and can be treated by counteracting medication. Loss of menstrual period is not necessarily serious, but the patient should be seen by a gynecologist and dose reduction considered. Patients with a history of epilepsy should take all antipsychotic drugs only under the careful supervision of their psychiatrist and neurologist.

If It Doesn't Work: Switching to a different drug is usually the best course of action if Trilafon is ineffective after four weeks.

If It Does Work: Patients with depression or mania who are given Trilafon should take it only until the psychotic symptoms resolve. Schizophrenia patients may have to take Trilafon indefinitely, but attempts to reduce the dose should be made periodically to determine the minimum dose that controls the psychotic symptoms.

Cost: Generic perphenazine is just as safe and effective as brand-name Trilafon and less expensive.

Special Comments: Trilafon is a kind of middle-of-the-road drug in terms of side effects between the very potent antipsychotics (Haldol, Stelazine, and Prolixin) and the lower-potency drugs (Thorazine and Mellaril). It produces all of the side effects of the other drugs but to a milder degree. Thus, it is more sedating than Haldol but less sedating than Thorazine. It is more likely than Thorazine but less likely than Haldol to produce neurological side effects (acute dystonia and Parkinsonian syndrome). Many psychotic patients find it is the most tolerable antipsychotic drug in terms of side effects. Like the other typical antipsychotic drugs, Trilafon was almost forgotten until the results of the large National Institute of Mental Health CATIE study were published in the *New England Journal of Medicine* in 2005. This study compared the atypical drugs to each other and to Trilafon, and Trilafon did surprisingly well. The dose of Trilafon was relatively low in the study and the study did not last long enough to see if tardive dyskinesia would occur (other studies strongly suggest that this is much less likely with atypical than typical antipsychotic drugs), so not everyone was that enthusiastic about Trilafon when the study results became public. Nevertheless, it is sobering to see how well a very old drug did compared to the modern ones, and given its very low cost Trilafon is likely to make something of a comeback.

THIOTHIXENE

Brand Name: Navane.

Used For: Psychosis in patients with schizophrenia, mania, or depression; psychotic symptoms in elderly patients with dementia.

Do Not Use If: You do not have psychotic symptoms. Navane may precipitate seizures in people with a history of convulsions.

Tests to Take First: None required.

Tests to Take While You Are on It: A physical examination called the AIMS test should be performed by the psychiatrist or nurse practitioner at least every six months to detect early signs of tardive dyskinesia. Weight should be monitored monthly.

Usual Dose: In emergency situations, the patient can be given 5 mg, and this is repeated as often as every fifteen minutes up to six doses to achieve rapid control of very agitated or violent behavior. In less urgent situations, the patient is usually started at 5 mg two or three times daily and then observed for several weeks. The dose of Navane can be raised as high as 60 mg, but the optimal dose is usually between 10 and 30 mg a day. Elderly patients should take much less, usually starting with 1 mg once or twice a day.

How Long Until It Works: The patient may feel calmer and less agitated after the first few doses, but complete control of psychotic symptoms usually takes up to four weeks.

Common Side Effects: Acute dystonia (sudden muscle stiffness), Parkinsonian syndrome (tremors and muscle stiffness), akathisia (jumpiness), akinesia (loss of interest and decreased movements)—all defined more fully earlier in this chapter; weight gain.

Less Common Side Effects: Neuroleptic malignant syndrome (serious increase in temperature and muscle rigidity—rare), tardive dyskinesia (involuntary movements after prolonged use), production of breast milk in men and women, seizures in people who already have epilepsy, loss of menstrual period and sex drive.

What to Do About Side Effects: At the same time Navane is started, patients under age forty should also be placed on one of the drugs listed in Table 26 to prevent dystonia, Parkinsonian syndrome, and akinesia. Patients over forty should be given these drugs only if the side effects actually occur. Akathisia is treated with Inderal, Valium, or Ativan. The only treatment for weight gain is a diet, which sometimes helps. Neuroleptic malignant syndrome is an emergency that requires immediate medical care. Tardive dyskinesia usually occurs only after years of taking these drugs; in most cases, it can be controlled by stopping the drug when the first signs occur. Production of breast milk is very rare and can be treated with special medication. Patients with a history of epilepsy should take all antipsychotic drugs only under the careful supervision of their psychiatrist and neurologist. Loss of menstrual period is not necessarily serious, but the patient should be seen by a gynecologist and dose reduction considered.

If It Doesn't Work: First, make sure the patient is actually taking the medicine. Psychotic patients have a habit of forgetting to take their pills, causing everyone to think the drug is ineffective. If nonadherence is not the problem and the patient has not responded after four weeks, it is usually best to change drugs.

If It Does Work: Patients with mania, depression, or dementia should take Navane only until the psychotic symptoms resolve. Schizophrenia patients may have to remain on Navane indefinitely, but attempts to lower the dose to the minimum required to control psychotic symptoms should be made periodically.

Cost: Generic thiothixene is not available, so expensive Navane must be prescribed.

Special Comments: Navane, like Stelazine and Prolixin, is very similar to Haldol and was generally used for psychotic patients who do not need to be sedated. Navane is rarely prescribed today in favor of the atypical antipsychotic medications.

LOXAPINE

Brand Name: Loxitane.

Used For: Psychosis in patients with schizophrenia, mania, or depression.

Do Not Use If: You do not have psychosis, have a history of seizures that your doctor doesn't know about, have an enlarged prostate gland, or have narrow-angle glaucoma.

Tests to Take First: None required.

Tests to Take While You Are on It: A physical examination called the AIMS test should be performed by the psychiatrist or nurse practitioner at least every six months to detect early signs of tardive dyskinesia. Weight should be monitored monthly.

Usual Dose: Patients are usually started at 10 mg twice a day and then increased to the optimal dose between 60 and 100 mg a day.

How Long Until It Works: The psychotic patient may feel some relief from severe agitation and become less violent after the first few doses, but full control of psychotic symptoms usually takes up to four weeks.

Common Side Effects: Mild sedation, mild dizziness from lowered blood pressure, dry mouth, constipation, difficulty urinating, blurry vision, akathisia (jumpiness), Parkinsonian syndrome (tremors and stiffness), akinesia (loss of motivation and decreased movements, weight gain, increased sensitivity to the sun.

Less Common Side Effects: Acute dystonia (sudden tightening of muscles), tardive dyskinesia (involuntary movements after prolonged use), neuroleptic malignant syndrome (severe muscle rigidity and fever—rare), loss of menstrual period and sex drive, breast milk production in men and women, seizures in people with a history of epilepsy.

What to Do About Side Effects: The only remedy for sedation and dizziness is reduction of the dose. The four anticholinergic side effects—dry mouth, constipation, difficulty urinating, and blurry vision—are usually annoying but not dangerous. Dry mouth is best relieved by mouthwash and sugarless hard candies, constipation by eating bran and using laxatives, difficulty urinating by bethanechol (Urecholine), and blurry vision by new glasses.

The best way to treat the neurologic side effects of Parkinsonian syndrome, acute dystonia, and akinesia is with one of the counteracting medications listed in Table 26, such as Cogentin or Benadryl. Some psychiatrists place the patient on these counteracting drugs as soon as Loxitane is started. Weight gain is controlled by diet, and sensitivity to the sun by using sunblock of at least SPF 30 and drinking plenty of fluids.

Tardive dyskinesia, the development of involuntary movements in some patients treated with Loxitane for prolonged periods, usually goes away if the drug is stopped after the first signs appear. Therefore, the patient should be checked by the doctor about once a month. Neuroleptic malignant syndrome is very rare and usually requires emergency treatment in the hospital. Breast milk production is similarly very rare and can be treated by counteracting medication. Loss of menstrual period is not necessarily serious, but the patient should be seen by a gynecologist and dose reduction considered. Patients with a history of epilepsy should take all antipsychotic drugs only under the careful supervision of their psychiatrist and neurologist.

If It Doesn't Work: The problem may be that the patient simply isn't taking the medication. If that is not true and Loxitane has not worked after four weeks, it is usually best to switch drugs.

If It Does Work: Patients with depression or mania should keep taking Loxitane only as long as needed to eliminate the psychotic symptoms. Schizophrenia patients may have to take Loxitane indefinitely, but frequent attempts should be made to reduce the dose to the lowest possible level that still controls psychotic symptoms.

Cost: Generic loxapine is not available, so expensive Loxitane must be prescribed.

Special Comments: Loxitane is similar to Trilafon and Moban in being a middle-of-the-road antipsychotic drug. It has less tendency than Haldol or Stelazine to produce acute dystonia (sudden muscle stiffness) but is more likely to do this than Thorazine or Mellaril. It is less sedating and causes less of a decrease in blood pressure than Thorazine and Mellaril, but more than Haldol or Stelazine. Nevertheless, Loxitane is rarely prescribed now in favor of the atypical antipsychotics.

MOLINDONE

Brand Name: Moban, Lidone.

Used For: Psychotic symptoms in patients with mania, depression, or schizophrenia.

Do Not Use If: You do not have psychotic symptoms, have an enlarged prostate, or have narrow-angle glaucoma.

Tests to Take First: None required.

Tests to Take While You Are on It: A physical examination called the AIMS test should be performed by the psychiatrist or nurse practitioner at least every six months to detect early signs of tardive dyskinesia. Weight should be monitored monthly.

Usual Dose: The usual starting dose is 50 or 75 mg a day. This is slowly increased over several days to 100 mg but can go as high as 225 mg to treat severe psychosis.

How Long Until It Works: Although there may be some calming after the first few doses, complete resolution of psychotic symptoms usually takes up to four weeks.

Common Side Effects: Mild sedation, mild dizziness from lowered blood pressure, dry mouth, constipation, difficulty urinating, blurry vision, akathisia (jumpiness), Parkinsonian syndrome (tremors and stiffness), akinesia (loss of motivation and decreased movements), increased sensitivity to the sun.

Less Common Side Effects: Acute dystonia (sudden tightening of muscles), tardive dyskinesia (involuntary movements after prolonged use), neuroleptic malignant syndrome (severe muscle rigidity and fever—rare), loss of menstrual period and sex drive, breast milk production in men and women.

What to Do About Side Effects: The only remedy for sedation and dizziness is reduction of the dose. The four anticholinergic side effects—dry mouth, constipation, difficulty urinating, and blurry vision—are usually annoying but not dangerous. Dry mouth is best relieved by mouthwash and sugarless hard candies, constipation by eating bran and using laxatives, difficulty urinating by bethanechol (Urecholine), and blurry vision by new glasses.

The best way to treat the neurological side effects of Parkinsonian syndrome, acute dystonia, and akinesia is with one of the counteracting medications listed in Table 26, such as Cogentin and Benadryl. Some psychiatrists place the patient on these counteracting drugs as soon as Moban (or Lidone) is started. Sensitivity to the sun is treated by use of a sunblock of at least SPF 30 and ingestion of plenty of fluids. Tardive dyskinesia, the development of involuntary movements in some patients treated with Moban for prolonged periods, usually goes away if the drug is stopped after the first signs appear. Therefore, the patient should be checked by the doctor about once a month. Neuroleptic malignant syndrome is very rare and usually requires emergency treatment in the hospital. Breast milk production is similarly very rare and can be treated by counteracting medication. Loss of menstrual period is not necessarily serious, but the patient should be seen by a gynecologist and dose reduction considered.

If It Doesn't Work: Assuming the patient has been taking the pills as prescribed, if there is no response to Moban after four weeks, it is usually best to switch to a different drug.

If It Does Work: Patients with depression or mania should stop taking Moban as soon as the psychotic symptoms resolve. Schizophrenia patients may have to remain on Moban indefinitely, but it is very important to reduce the dose to the lowest possible level that still controls the psychotic symptoms.

Cost: Generic molindone is not available, so expensive Moban must be prescribed.

Special Comments: Moban is very much like Trilafon and Loxitane in having a middle-of-the-road side effect profile between the high-potency antipsychotics (Haldol and Prolixin) and the low-potency antipsychotics (Thorazine and Mellaril). Moban has two other interesting features. First, like Prolixin, it is less likely than the other antipsychotic drugs to cause seizures in a patient who has a history of epilepsy. Second, Moban is said to cause less weight gain than the other antipsychotic drugs. However, there have always been questions about how effective Moban is and it is rarely prescribed now, in favor of the atypical antipsychotic medications.

PIMOZIDE

Brand Name: Orap.

Used For: The neurological condition Tourette's syndrome, which often begins in childhood and is characterized by uncontrollable tics and a variety of involuntary noises. Occasionally, Orap is used to treat psychotic conditions; it is claimed to be especially useful for patients with the specific delusion that they have a serious abnormality with their physical health (called a somatic delusion). A research study is being conducted to evaluate the theory that pimozide can enhance the effects of clozapine in patients for whom clozapine has not been sufficiently effective.

Do Not Use If: You do not have Tourette's syndrome or psychosis, or if you have a heart condition. Pimozide has many drug interactions, so your doctor needs to go over the drugs you are taking. Pimozide is usually used only after another dopamine-blocking drug, like Risperdal, is used first and doesn't work.

Tests to Take First: Patients must have an electrocardiogram (ECG) before starting Orap because this drug can exacerbate a rare cardiac problem.

Tests to Take While You Are on It: The electrocardiogram should be repeated at regular intervals to make sure Orap is not causing an abnormality. About 10 percent of patients treated with Orap show changes on the electrocardiogram, called QT or QTc prolongation, but most of these changes are not clinically significant. Actual heart problems caused by Orap are probably very uncommon, but they can be serious. A physical examination called the AIMS test should be performed by the psychiatrist or nurse practitioner at least every six months to detect early signs of tardive dyskinesia. Weight should be monitored monthly.

Usual Dose: Patients are usually started at 1 mg at night and the dose is raised about once a week by 1 mg until symptoms are controlled. The usual effective dose ranges between about 2 and 10 mg daily.

How Long Until It Works: For treatment of Tourette's, it may take weeks until the proper dose is reached and the tics are under control. For treatment of psychotic conditions, such as somatic delusions, it may also be several weeks before improvement is realized.

Common Side Effects: Acute dystonia (sudden muscle stiffness), Parkinsonian syndrome (tremors and muscle stiffness), akathisia (jumpiness), akinesia (loss of interest and decreased movements)—all defined more fully earlier in this chapter; weight gain.

Less Common Side Effects: Neuroleptic malignant syndrome (serious increase in temperature and muscle rigidity—rare), tardive dyskinesia (involuntary movements after prolonged use), production of breast milk in men and women, seizures in people who already have epilepsy, loss of menstrual period and sex drive, changes in the electrocardiogram.

What to Do About Side Effects: At the same time Orap is started, patients under age forty should also be placed on one of the drugs listed in Table 26 to prevent dystonia, Parkinsonian syndrome, and akinesia. Patients over forty should be given these drugs only if the side effects actually occur. Akathisia is treated with either Inderal, Valium, or Ativan. The only treatment for weight gain is a diet, which sometimes helps. Neuroleptic malignant syndrome is an emergency that requires immediate medical care. Tardive dyskinesia usually occurs only after years of taking these drugs; in most cases it can be controlled by stopping the drug when the first signs occur. Production of breast milk is very rare and can be treated with special medication. Orap is said to produce a change in the electrical activity of the heart, reflected in a change in the electrocardiogram. This is probably rarely of clinical significance and nothing to worry about for most patients, but in a small number of people it can be very serious. Most doctors require periodic electrocardiograms to ensure that no harm is being done; stopping the drug returns the electrocardiogram to normal.

If It Doesn't Work: Tourette's syndrome is very difficult to treat, and a great deal more research is needed to understand what causes it. Orap is usually used in psychotic patients only if they have not responded to other drugs for psychosis. If it also doesn't work, the doctor will probably try something else.

If It Does Work: Tourette's syndrome tends to worsen and improve on its own periodically. Also, when the patient with Tourette's reaches adulthood, the symptoms sometimes improve. Therefore, frequent attempts should be made to lower the dose or even discontinue Orap. Some patients, however, must remain on Orap almost continuously to maintain control over their symptoms. The same is true of patients with psychotic illnesses treated with Orap; to reduce the risk of tardive dyskinesia, the doctor should constantly try to reduce the dose as much as possible.

Cost: Generic pimozide is not available, so expensive brand-name Orap must be prescribed.

Special Comments: I have included pimozide (Orap) in this chapter because it is sometimes used to treat patients with psychotic conditions, especially those who develop somatic delusions, and it may be effective when added to clozapine for patients who have not had a sufficient response to clozapine. In almost every way, Orap looks and acts like the other antipsychotic drugs, but its main use is the treatment of patients with Tourette's syndrome, not psychosis.

CLOZAPINE

Brand Name: Clozaril.

Used For: Schizophrenia (both positive and negative symptoms) in patients who do not respond to other antipsychotic drugs or who have developed severe neurological side effects from other antipsychotic drugs, especially tardive dyskinesia. May also be used in bipolar mood disorder patients who fail to respond to everything else.

Do Not Use If: You cannot comply with the absolute need to have blood counts weekly for the first six months and then every other week thereafter. Patients with a history of convulsions (seizures) may be told not to take clozapine by their doctor.

Tests to Take First: A complete blood count (CBC) is obtained before initiation of clozapine. In addition, most physicians require a physical examination, blood tests of liver function, blood sugar, cholesterol, and triglycerides, and an electrocardiogram (ECG).

Tests to Take While You Are on It: A patient on clozapine is required to have a CBC every week for the first six months and then every other week for the rest of the time he or she takes the drug. Procurement of the next supply is contingent on the doctor's review of the previous CBC and confirmation of the absence of abnormalities. Repeat blood tests of liver function may also be obtained several times in the first few months of treatment. Blood sugar, cholesterol, and triglyceride blood tests are regularly obtained (at least every six months and more often if weight gain is substantial (which it almost always is). Weight should be monitored at least monthly.

Usual Dose: Most patients are started on relatively low doses (25 or 50 mg a day) and gradually increased to between 300 and 600 mg per day over the next several weeks. The recommended top dose is 900 mg.

How Long Until It Works: As with all antipsychotic medications, there may be some immediate relief of severe agitation, but a true decrease in psychotic symptoms may take two to four weeks.

Common Side Effects: Sedation, increased salivation and drooling, rapid heart rate, dizziness caused by lowered blood pressure, fever, nausea and vomiting, constipation, dry mouth, weight gain.

Less Common Side Effects: Blood abnormality involving the white blood cells, technically called agranulocytosis. If not detected and treated by immediate discontinuation of medication, agranulocytosis is fatal. For this reason, patients on clozapine must have a CBC, which includes a count of the white blood cells, every week for the first six months and then every other week. The risk of agranulocytosis may be as high as 1 percent, although since the drug was reintroduced in 1990 the rate is lower, about 0.4 percent. Because of the careful CBC monitoring, there have been no deaths in the United States from agranulocytosis caused by clozapine. The risk of seizures while taking clozapine is about 4 percent, higher than with the other antipsychotic drugs. Sudden loss of muscle strength lasting a few moments, called periodic cataplexy; bed-wetting (enuresis); diabetes; abnormalities in the function of heart, liver, or pancreas.

What to Do About Side Effects: There is no question that clozapine is a hard drug to take. Sedation, dizziness, nausea, vomiting, and fever are generally transient. Drooling (technically called sialorrhea) is a mysterious side effect, the cause of which remains unknown. There is no cure for this side effect, which, according to the manufacturer, occurs in about 5 percent of patients treated with clozapine. Fortunately, it is not serious in most cases. Constipation can be treated by drinking extra fluids or using stool softeners. Dry mouth is treated with mouthwash or sugarless hard candies. Increases in heart rate caused by clozapine are also generally not serious, although sometimes counteracting medication is prescribed. Weight gain is the most troubling of the common side effects and unfortunately leads some patients to discontinue the drug. From the moment a patient starts taking clozapine, he or she should be counseled about weight gain, placed on a low-calorie diet (unless he or she is already underweight, in which case this is postponed until the patient has gained weight), and given an exercise regimen. This must be reinforced regularly.

The less common side effects are clearly more serious. A decrease in white blood cell count is potentially fatal. The blood count must be checked regularly and the drug stopped immediately if this anemia occurs. Because seizures can be provoked by clozapine, patients with a history of convulsions or epilepsy need to be carefully monitored and take anticonvulsant medications if placed on clozapine. Sudden loss of muscle strength, which can result in falls, is very rare. Bed-wetting occurs in less than 1 percent of patients; restricting fluids before bedtime is helpful. In order to guard against diabetes, it is important to try to keep the patient's weight under control as much as possible. The risk for diabetes is greatest in people who gain a lot of weight and/or have a family history of diabetes. Checking the blood sugar level regularly is important. Other blood tests and the EKG can alert patient and doctor to problems with the functioning of organs such as liver, heart, and pancreas.

If It Doesn't Work: Clozapine sometimes produces dramatic improvements in patients with schizophrenia who have failed to respond to many other antipsychotic drugs. It is not a "miracle drug," and such dramatic reversals in previously refractory patients probably occur only a little over one-fourth of the time. If clozapine does not work, it should be discontinued.

If It Does Work: Patients should remain on clozapine indefinitely, because they are likely to have long-standing schizophrenia that has failed to respond to many other attempts at treatment. If clozapine doesn't work or the patient cannot tolerate the less serious side effects, the drug should be gradually discontinued over several weeks.

Cost: Generic clozapine is as safe and effective as brand-name clozaril and cheaper. Part of the cost of taking clozapine is the many blood tests required.

Special Comments: Clozapine was the first true advance in the treatment of schizophrenic patients in almost thirty years. It was approved by the Food and Drug Administration in 1989. It has potentially serious side effects and therefore is now recommended for use in schizophrenia and bipolar disorder patients who have failed to respond to other medications or who have developed tardive dyskinesia and therefore should no longer take the other currently marketed drugs. The recent CATIE study confirmed that clozapine is the most effective of all antipsychotic medications and therefore it is a tragedy if a patient who has not responded to anything else is not offered a trial of clozapine. Clozapine does not cause the neurological side effects of dystonia, Parkinsonian syndrome, akinesia, akathisia, and tardive dyskinesia that are common to the typical antipsychotic drugs. It is also weaker than the older antipsychotics at blocking dopamine and has strong serotonin-blocking properties. For these reasons, clozapine was called the first of the atypical antipsychotics. Clozapine has truly had a dramatic effect on the treatment and understanding of schizophrenia. Some patients previously untouched by antipsychotic drugs are now doing well and the drug seems helpful even for negative symptoms. Basically, any patient who has schizophrenia and has either not responded to or has severe side effects from other antipsychotic drugs deserves a try on clozapine. Patients with bipolar disorder who have had exhaustive trials with other medications without getting any help may also respond to clozapine.

RISPERIDONE

Brand Names: Risperdal, Risperdal Consta, Risperdal M-Tab.

Used For: Schizophrenia (both positive and negative symptoms—see below) and the manic phase of bipolar disorder. Also used to enhance the effects of antidepressants in patients who have not had a sufficient response, and to treat psychotic depression, psychosis, and disruptive behavior in children with autism, Tourette's syndrome, and extreme agitation and psychosis in elderly patients with dementia.

Do Not Use If: There are very few absolute reasons not to take Risperdal.

Tests to Take First: For most people, there are no required tests before taking Risperdal. It can cause changes in the electrocardiogram that might be harmful to people who already have heart conditions, so if you fall into that category an electrocardiogram (ECG) should be taken first. Also, Risperdal can lower blood pressure, so it is a good idea for elderly people to have their blood pressure checked before starting Risperdal.

Tests to Take While You Are on It: Blood pressure should be checked a few times in the weeks after starting Risperdal, although except for elderly people there usually is not much of a problem. A physical examination called the AIMS test should be performed by the psychiatrist or nurse practitioner at least every six months to detect early signs of tardive dyskinesia. Weight should be monitored monthly.

Usual Dose: Risperdal can be given once a day, usually starting at 1 mg and increased as fast as 1 mg a day to 3–4 mg, doses that often are sufficient. Doses of 6 mg or more are sometimes needed, but as the dose gets higher, the risk of neurological symptoms called EPS (dystonia, Parkinson's syndrome, and akathisia) gets greater. In elderly patients and children, the dose is usually started at a much lower level, 0.25 or 0.5 mg a day, and not advanced beyond 1–3 mg a day. Risperdal Consta is the long-acting depot formulation of risperidone, which is given by injection, 25 or 50 mg every two weeks. Risperdal M-Tab is the melt-in-your-mouth version.

How Long Until It Works: In situations of very acute psychosis, with hallucinations, delusions, and a great deal of behavioral disturbance, antipsychotic drugs like Risperdal often have an immediate effect. After even just one or two doses, the patient may become calmer and less confused. Usually, however, it takes four to six weeks before a complete effect occurs with antipsychotic drugs. There is some evidence that Risperdal may reduce psychotic symptoms more quickly: Studies done with Risperdal prior to its approval by the FDA suggest that after one week the drug was already exerting an antipsychotic effect. It is still a good idea, however, to give it at least a month before deciding how well Risperdal is working.

Common Side Effects: One of the main reasons for prescribing Risperdal instead of the original typical antipsychotic drugs like Thorazine and Haldol is that Risperdal has fewer side effects. Most important, if the dose of Risperdal is kept under 6 mg a day, it seems to have a lower potential than the older drugs to cause the neurological EPS side effects, dystonia, Parkinsonian syndrome, akathisia, and akinesia (described in detail on pages 229–230). These neurological side effects are uncomfortable and often lead to patient refusal to take antipsychotic medications. Clozapine also has low potential to cause EPS, but the need to have weekly or biweekly blood tests is a clear drawback to using it. Blood monitoring is not necessary for Risperdal; it does not cause the serious blood cell abnormality called agranulocytosis that occurs in approximately 1 percent of patients who take clozapine. Hence, Risperdal has a clear side effect advantage over the other antipsychotic drugs. It is important to emphasize that if the dose of Risperdal is raised above 6 mg, the drug does start to produce EPS and much of the side effect advantage over the traditional antipsychotic drugs is lost. At that point, some cynics have called Risperdal "expensive Haldol."

Risperdal does, of course, have side effects. The most common are insomnia, anxiety, headache, and runny nose. It also causes weight gain, but usually less than other antipsychotic drugs like clozapine, Zyprexa, and Seroquel.

Less Common Side Effects: Sedation, nausea, dizziness, constipation, and rapid heartbeat. There are a few reports of Risperdal causing compulsions or mania. A major question is whether Risperdal will produce the very serious neurological condition tardive dyskinesia (described on pages 230–231). Tardive dyskinesia involves involuntary movements that occur in 20 percent to 40 percent of patients who take the traditional antipsychotic drugs for prolonged periods of time (usually years). TD usually begins with movements of the mouth, lips, and tongue that the patients cannot control; these can also occur in other parts of the body, including the head, arms, legs, and trunk. Usually the movements go away if the drug is stopped, but in some cases they can become permanent. Studies have shown that the risk of TD with Risperdal is less than for the typical antipsycotics, but it still can happen. Therefore, it is important that patients be monitored for the emergence of any involuntary movements while taking Risperdal.

In elderly patients with dementia, there is a small but definite increased risk of death, usually from heart problems or infections.

What to Do About Side Effects: In general, side effects are mild with Risperdal when the dose is kept low. More common ones like headache, insomnia, anxiety, and runny nose are usually not severe enough to cause the patient to want to stop taking the drug. Patients can be given low doses of antianxiety drugs like Xanax (alprazolam) or Ativan (lorazepam) to combat anxiety and to help with sleep. There is little that can be done to prevent weight gain except to try and keep calorie intake as low as possible and get exercise. The best treatment for orthostatic hypotension (dizziness from a drop in blood pressure when getting up from a sitting or lying position) is to get up slowly and to drink plenty of fluids. The less common side effects are also usually not severe and can go away without any intervention. A patient who feels sleepy from Risperdal can try to lower the dose and take most of it at bedtime. Increase in heart rate is usually not serious and does not require any intervention, although the doctor should keep an eye on it by taking the patient's pulse from time to time.

If a patient does develop EPS side effects while taking Risperdal, the antidotes described in Table 26 on page 232 can be given. These include drugs like Cogentin (benztropine), Artane (trihexyphenidyl), and Symmetrel (amantadine).

The best thing to do about tardive dyskinesia is to watch for its development and stop the drug if at all possible if it appears. Again, we think that Risperdal has a low chance of causing tardive dyskinesia, but not a zero chance. A rating scale called the AIMS scale should be used on a regular basis to check the patient for early signs of TD.

The risk for death in elderly patients treated with Risperdal is mysterious and some experts doubt it is a real problem. However, studies are very clear that this occurs in a small percentage of patients (under 5 percent). Hence, the decision to put an elderly patient on Rispderal should be made only if agitation and/or psychotic symptoms are so severe that it would be inhumane not to. Then, the patient should be placed on the smallest possible dose for the shortest period of time and monitored carefully.

If It Doesn't Work: If a patient fails to respond to Risperdal, it is probably best to try a different antipsychotic drug. My impression is that some patients who don't get better with Risperdal may respond to another atypical antipsychotic drug, like Zyprexa, or to a typical drug, like Trilafon. However, many patients who do not get better with Risperdal won't respond to those drugs either and therefore become candidates for treatment with clozapine.

If It Does Work: Patients with schizophrenia need prolonged treatment to decrease the chance of relapse. Following a first psychotic episode, many clinicians stop the drug after about one year of remaining symptom free because there is a chance psychosis will never recur. After a second psychotic episode, however, patients with schizophrenia probably do best if treated for several years. After a third episode, lifelong therapy may be necessary, although it is a good idea to try and keep the dose of medication as low as possible. Many studies have shown that the chance of relapse and rehospitalization is substantially lowered when patients with schizophrenia continue to take their medicine. When Risperdal is used to treat adults with the manic phase of bipolar disorder or psychotic depression, it is usually discontinued when mood stabilizers in the former case or antidepressants in the latter begin to work. When treating children with Tourette's syndrome or autism, there are as yet no clear guidelines for how to treat a patient with Risperdal, so the standard rule of as short a time as possible holds. As stated earlier, this is also especially the case when treating elderly patients with dementia.

Cost: No generic form of Risperdal or Risperdal Consta is available, so the drug is expensive. Risperdal M-Tabs are rarely necessary (most people can swallow a pill). Risperdal will be off patent in a year or two and then generic risperidone will become available and be cheaper. The manufacturer is already working on a "new and improved" version of Risperdal, which of course will be a patented drug and therefore more expensive than generic risperidone. Whether it will really be better than risperidone has been met with considerable skepticism but remains to be seen.

Special Comments: Risperdal was the second atypical antipsychotic drug introduced in the United States. Like the first atypical drug, clozapine, it has effects on both the dopamine and serotonin brain neurotransmitter systems. Also like clozapine, Risperdal produces relatively fewer side effects than the typical antipsychotics in most patients. Another very important aspect of atypical drugs is that they seem to treat both the positive and the negative symptoms of schizophrenia. The positive symptoms of schizophrenia, described on page 216, include hallucinations (like hearing voices), delusions (such as believing strangers are plotting to harm one), thought disorder (when thoughts and speech are so disorganized that one cannot communicate logically to others), and markedly disturbed behavior (like undressing in public). All of the traditional antipsychotic drugs are fairly effective at treating these positive symptoms. They are not good, however, at treating the negative symptoms, which often begin only years after the positive symptoms appear and may even be worsened by the traditional antipsychotic drugs. Negative symptoms include apathy, social withdrawal, and loss of motivation. Clozapine and Risperdal not only do not worsen negative symptoms, they appear to improve them. Hence, patients with prominent negative symptoms may be especially good candidates to receive Risperdal. Some studies also suggest that Risperdal improves the cognitive symptoms (mostly subtle memory deficits) in patients with schizophrenia, something again not helped by traditional typical antipsychotic medications.

There are important differences between Risperdal and clozapine. The use of clozapine is limited because patients must have a weekly or biweekly blood test to warn if they are about to develop the potentially fatal side effect called agranulocytosis that occurs in about 1 percent of patients. Risperdal does not cause agranulocytosis and therefore is obviously much safer than clozapine. On the other hand, clozapine has been shown to be effective in many patients (but by no means all) who fail to respond to any of the antispychotic drugs; this does not appear to be true for Risperdal. That is, a patient who does not respond to Haldol, Thorazine, Prolixin, or Stelazine may still respond to clozapine but will probably not respond to Risperdal. On the other hand, patients who do respond to Haldol, Thorazine, Prolixin, or Stelazine will probably also respond to Risperdal and have fewer side effects and fewer negative symptoms.

Because of this profile, and the fact that it causes less weight gain than Zyprexa or Seroquel, many clinicians now believe that Risperdal should be the first choice for treating patients with schizophrenia and should also be given to patients who respond to the traditional antipsychotic drugs but experience many side effects. On the other hand, if higher doses are needed to control symptoms, Risperdal can cause EPS at the same rate as the traditional drugs, a bigger problem than with any of the other atypical drugs. Risperdal Consta is the first and only depot formulation of an antipsychotic medication. For patients who cannot remember or are unwilling to take their medications and have frequent relapses, these every-other-week injections can be a terrific solution. However, there is no guarantee that the patient will return to the clinic or doctor's office to get the shot every two weeks. Also, Haldol Decanoate is cheaper and has to be injected only every four weeks. It is unclear whether Risperdal Consta works better or has fewer side effects than Haldol Decanoate and is therefore worth the extra cost, although patients do say that injections of Risperdal Consta are less painful. Unfortunately, the miserable American health care system has not figured out how to deliver depot antipsychotic medications to patients, so for some patients it is difficult to find a physician or nurse available to give them on a regular basis.

OLANZAPINE

Brand Names: Zyprexa, Zyprexa Zydis.

Used For: Schizophrenia and bipolar disorder (both acute mania and as a mood stabilizer). Also used to increase the effects of antidepressants for patients with depression or anxiety disorder when the response has been inadequate.

Do Not Use If: There are no absolute contraindications for olanzapine. However, patients who are obese or have a personal or family history of diabetes need to be very careful.

Tests to Take First: Weight and height should be recorded.

Tests to Take While You Are on It: A physical examination called the AIMS test should be performed by the psychiatrist or nurse practitioner at least every six months to detect early signs of tardive dyskinesia. Weight should be monitored monthly. In order to guard against diabetes, it is important to try to keep the patient's weight under control as much as possible. The risk for diabetes is greatest in people who gain a lot of weight and/or have a family history of diabetes. Checking the blood sugar level regularly is important.

Usual Dose: Patients are started on a single 10-mg tablet, usually at bedtime. This is the effective dose for most patients, although some people do better with 5 mg and some may need to go up to 30 mg to get the full benefit.

How Long Until It Works: Some decrease in psychotic symptoms, like hallucinations and delusions, may be seen in a matter of hours to days, but the full benefit may take several weeks. Zyprexa tends to have a fairly rapid calming effect, making it an attractive choice for very agitated patients.

Common Side Effects: Dizziness and sedation sometimes occur, but they usually do not last. Some patients complain about anticholinergic side effects like dry mouth and constipation, but these tend not to be severe. The biggest problem with Zyprexa is weight gain. Some patients gain forty or more pounds over the first few months, putting them at risk for all the complications of obesity.

Less Common Side Effects: There is a very small chance of a minor effect on the liver, but this is probably not of any real significance. As mentioned above, it is possible that olanzapine will cause tardive dyskinesia, but the risk of this is much less than with the older antipsychotic drugs like Haldol and Prolixin. The biggest worries are the complications of obesity, such as diabetes and heart disease. Also, in elderly patients with dementia there is an increased risk of death, usually due to heart problems or infections.

What to Do About Side Effects: The main side effect of concern is weight gain, about which there is not a lot that can be done. Diet and exercise will help. Sedation is usually not a major problem, and most patients find that by taking the drug at night there is not too much daytime sleepiness.

If It Doesn't Work: You will probably need to try a different antipsychotic drug. Risperidone is a possibility. Clozapine is another choice.

If It Does Work: The question of how long people with schizophrenia should stay on an antipsychotic medication has never been answered completely. Most say that after a first episode, it may be possible to try to stop the medication after six months to a year, but the risk of developing another psychotic episode is great. Because olanzapine is well tolerated and seems to have a very low risk for tardive dyskinesia, most doctors recommend that their patients with schizophrenia who respond to the medication stay on it for an indefinite period of time. However, severe weight gain may force a switch to a different drug.

Cost: Generic Zyprexa is not available and hence it is an expensive medication. Zyprexa Zydis is the melt-in-your-mouth version, also quite expensive.

Special Comments: Olanzapine was the third atypical antipsychotic drug introduced into the United States. It came out in 1996 and rapidly became neck and neck with Risperdal for the most popular medication for schizophrenia. It is also one of only a handful of drugs that are approved by FDA for maintenance treatment of bipolar disorder (that is, to prevent future highs and lows). It is similar in some ways to clozapine but does not cause the serious blood abnormality agranulocytosis; therefore, weekly blood monitoring is not required. It is very easy to prescribe—most patients need just one 10-mg pill a day. In the large National Institute of Mental Health CATIE study that compared antipsychotic drugs, Zyprexa did a bit better than the other atypicals and the typical drug Trilafon, but caused the most weight gain. When a patient first presents with psychosis or is very agitated, Zyprexa is a very attractive choice because it works quickly and well. However, after a few weeks, as the patient begins to gain a lot of weight, he or she may be sorry to be taking it. For this reason, I have a preference for Risperdal, but that is not shared by many psychiatrists.

QUETIAPINE

Brand Name: Seroquel.

Used For: Schizophrenia and acute mania in patients with bipolar disorder. Also often used as a sedative for very anxious patients with other psychiatric illnesses, like generalized anxiety disorder or depression.

Do Not Use If: There are no absolute contraindications for Quetiapine. However, patients who are obese or have a personal or family history of diabetes need to be very careful.

Tests to Take First: Weight and height should be recorded.

Tests to Take While You Are on It: A physical examination called the AIMS test should be performed by the psychiatrist or nurse practitioner at least every six months to detect early signs of tardive dyskinesia. Weight should be monitored monthly. In order to guard against diabetes, it is important to try to keep the patient's weight under control as much as possible. The risk for diabetes is greatest in people who gain a lot of weight and/or have a family history of diabetes. Checking the blood sugar level regularly is important.

Usual Dose: Seroquel lasts a relatively short time in the body (technically, it has a short half-life) and needs to be taken twice a day. Usually, it is started at 25 or 50 mg twice daily, but patients who are extremely agitated may be started at even higher doses. For schizophrenia, it usually takes at least 300 mg twice daily to work, and it can take a week or more to get the patient to that level. The highest dose is 800 mg a day, which requires that the patient take a 100-mg and 300-mg pill in the morning and the same thing in the evening. When it is used for its calming and sedative properties in patients with anxiety disorder or depression, much lower doses are usually used and it is often given only at night, with 100 or 200 mg generally being tops.

How Long Until It Works: Seroquel tends to have a fairly rapid calming effect, making it an attractive choice for very agitated patients. However, it can take a week or more to get to a therapeutic dose for patients with schizophrenia.

Common Side Effects: Seroquel is a very sedating drug, which is a benefit for very agitated patients or those with insomnia but difficult for others who find it makes them sleepy during the day. It can also cause dizziness, but this is usually transient. The biggest problem with Seroquel is weight gain. Some patients gain twenty or more pounds over the first few months, putting them at risk for all the complications of obesity.

Less Common Side Effects: As mentioned above, it is possible that quetiapine will cause tardive dyskinesia, but the risk of this is much less than with the older antipsychotic drugs like Haldol and Prolixin. The biggest worries are the complications of obesity, such as diabetes and heart disease. Also, in elderly patients with dementia there is an increased risk of death, usually due to heart problems or infections. Seroquel caused cataracts in animal studies during initial testing and therefore it is recommended that patients see an ophthalmologist every six months for an eye exam. However, cataract formation has not actually been seen in human patients.

What to Do About Side Effects: The main side effect of concern is weight gain, about which there is not a lot that can be done. Diet and exercise will help. Sedation can be a problem and some patients try to take more of the medication at bedtime than during the daytime, although this means that a smaller dose is at work during the day.

If It Doesn't Work: You will probably need to try a different antipsychotic drug. Risperidone and Zyprexa are possibilities. Clozapine is another choice.

If It Does Work: The question of how long people with schizophrenia should stay on an antipsychotic medication has never been answered completely. Most say that after a first episode, it may be possible to try to stop the medication after six months to a year, but the risk of developing another psychotic episode is great. Because quetiapine is generally well tolerated and seems to have a very low risk for tardive dyskinesia, most doctors recommend that their patients with schizophrenia who respond to the medication stay on it for an indefinite period of time. However, severe weight gain may force a switch to a different drug.

Cost: Generic Seroquel is not available and hence it is an expensive medication.

Special Comments: Seroquel is a very frequently prescribed drug, but although its first official indication was for schizophrenia, it is not often prescribed for it. This is because the need to titrate up to a high dose, the sedation, and the twice-a-day schedule make it difficult to get good effects for patients with schizophrenia. On the other hand, Seroquel's calming and sedating properties have led it to be an add-on drug, that is, a drug that is added on to other medications, often instead of sleeping pills like Ambien or Lunesta or antianxiety medications like Xanax and Klonopin. Physicians believe that Seroquel is less habit-forming than those drugs, although there is as yet no proof that this is true. Because of this belief, Seroquel is often prescribed to patients recovering from alcohol or drug addiction who get anxious or can't sleep. It is a very useful medication, although not so much for its originally intended purpose.

ZIPRASIDONE

Brand Name: Geodon.

Used For: Schizophrenia and the manic phase of bipolar disorder.

Do Not Use If: You have an abnormality on your electrocardiogram known as QT or QTc prolongation or you are taking medications known to cause this.

Tests to Take First: Weight and height should be recorded.

Tests to Take While You Are on It: A physical examination called the AIMS test should be performed by the psychiatrist or nurse practitioner at least every six months to detect early signs of tardive dyskinesia. Weight should be monitored monthly.

Usual Dose: Patients are usually started at 20 mg twice a day and then the dose can be increased as needed to a maximum of 80 mg twice daily. Geodon also comes in an injectable form for use in emergencies for very agitated or violent patients.

How Long Until It Works: Some decrease in psychotic symptoms, like hallucinations and delusions, may be seen in a matter of hours to days, but the full benefit may take several weeks, particularly if the dose needs to be titrated up, which it frequently does.

Common Side Effects: Dizziness, constipation, dry mouth, agitation and sedation sometimes occur, but they usually do not last. Weight gain is also possible, but it appears to be much less of a problem than with Zyprexa, Seroquel, and Risperdal.

Less Common Side Effects: As mentioned above, it is possible that ziprasidone will cause tardive dyskinesia, but the risk of this is much less than with the older antipsychotic drugs like Haldol and Prolixin. Also, in elderly patients with dementia there is said to be an increased risk of death, usually from heart problems or infections.

What to Do About Side Effects: Very few of the side effects of Geodon are severe and most go away on their own. Sometimes a reduction in dose is needed. If agitation is a problem, antianxiety drugs like Valium or Klonopin or the atypical antipsychotic drug Seroquel are sometimes added until it subsides.

If It Doesn't Work: You will probably need to try a different antipsychotic drug. Risperidone and Zyprexa are possibilities. Clozapine is another choice.

If It Does Work: The question of how long people with schizophrenia should stay on an antipsychotic medication has never been answered completely. Most say that after a first episode, it may be possible to try to stop the medication after six months to a year, but the risk of developing another psychotic episode is great. Because ziprasidone is well tolerated and seems to have a very low risk for weight gain or tardive dyskinesia, most doctors recommend that their patients with schizophrenia who respond to the medication stay on it for an indefinite period of time. For bipolar patients with mania, it is usually tapered and discontinued after the patient is calm and can be managed with mood stabilizers like lithium, Depakote, or Lamictal alone.

Cost: Generic Geodon is not available and hence it is an expensive medication.

Special Comments: Before approval by the FDA, some research studies suggested that Geodon might have a serious adverse effect on the heart, called QT or QTc prolongation. This can cause sudden death. The FDA held off approval until further tests were done; these revealed that Geodon does not seem to cause this problem to any significant extent. Moreover, it has not been a problem in the thousands of patients who have taken it since it was approved, so clinicians do not consider it a risk. Unfortunately, a competing drug company highlighted the issue even before Geodon was officially approved, scaring away many physicians. Now that the heart issue has been resolved, the major question about Geodon is how well it works. It has a very good side effect profile, so everyone would like it to work, but it does not seem to be as potent, at least until the dose gets to 80 mg twice a day, as either Zyprexa or Risperdal.

ARIPIPRAZOLE

Brand Name: Abilify.

Used For: Schizophrenia and bipolar disorder (both acute mania and as a mood stabilizer). It is sometimes added onto other antipsychotics in an attempt to reverse the weight gain that they cause.

Do Not Use If: There are no absolute contraindications for aripiprazole.

Tests to Take First: None are required.

Tests to Take While You Are on It: A physical examination called the

AIMS test should be performed by the psychiatrist or nurse practitioner at least every six months to detect early signs of tardive dyskinesia.

Usual Dose: Patients are started on a single 10- or 15-mg tablet, usually in the morning. This is the effective dose for many patients, although some people will do better at 30 mg a day.

How Long Until It Works: Some decrease in psychotic symptoms, like hallucinations and delusions, may be seen in a matter of hours to days, but the full benefit may take several weeks.

Common Side Effects: Headache, insomnia, and agitation can occur. In some people this is mild, in others it is quite bothersome.

Less Common Side Effects: As mentioned above, it is possible that aripiprazole will cause tardive dyskinesia, but the risk of this is much less than with the older antipsychotic drugs like Haldol and Prolixin.

What to Do About Side Effects: Lowering the dose can help. Sometimes a calming medication is needed, such as the atypical antipsychotic drug Seroquel or a benzodiazepine antianxiety drug like Klonopin.

If It Doesn't Work: You will probably need to try a different antipsychotic drug. Risperidone or Zyprexa are possibilities. Clozapine is another choice.

If It Does Work: The question of how long people with schizophrenia should stay on an antipsychotic medication has never been answered completely. Most say that after a first episode, it may be possible to try to stop the medication after six months to a year, but the risk of developing another psychotic episode is great. Because ziprasidone is well tolerated and seems to have a very low risk for weight gain or tardive dyskinesia, most doctors recommend that their patients with schizophrenia or bipolar disorder who respond to the medication stay on it for an indefinite period of time.

Cost: Generic Abilify is not available and hence it is an expensive medication.

Special Comments: Abilify has a unique mechanism of action. All of the previous antipsychotic medications, both typical and atypical, block the D2 receptor in the brain for the chemical dopamine. Abilify, on the other hand, actually stimulates the D2 receptor. Given the fact that studies have persistently shown that increasing dopamine activity in the brain *causes* psychosis, it seems counterintuitive that an antipsychotic drug should stimulate a dopamine receptor. The trick is that there is also evidence that if dopamine levels are too low, negative and cognitive symptoms may result. Animal studies suggest that Abilify increases dopamine activity when the brain's own dopamine activity is abnormally low and blocks dopamine activity when it is too high. At the same time, it, like Geodon, has a very favorable side effect profile compared to other atypicals, with very little weight gain or the neurological side effects called EPS. Once again, however, there are questions about effectiveness. Abilify tends to be an activating drug, so some patients get agitated from it, while others get better. It is very hard to predict for whom it will work, not work, or cause worsening. This is a very interesting drug that requires more time to know exactly where it fits in for the treatment of schizophrenia and bipolar disorder.

INVEGA (PALIPERIDONE)

Invega was just approved as the fourth edition of *The Essential Guide to Psychiatric Drugs* was nearing completion. Paliperidone is a metabolite of risperidone (Risperdal), which means that risperidone is turned into paliperidone by the liver. The unique property of Invega is that it is an extended release drug, which means it has to be taken only once a day, usually in the morning. The dose is 6 to 12 mg daily.

ON THE HORIZON

Pharmaceutical companies are very actively researching potential new ways to treat schizophrenia. One drug nearing FDA approval at the time this edition of *The Essential Guide to Psychiatric Drugs* was written is bifeprunox. Bifeprunox seems close to Abilify. Many companies are specifically targeting negative and cognitive symptoms, attempting to develop drugs that can be added on to current antipsychotics to improve those symptoms in addition to positive symptoms. It is too early to know how any of these will actually work, but it is encouraging that there is a tremendous amount of activity in the search for better ways to treat schizophrenia.

Chapter 11

Sleeping Pills

For most of us, about two-thirds of Americans, in fact, our only sleep problem is the morning alarm clock. We work and play hard, get tired at night, and can't wait to get into bed for a good night's sleep.

According to a recent survey, however, about one-third of Americans have some degree of insomnia—inability to get enough sleep—and almost one-fifth find the insomnia severe. People with insomnia often dread getting into bed, anticipating the long and lonely hours of lying awake, tossing and turning, and worrying. The most common serious effect of insomnia is daytime sleepiness or anxiety: If you cannot sleep well at night you probably will not function well during the day either. Other serious consequences include automobile and other accidents and poor performance in school or at work.

FACTS ABOUT SLEEP

Many myths about sleep need clarification. Some people believe, for example, that not sleeping will drive them crazy or cause severe physical damage. It is true that people who are kept awake for many days, as done in research experiments many years ago, do show bizarre mental behavior, like hearing and seeing things; however, the insomnia most people suffer from does not seriously harm the brain or the rest of the body. Insomnia is very unpleasant and disruptive but not life threatening. Unless, of course, you fall asleep at the wheel of your car.

People are said to need at least eight hours of sleep to function properly. This, too, is only partly true. Sleep requirements vary with age and among individuals. A newborn infant sleeps up to twenty hours a day, whereas young children may need ten to twelve hours to function well during the day. Basically, adults should sleep about one-third of the time.

Parents often tell their children that unless they get to bed on time and sleep through the night they won't grow to be big and strong. Interestingly, there may be some scientific truth to this statement. Growth hormone, a chemical messenger secreted by the pituitary gland in the brain, is typically produced in the largest amounts in growing children during the early phases of sleep each night. Although lack of sleep has not been shown to disturb growth, some parents (me included) feel they are on somewhat solid scientific ground when cajoling their children to bed by telling them sleep is needed for proper growth.

The adult's need to sleep is extremely variable and probably is determined by an internal clock located in the part of the brain called the hypothalamus. This internal clock is highly individualized; some people need ten hours of sleep and others do fine with just five. The times at which a person should go to bed and wake up also vary greatly; the internal clock may not be set in the same way as the real clock. For example, some people seem to have an internal clock that operates in a time zone different from the one in which they live. For these people, the day might start naturally when the alarm clock says 4 A.M., and by 8 P.M. they are tired and ready to sleep. If they are forced to stay in bed until 7 A.M. and remain awake until 11 P.M., they will spend three hours in the morning lying awake and three hours at night intolerably drowsy. For others, the internal clock may tick to a day that is shorter or longer than twenty-four hours. These people can become permanently out of sequence with social convention and may constantly feel tired.

Elderly people generally need and obtain less sleep than younger people. Furthermore, the sleep of older people is often routinely disrupted; a few hours of sleep are interrupted by a few hours of being awake several times through the night. This is normal, but many elderly people who have been taught for years that a person is "supposed" to sleep eight hours every night believe there is something wrong with them. They become so worried about sleep that their anxiety keeps them awake. Often, doctors place elderly people on sleeping pills when the proper action would be to reassure them that less sleep is normal with increasing age.

The proper amount of sleep for an adult is the amount that makes it possible to remain awake and alert during the day. That is usually somewhere between five and ten hours. No one should be treated for insomnia unless the failure to sleep at night results in an inability to function during the day.

The next myth about sleep has to do with dreaming. Some people think that dreaming is necessary for a night's sleep to be truly restful. Others think that too much dreaming means the sleep has been disturbed and too active to give the body a good rest.

In fact, there is little evidence that the amount of dreaming has anything to do with how restful a night's sleep actually is. Many psychiatric medications, including most antidepressants, reduce or even eliminate dreaming, but patients whose depression is cured by these drugs find the quality of their sleep much improved.

THE NORMAL STAGES OF SLEEP

Before discussing the remedies for insomnia, a characterization of normal sleep would be helpful. Normal sleep comprises two main phases: REM sleep and non-REM sleep. During the REM (rapid eye movements) phase, the sleeper's eyes dart back and forth. It is during this phase that dreaming occurs. The first REM period usually begins about ninety minutes after a person first falls asleep at night and lasts about ten minutes. As the night progresses, the REM periods typically grow longer and longer. That is why the alarm clock usually rings in the middle of a dream. Adults spend about 25 percent of the night in the REM phase.

The remaining 75 percent of the night is spent in the phase called non-REM sleep. Non-REM sleep is itself divided into four stages. Stages 3 and 4 are also called deep sleep. There is more deep sleep in the first half of the night than in the second half. For this reason, waking someone suddenly in the very early hours of the morning is especially disturbing; a person usually feels disoriented and confused if suddenly aroused from stage 3 or 4 sleep. When I was an intern, I learned that it was better to remain awake between one and three in the morning instead of getting a few minutes of sleep, because it is especially difficult to be alert and ready to work if awakened during those hours.

Two sleep disturbances can be understood on the basis of these different stages of sleep. *Nightmares* are bad dreams and occur only during the REM phase. *Night terrors* (or *pavor nocturnes*), on the other hand, usually affect young children; the sleeper suddenly awakens, feeling suffocated and terrified, but not in the middle of a dream. Night terrors occur during stages 3 and 4 of non-REM sleep. Nightmares may reflect daytime worries and fears; night terrors are probably a biological phenomenon and often require drug treatment.

Other sleep-related problems of childhood, like bed-wetting and sleepwalking, also occur during non-REM sleep and consequently have absolutely nothing to do with bad dreams.

CAUSES OF INSOMNIA

Insomnia is often a complex problem with several possible causes. Many people, perhaps reinforced by what they see on TV, think that reaching for a sleeping pill is the first thing to do if they cannot fall asleep. Taking a sleeping pill sounds so safe and people so badly want to sleep well at night that it may appear simple and harmless.

Now that I have described the different phases of sleep and the many highly individual variations in sleep behavior from person to person, it should be obvious that sleep patterns are a highly regulated physiological function controlled by very complex brain circuits. All sleeping pills, even those bought over-the-counter without a prescription, disrupt the normal patterns of sleep. Eventually, it becomes pill against brain as the sleep medication attempts to fend off the body's own sleep schedule. Sooner or later, the brain wins and a person who tries to take sleeping pills every night for several weeks may end up with the original problem: insomnia.

There are many situations in which sleeping pills, which doctors call hypnotics, are the only solution to disabling sleep problems. In those cases they should be prescribed and used as long as they are needed and continue to work. Before sleeping pills are prescribed, all other means of conquering insomnia should first be tried. Sleeping pills are a last resort but not a disastrous resort.

What are the possible causes of insomnia? They range from simple and seemingly obvious to some very obscure disorders that require special diagnostic equipment and skills. The following is what goes through the doctor's mind when a person complains that he or she cannot fall asleep or stay asleep through the night:

1. Nothing is wrong; the patient only *thinks* he can't sleep. It is hard to say why, but some people who claim they can't sleep are just simply mistaken. One way to show this is to ask the person to write down the time he gets into bed and then to make a mark on the paper every hour he remains awake after that. Surprisingly, many people come back a week later with blank space after the bedtimes they recorded. They have actually slept. Perhaps they had vivid dreams that made them feel they weren't sleeping, or maybe they thought it had taken longer than ten or fifteen minutes to fall

asleep. Whatever the reason, nothing is wrong here and the doctor should not prescribe or recommend sleeping pills.

2. The patient is temporarily worried about something. This is a leading cause of not being able to fall asleep. Once the lights are off, the room is quiet, and there are no distractions, an anxious person is left alone with her thoughts. If she is worried, she will not fall asleep. Then she will start to worry about not being able to fall asleep, and things will get worse. Worries can even wake a person up in the middle of the night. Surprisingly, many people are completely unaware that worries are keeping them awake at night. Simply pointing this out sometimes gives the patient an explanation for the insomnia and the problem disappears.

3. The patient has bad sleep habits. Some of these bad habits may seem obvious, but again it is surprising how often people overlook them and come to the doctor looking for sleeping pills. Drinking black coffee an hour before bedtime is almost guaranteed to keep you up. It is best to avoid any beverage containing caffeine up to three hours before bedtime. Other stimulants, like cold remedies and sinus tablets, can also cause insomnia and should be avoided right before bedtime if possible.

Another big mistake is to drink alcohol before bed. Alcohol will make you sleepy, but the effect is very short-lived. After two or three hours when the alcohol is eliminated from the body, there will occur a sudden, often jolting awakening. Then you will lie awake for an hour. It is best not to drink alcohol for several hours before going to bed. Exercise at night is tricky, too. Getting a good workout two or more hours before trying to sleep actually improves your chances of falling asleep, but exercising immediately before sleep often has the opposite effect. Immediately after exercising, a person is usually aroused and adrenaline is still pouring through the bloodstream. The doctor should take a history to learn what you eat, drink, and do in the evening and thus determine if some bad sleep habit is keeping you awake.

4. A bad sleep environment is less commonly a cause of insomnia, but of course the room in which you sleep should be quiet and at the proper temperature. If you wake up drenched in sweat every night, an internist might worry that you have tuberculosis, and a psychoanalyst may think you are suffering from nightmares; but it also could be that your bedroom is too warm.

5. Sleep changes with aging. As I mentioned earlier, it is perfectly normal for people to sleep less as they get beyond age sixty. Many older people do fine with just four or five hours of sleep. Often, they fall asleep with no difficulty and then wake up at 4 A.M. This is not abnormal and not dangerous.

The best remedy is to get out of bed and be active. Elderly people will find that they are alert and awake at 4 A.M. and can get a lot of reading done. Giving them sleeping pills to prolong their sleep in this case is almost guaranteed to produce daytime drowsiness and even more serious sleep disturbances.

6. I recall one patient who complained that he could not fall asleep until 2 A.M. I couldn't find any reason until I took a detailed history of his regular daily routine. It turned out that he took a two-hour nap every day after work. The problem at bedtime simply was that he wasn't sleepy. Sleeping during the day often makes it impossible to fall asleep at a "conventional" bedtime. Either eliminate the naps or don't try to fall asleep at night until you really feel tired.

7. Sleeping pills themselves can be the cause of insomnia. Here's how it works: You can't fall asleep for a few nights for whatever reason. So you buy over-the-counter sleeping pills or take some Valium from the medicine cabinet. You sleep fine for a week. Then the effect starts wearing off, so you take a second sleeping pill in the middle of the night when you wake up. Soon, your body becomes trained to expect a middle-of-the-night sleeping pill and you automatically wake up for it. Before long, you awaken regularly several times through the night. You tell the doctor that you can't sleep "even though I am taking sleeping pills." The real danger here is that you and your doctor become misled into thinking that the insomnia is so bad it is breaking through the sleeping pills, and you both conclude incorrectly that stronger sleeping pills are needed. In fact, sleeping pills often disrupt a normal sleep cycle and therefore cause insomnia. The only solution is to bite the bullet, taper off the sleeping pills, and suffer a few sleepless nights. This allows the body to reestablish its own normal sleep schedule.

8. Many medical disorders specifically worsen at night and disrupt sleep, for example, congestive heart failure and some respiratory (breathing) disorders. Even a bad cold or hay fever can disrupt sleep; when a person lies down, postnasal drip worsens and induces more coughing. Also, a stuffy nose may cause otherwise reasonable people to worry that they will quietly suffocate in the middle of the night. Many of these problems are relieved by sleeping with three or four pillows so the head is propped up and by keeping the room well humidified. Sleeping pills are sometimes advisable, but careful monitoring is needed for people with serious medical problems.

9. Almost all psychiatric illnesses produce insomnia. One of the cardinal symptoms of depression, for example, is inability to sleep through the night. People with major depressive disorder commonly exhibit early-morning awakening. Anxiety disorders usually make it very difficult to fall asleep.

Manic patients feel they don't need sleep at all. A careful psychiatric history often reveals a psychiatric problem requiring treatment to be the cause of the sleep disturbance.

The best treatment for insomnia in these cases is treatment of the underlying psychiatric problem. Short-term use of sleeping pills, however, is often recommended because the psychiatric treatment may take a few weeks to be effective. For example, if a diagnosis of depression is established and an antidepressant recommended, it may be four to six weeks before the medication works to relieve the depression and therefore reverse the insomnia. There is nothing wrong in prescribing sleeping pills for that waiting period. It is still best to avoid taking them every night so that it is easy to stop use once the antidepressant starts to work.

What if you and the doctor cannot find any obvious reason for insomnia, like minor worries or bad habits, and no medical or psychiatric illness exists? More and more often, patients with long-standing insomnia who fall into this category are being referred to sleep laboratories for a full evaluation. Sleep laboratories are cropping up in many medical centers and hospitals. Essentially, these laboratories give doctors an opportunity to fully evaluate a patient's sleep patterns. You usually must sleep in the laboratory two or three nights. During that time, a trained sleep technician records and videotapes the amount of time you remain awake, unusual body movements during sleep, and all nighttime awakenings. A continuous recording of brain waves (electroencephalogram, or EEG) is made to determine how much time you spend in each stage of sleep. Breathing patterns during sleep are also recorded. Many health insurance plans now reimburse patients for the cost of a full sleep laboratory evaluation.

Several disorders can be detected in the sleep laboratory. *Nocturnal myoclonus* is a condition in which the body suddenly undergoes involuntary jerking movements in the middle of the night. This movement will awaken the person with a start and may disrupt sleep several times throughout the night. The patient almost always feels tired during the day because of this sleep disruption. Patients with *sleep apnea* actually stop breathing during sleep and wake up immediately. Often, the patient is unaware that he has awakened ten or twenty times during the night because each awakening lasts only seconds. But he has the impression that he did not sleep well the next morning and feels tired all day. Patients with sleep apnea often snore at night and suffer from headaches when they wake up in the morning. It is most common in obese men. Conditions such as nocturnal myoclonus and sleep apnea cause insomnia, can usually be diagnosed only in a sleep laboratory, and require specialized medical treatment. A sleep laboratory evaluation can also detect those people whose biological clock is not synchronized with the real time clock. Such people may think it is nighttime at 12 noon and time to wake up at 1 A.M. Sleep experts have worked out a complex but often successful treatment that resets the biological clock more in line with the conventional clock.

Sometimes, however, the sleep laboratory evaluation reveals only what the patient knew all along—he can't fall asleep or stay asleep. No cause is found and no specialized treatment is recommended. In this case, sleeping pills may be the only treatment that works. (Table 28 summarizes the preceding points.)

The reason I have explained how sleep works and what causes insomnia is to make it clear that sleeping pills are always the last resort. In other chapters I encouraged the reader to view psychiatric medication as not dangerous and often beneficial; however, sleeping pills are clearly overprescribed in this country and often cause more harm than good. It is so easy to take a pill to

---

Table 28.

Ten Causes of Insomnia

1. Nothing	The patient only thinks he or she is not sleeping at night.
2. Minor worries	
3. Bad sleep habits	Ingestion of alcohol or stimulants or exercising immediately before bedtime.
4. Bad sleep environment	Excessive noise, increased or decreased temperature.
5. Aging	Older people normally do not sleep as much.
6. Daytime napping	A person cannot sleep if he or she isn't sleepy.
7. Sleeping pills	Interrupt the normal sleep cycle and may cause insomnia.
8. Medical illness	Even colds.
9. Psychiatric illness	Most psychiatric problems cause insomnia.
10. Sleep disorders	Diagnosis may require a few nights in a sleep laboratory.

fall asleep that many patients and doctors do not bother to find the cause of the insomnia, resulting in two new problems. First, the patient may never have the opportunity to find out what is wrong, such as some unnecessary worries or a psychiatric illness and, therefore, will never get proper treatment. Second, almost all sleeping pills are habit-forming. The body becomes conditioned to their use and eventually refuses to sleep without them. People then have trouble stopping sleeping pills because each time an attempt is made, the insomnia is worse than it was initially. I feel strongly that sleeping pills should be prescribed only if no other solution is possible.

NONDRUG SOLUTIONS FOR INSOMNIA

What solutions can be offered for insomnia other than drugs? Studies have shown that psychological interventions based on cognitive and behavioral therapy principles can be very helpful. This is sometimes called "sleep hygiene therapy." Some of the elements:

1. If you can't fall asleep, don't stay in bed worrying about it. Get up, go into a different room, do something else for a while, and try again. There is a good chance that eventually your brain and body will get it together and you will finally fall asleep.

2. The bedroom should be reserved for two things: sex and sleeping. If you can't sleep at night, don't nap during the day. This only results in more nighttime insomnia.

3. Don't drink alcohol or caffeinated beverages, take stimulant medications like cold remedies, or exercise vigorously less than two or three hours before bedtime.

4. Make sure your bedroom is quiet and not too hot or cold. Use a blanket or fan. Insulate your room against noise. Use a white noise machine if necessary.

5. Force yourself to put your worries out of your mind when you get into bed. Tell yourself that you can't do anything at midnight, so you might as well get some rest and be ready to tackle your worries in the morning. Most of the time, the worries seem a lot less important the next day. (See Table 29.)

If you still have insomnia despite your best efforts at improved sleep "hygiene," definitely consult your doctor. He or she should take a general

Table 29.

Before You Take Sleeping Pills for Insomnia

1. Remember, insomnia will not hurt you physically or mentally. It can, however, worsen your job or school performance and increase your risk for car and other types of accidents.
2. Do not take naps during the day so you will be sleepy at night.
3. Stop taking alcohol, stimulants, or caffeine and stop exercising three hours before bedtime.
4. Make your bedroom as quiet and as comfortable (not too hot or cold) as possible.
5. Try to get all your worries taken care of before you lie down.

medical history, perform a physical examination, and get laboratory tests if indicated.

What if your family doctor wants to prescribe a sleeping pill? Or what if the doctor says nothing is wrong but tells you it is all right to take an over-the-counter sleeping pill?

I certainly do not claim that no one should ever take a sleeping pill without first consulting a psychiatrist. There aren't enough psychiatrists in the United States to see all the people who think they should take a sleeping pill for a few nights. But there is a very good chance that the sleep problem represents an anxiety disorder or depression or some other psychiatric condition. So I advise two things. First, taking a sleeping pill for two or three nights with the doctor's advice won't hurt. Second, review the chapters in this book on depression, anxiety, and bipolar disorder (manic depression). Be honest with yourself. Is there any chance you are suffering from even a mild form of one of these disorders? If so, you should definitely see a psychiatrist before getting started on sleeping pills.

WHEN SHOULD SLEEPING PILLS BE TAKEN?

The reasons a person should take a sleeping pill can be summarized as follows:

1. You are temporarily under tremendous and unavoidable stress and your insomnia makes you so tired during the day that you cannot function

properly. This is making your life miserable and your problems worse. You have tried everything to relax and fall asleep, but nothing works. You know this stressful time will pass in a week or so, but in the meantime you absolutely have to get at least one good night's sleep. In this case, taking a sleeping pill for a few nights is probably a very wise choice. Take one and don't worry about it.

2. You are suffering from depression or anxiety disorder and your psychiatrist recently began a program of therapy and medication. However, it may be weeks before the treatment works and in the meantime you want to sleep at night. Once again, a few nights of sleeping pills won't hurt. You can stop taking them when the underlying psychiatric condition is relieved.

3. You are suffering from a chronic medical problem that regularly makes your nights miserable. You have thoroughly discussed this with your medical doctor, who knows your physical condition well and also knows all of the other drugs you are taking. It is decided that taking a sleeping pill a few nights per week will not make your medical condition any worse and may make you feel better. Patients suffering from terminal illnesses should almost always be given as much medication as they need to sleep at night.

4. You are suffering from a sleep disorder like nocturnal myoclonus, or you have chronic insomnia, that is, insomnia lasting months or years, and absolutely no cause has been found. In this case it may be necessary to use sleeping pills regularly.

Table 30.

Reasons to Take Sleeping Pills

- Severe stress produces insomnia and that nothing else can resolve.
- To relieve insomnia due to an underlying psychiatric disorder while waiting for treatment to work.
- A medical problem gets worse at night and keeps you awake.
- Chronic insomnia of unknown cause that no other remedy resolves.

TYPES OF SLEEPING PILLS

So far, I have used the term *sleeping pills* as if all drugs that make someone sleep are more or less the same. This is not true. There are different kinds of sleeping pills (Table 31).

Benzodiazepines and Related Drugs

Benzodiazepines are among the sleeping pills most commonly prescribed. This class also includes many of the drugs used to treat generalized anxiety disorder and panic disorder (discussed in Chapter 8). I am including in this category three very popular prescribed medications, Ambien (zolpidem), Sonata (zaleplon), and Lunesta (eszopiclone), that technically are not benzodiazepines. They have a chemical structure that is distinct from benzodiazepines but they bind to a receptor in the brain called the benzodiazepine receptor and hence have the same actions as the regular benzodiazepines. The four ordinary benzodiazepines sold specifically for insomnia are Dalmane (flurazepam), Restoril (temazepam), Halcion (triazolam), and ProSom (estazolam).

All drugs in this class decrease the amount of time it takes to fall asleep and increase the amount of total sleep time. They also suppress stage 4 sleep, the deepest sleep, and therefore usually eliminate such abnormal sleep events as night terrors and sleepwalking, which occur only in this stage of sleep.

Dependency may develop to benzodiazepines when taken for sleep. This means that your body becomes used to them and eventually requires them to fall asleep. Some people who discontinue benzodiazepines, especially after having taken them continuously for more than two weeks, experience rebound insomnia, that is, very bad insomnia usually lasting several nights, until a normal sleep pattern is reestablished. The longer the sleeping pills are continuously used, the more severe will be the rebound insomnia. For this reason, these sleeping pills should be used sparingly when possible. You should try to fall asleep on your own at least an hour before taking a benzodiazepine sleeping pill and should try not to take one every night.

Benzodiazepine sleeping pills are *not*, however, addicting. There is no physical craving, and no life-threatening events occur after discontinuation. Some patients with chronic insomnia wind up taking benzodiazepine sleeping pills more or less continuously. This is not medically harmful, although it may not work to resolve insomnia after several months. In general, benzodiazepine sleeping pills are safe and effective medications for insomnia, but they must be used judiciously and only under medical supervision.

The newer sleeping pills, Ambien, Sonata, and Lunesta, have surpassed the ordinary benzodiazepines in popularity. These three are thought by many to have lower risk of dependency, rebound anxiety, and rebound insomnia than the traditional benzodiazepine sleeping pills. Lunesta is approved by FDA for long-term treatment of insomnia. However, it is not clear that these three are free of these risks.

Over-the-Counter Sleeping Pills

Many drugs that do not require a doctor's prescription and are claimed to relieve insomnia are sold in drugstores, health food stores, and supermarkets. Some are simply vitamins and minerals that have no effect on sleep at all. They probably help a person sleep only if he or she is convinced that vitamins and minerals are good for the body and general health. I feel that if it is so easy to convince someone he can sleep at night, he probably doesn't need pills at all.

Most of the over-the-counter (that is, not requiring a prescription) sleep products contain antihistamines. These drugs, including Sominex, Nytol, and Nervine, will definitely produce sleepiness. Antihistamines are usually prescribed to relieve allergies and rashes, but long ago most of these drugs were noted to produce the side effect of drowsiness. This side effect, usually unwanted in treatment for hay fever or poison ivy, was exploited by drug companies in formulating over-the-counter sleeping pills. Actually, I think these over-the-counter sleeping pills have more side effects and are less effective than benzodiazepine sleeping pills. Furthermore, if taken several weeks in a row to combat insomnia, they are just as likely to become habit-forming. In general, therefore, I feel that over-the-counter sleeping pills should be avoided. If medication is needed, prescription medication is usually superior.

Melatonin

A relatively new drug, Rozerem (ramelteon), stimulates the receptor in the brain to which melatonin binds. Melatonin is a hormone naturally secreted by the pineal gland during sleep. Exposure to light shuts off pineal gland production of melatonin. It is clear that melatonin makes many people sleepy when taken as a pill. Consequently, melatonin itself, which does not require a prescription and has been sold for many years in health food stores, is now used by many people to treat jet lag and insomnia. Does it work?

This is hard to know for sure because melatonin has never been subjected to the rigorous testing that is required for a new prescription medicine. One study failed to find any benefit for melatonin in the treatment of jet lag. The effectiveness of melatonin is largely word of mouth, which means it could all be a placebo effect. Is it safe? Melatonin does not appear to be dangerous and we have not received any horror stories about it yet, but keep in mind again that it has not been rigorously tested in a medical setting. We do not know, for example, if large doses of melatonin interact badly with other drugs, like antihistamines or antidepressants. My recommendation is that it is probably okay to try it for people who are not on other medications and do not have psychiatric illnesses like depression. It may not work as well as prescription sleeping pills or as well as the books about it say it does, but it is probably not harmful.

Rozerem, on the other hand, is a prescription medication. Its major advantage over benzodiazepine sleeping pills is that it seems to have no risk for dependency, withdrawal effects, or rebound anxiety. Because it is relatively new, the only thing I can say about its effectiveness is that it was sufficiently better than placebo in studies that convinced the FDA to approve it for insomnia. It may increase the risk for depression.

Prescription Antihistamines

Some antihistamines require a prescription and are occasionally prescribed for insomnia. These include Atarax and Vistaril. They are no different from the over-the-counter antihistamines like Sominex and Nytol.

Sedating Antidepressants

Several antidepressant drugs, especially Elavil (amitriptyline), Sinequan (doxepin), and Desyrel (trazodone), also make patients feel sleepy. This is usually regarded as an unwanted side effect, but low doses of these sedative antidepressant drugs, especially trazodone, are increasingly being prescribed for the treatment of insomnia. Although 50 mg of Elavil or Desyrel is too small a dose to treat depression, it will induce sleep in most people. There is some suggestion that sedative antidepressants are less habit-forming than benzodiazepine sleeping pills. Therefore, low doses of sedative antidepressants are often a good choice for a patient with chronic insomnia who requires long-term treatment. Desyrel is clearly the best choice. It has relatively few side effects (see Chapter 7 for a full discussion). Desyrel is sometimes prescribed to patients with depression who are taking one of the antidepressants like Prozac, Zoloft, Effexor, or Wellbutrin that sometimes cause insomnia. It is available in an inexpensive generic preparation. Its main drawback is that it has a long length of action in the body (that is, a long half-life), and therefore some patients complain about sleepiness during the day after taking it.

Sedating Antipsychotics

It was considered improper to use antipsychotic drugs just for insomnia until the newer atypical antipsychotic drugs became available. The old drugs carried the risk for the potentially permanent neurological problem tardive dyskinesia, but the new drugs have a much reduced risk for TD. Of the atypical antipsychotic drugs, Seroquel and Zyprexa are very sedating. Seroquel especially in low doses, between 25 and 100 mg at bedtime, can be used for patients with bipolar or anxiety disorders who cannot sleep. It has a short length of action in the body and therefore does not usually cause sleepiness the next day. It is not habit-forming and there are no withdrawal effects. However, it is prone to causing significant weight gain and therefore may not be a good choice for long-term use. A longer description of Seroquel can be found in the chapter on treating schizophrenia.

Other Sleeping Pills

A large number of prescription sleep medications should generally be avoided, even though they can still be legally prescribed. These drugs are not described individually in the next section because there is almost no instance in which they should be administered, and doctors who prescribe them should become better informed. These medications include barbiturates like phenobarbital and Seconal (although barbiturates may have other legitimate uses besides sedation), Noludar, Placidyl, and Doriden. Chloral hydrate is a sleeping medication sometimes properly used for hospitalized psychiatric patients, but it has little use in the treatment of insomnia in outpatients.

If drugs are to be prescribed, the best choices for short-term treatment are probably trazodone (Desyrel), Ambien, Lunesta, or possibly Rozerem. For longer-term use, Desyrel and sometimes Seroquel (quetiapine), are good choices, although for many people chronic use of Ambien or Lunesta is the best treatment. A new drug to treat insomnia, Indiplon, was given tentative approval by the FDA in 2006. With some changes to the label (information and prescribing information for physicians), Indiplon–immediate release will probably get final approval and be available for prescription sometime in

2007. The medication belongs to a new class of sedative medications that is not related to the benzodiazepines. An extended-release formulation of Indiplon, however, raised safety and effectiveness concerns and the FDA did not grant tentative approval. Because Indiplon is so new and not yet prescribable, it is not possible to give guidelines for it yet.

Follow these six rules with respect to sleeping pills:

1. Don't take them if there is another way to treat your sleep problem.

2. Don't take over-the-counter drugs more than once or twice. If you need sleeping pills longer than this, see your doctor.

3. If Ambien, Sonata, Lunesta, or a benzodiazepine sleeping pill is prescribed, take the lowest dose effective for the fewest number of nights possible. Always try to fall asleep before you take the pill and try to skip nights.

4. A low dose of a sedative antidepressant such as Desyrel should be considered for long-term treatment of insomnia.

Table 31.

Drugs for Insomnia

Benzodiazepine sleeping pills	Dalmane, Restoril, Halcion, ProSom
Ambien, Ambien CR, Sonata, Lunesta	
Over-the-counter sleeping pills	Nervine, Nytol, Sleep-Eze, Sleepinal, Sominex, Unisom, and others
Melatonin	Rozerem
Prescription antihistamines	Vistaril, Atarax
Sedating antidepressants	Elavil, Desyrel, Sinequan, Adapin
Sedating antipsychotics	Seroquel, Zyprexa
Drugs to avoid for insomnia	Doriden, Noludar, Seconal, phenobarbital, chloral hydrate, Placidyl

5. Generally, it is safe to take sleeping pills if you are on other psychiatric medication, as long as you do so under medical supervision.

6. If you are taking sleeping pills, do not drink alcoholic beverages.

Do not let anyone make you feel guilty about taking a sleeping pill. Sleeping pills may not always work, but they are generally safe. Certainly, it is better to take a sleeping pill than to get drunk to sleep or to be so sleep deprived that you crack up your car.

TREATMENT OF JET LAG

Before describing each individual sleeping pill, a word about a popular use for sleeping pills is in order. Many people now use sleeping pills to treat jet lag. The idea here is simple: If you have to fly from one time zone to the next, why not take a sleeping pill to help you sleep in the new time zone? This should help you adjust to the new time zone more quickly. Or, if you are flying overnight, why not take a sleeping pill on the plane and sleep through the trip? You will be wide awake when the plane lands in the morning at your destination.

This type of use makes some doctors uncomfortable, because it represents the use of medication for a "nonillness." Jet lag is not a medical disorder and people should not be encouraged to take medicine under these conditions.

There probably is no harm in taking a short-acting sleeping pill, like Ambien, Sonata, or Lunesta, for this purpose. I have heard several anecdotes of people who missed the next plane connection because they forgot where they were going after taking a sleeping pill on the first part of their trip. Personally, I think these stories are somewhat exaggerated. In general, it is safe to take a sleeping pill for the "red eye" or "jet lag," but a doctor may be uncomfortable prescribing one specifically for that purpose.

DRUGS USED TO TREAT INSOMNIA

There are five types of drugs in this section: benzodiazepines, the newer benzodiazepinelike drugs (Ambien, Sonata, and Lunesta), over-the-counter drugs, prescription antihistamines, and Rozerem.

Information about Desyrel (trazodone) can be found in the chapter on antidepressants and about Seroquel (quetiapine) in the chapter on antpsychotics.

Benzodiazepine Sleeping Pills

FLURAZEPAM

Brand Name: Dalmane.

Used For: Insomnia.

Do Not Use If: You have a history of addiction to drugs or alcohol or if you think your doctor has overlooked the cause of your sleeping problem.

Tests to Take First: None required.

Tests to Take While You Are on It: None required.

Usual Dose: Most people take one 30-mg capsule about thirty minutes before going to sleep. Elderly people should try to take half that dose (15 mg) to see if it works.

How Long Until It Works: You should fall asleep about a half hour after taking Dalmane. The drug remains effective if taken every night for at least a month and in many people continues to be effective in inducing sleep indefinitely.

Common Side Effects: You may be drowsy the day after because Dalmane has a very long length of action and remains in the body at least a day. You may experience withdrawal symptoms after taking Dalmane nightly for several weeks and then stopping it. The withdrawal syndrome includes anxiety, restlessness, sweating, and insomnia, and is very severe in some people and not so bad in others. It always goes away by itself but can last as long as two weeks. It is not life threatening but can be very disturbing and uncomfortable.

Less Common Side Effects: Elderly people who take Dalmane, particularly for several weeks, may experience dizziness, confusion, and unsteadiness when they walk. Falls have occurred.

What to Do About Side Effects: If Dalmane makes you feel too sleepy the next day, it is probably better to switch to one of the shorter-acting sleeping pills, like Ambien, Sonata, or Lunesta. To avoid a withdrawal syndrome, it is best not to take Dalmane every night for longer than two weeks. Always try to skip a night here and there and test yourself before taking it by attempting to sleep without it at least one hour before reaching for the pill. Some people with insomnia are surprised to find the pill still on the night table the next morning. Sleeping pills should be given very carefully to elderly people. The presence of very serious pain or medical problems that make insomnia insurmountable by any other remedy are valid reasons to give an elderly person small doses of sleep medication. Elderly people who take Dalmane should be cautioned to get out of bed the next day very slowly and to sit down if they have the slightest sensation of dizziness or unsteadiness. Elderly people with low blood pressure, poor eyesight, or medical problems that make them weak are especially likely to fall if they take sleeping pills. Sleeping pills should be given only with the greatest of care to people with past or present history of alcohol or drug abuse or older people without very strict medical supervision.

If It Doesn't Work: If you cannot fall asleep even after you take Dalmane, it is unlikely that any other sleeping pill will do much better, although one of the newer sleeping pills is worth trying. Staying awake even after you have taken a drug like Dalmane should alert you that there is a cause of your insomnia that is being overlooked and that a sleeping pill can't cure. You should ask your doctor to refer you to a sleep disorder expert.

If It Works: After you have had a few nights of good sleep, try doing without the pill. An occasional restless night is preferable to getting dependent on sleeping pills.

Cost: Generic flurazepam is as safe and effective as brand-name Dalmane and less expensive.

Special Comments: Dalmane was the first of the benzodiazepine sleeping pills introduced onto the American market. It is chemically related to other benzodiazepine drugs described in Chapter 8, like Valium and Xanax that are used to treat anxiety disorder. Dalmane is very safe and highly effective in treating insomnia. It can be used to relieve insomnia experienced by people with depression while they wait for the antidepressant to work. It can also be used to treat a wide variety of sleep problems, including insomnia caused by stress and worry. The major drawback is that, like any sleeping pill, it is habit-forming. Your body will come to depend on Dalmane to fall asleep, so that if you take it a long time and then stop, your insomnia may be even worse than it was originally. It should be used judiciously and as sparingly as possible.

TEMAZEPAM

Brand Name: Restoril.

Used For: Insomnia.

Do Not Use If: You have a history of drug or alcohol addiction or if you think your doctor may have overlooked the cause of your insomnia.

Tests to Take First: None required.

Tests to Take While You Are on It: None required.

Usual Dose: Most people take one 30-mg capsule about an hour before bedtime. Elderly people should take 15 mg and see if it works. Patients should not take more than 30 mg at night except in very special circumstances under medical supervision.

How Long Until It Works: You should fall asleep an hour after taking Restoril. The drug remains effective if taken every night for about one month, and longer in most people, but it is always best to avoid taking it every night.

Common Side Effects: You may feel drowsy the next day, but Restoril is shorter acting than Dalmane so this is less of a problem. After taking Restoril night after night for many weeks and then stopping it, you will probably experience a withdrawal syndrome, characterized by anxiety, insomnia, restlessness, and sweating. This is uncomfortable but not medically dangerous. It will go away by itself but can last up to two weeks. Some people may feel anxious the next day after taking Restoril.

Less Common Side Effects: Elderly people who take sleeping pills like Restoril may experience dizziness, confusion, and unsteadiness when they walk. Falls may result.

What to Do About Side Effects: If Restoril makes you feel sleepy during the day, you might switch to an even shorter-acting pill, like Ambien, Sonata, or Lunesta. The best way to minimize withdrawal symptoms is never to get into the habit of taking Restoril every night for more than a few nights in a row. Suffering through a sleepless night here and there is better than getting hooked on a sleeping pill. People who feel anxious the day after taking Restoril should switch to a different drug. Sleeping pills like Restoril should be given with great caution to elderly people, who may become confused and disoriented when given the drug for prolonged periods.

If It Doesn't Work: If Restoril doesn't help you to sleep, it is unlikely any sleeping pill will do much better, although switching to a newer drug like Ambien or Lunesta is worth trying. Do not increase the dose. It is better to ask your doctor to refer you to a specialist in sleep disorders and to consider the possibility that there is a reason for your insomnia that cannot be resolved by a sleeping pill.

If It Does Work: After you have slept two or three nights, try taking at least a night off from the pill. Remember, insomnia is unpleasant but usually not dangerous, and staying awake is better than getting dependent on sleeping pills.

Cost: Generic temazepam is as safe and effective as brand name Restoril and cheaper.

Special Comments: Restoril is intermediate between Dalmane and Halcion in its length of action. The drug remains active about twelve hours, not as long as Dalmane but longer than Halcion. Originally, there were problems with the capsule material that Restoril was packaged in and the drug was not absorbed rapidly into the blood. This meant that it took hours for a patient to fall asleep. This problem has been corrected and Restoril now works about as rapidly as Dalmane to induce sleep. It is medically safe and does not become habit-forming until taken every night for several weeks. Restoril, like all sleeping pills, is likely to be more habit-forming in alcoholics and people with drug abuse problems. They should be given Restoril only in special circumstances and then only under strict medical supervision.

TRIAZOLAM

Brand Name: Halcion.

Used For: Insomnia.

Do Not Use If: You have history of addiction to drugs or alcohol or if you think your doctor has overlooked the reason for your insomnia. Halcion has interactions with some other drugs, so be sure your doctor knows everything else you are taking, including over-the-counter medications. Grapefruit juice may increase blood levels of Halcion.

Tests to Take First: None required.

Tests to Take While You Are on It: None required.

Usual Dose: Most people will fall asleep after taking a single tablet of 0.125 mg.

How Long Until It Works: Halcion will make you fall asleep in less than thirty minutes.

Common Side Effects: Halcion is very powerful and the morning after taking it, some people find that they have forgotten what happened the night before and are a bit disoriented or even irritable. The drug does not produce permanent memory loss or brain damage as far as is known, and not everyone experiences the effect on memory. Also, some of the memory problems probably arose in persons who took the 0.5-mg dose of Halcion. This dose has been discontinued by the manufacturer and the recommended top dose is 0.125 mg. After taking Halcion every night for several weeks and then stopping it, you will probably experience some degree of withdrawal syndrome, the most pronounced component of which is rebound insomnia. Your body will become so used to sleeping with Halcion that it will refuse to sleep without it. You may also experience some anxiety and restlessness. None of this is dangerous to your health, and the withdrawal syndrome will go away on its own, although it may take a few days if you have been taking Halcion nightly for many months. Some people feel anxious the morning after taking Halcion.

Less Common Side Effects: Daytime drowsiness is uncommon because Halcion is so short acting and is eliminated from the body by the next morning. Elderly people are prone to develop confusion, dizziness, disorientation, and unsteadiness when they walk if given Halcion or any other sleeping pill.

What to Do About Side Effects: If memory problems occur after taking Halcion or any other sleeping pill, the medication should be discontinued. The best way to avoid a withdrawal syndrome is not to take Halcion too many nights in a row. Always give your body a chance to reestablish its normal rhythm. You may find that after a night or two of taking Halcion you will be able to sleep just fine without it. Try very hard not to convince yourself that the only way you will ever fall asleep is to take the pill. Your body might start to believe you. Elderly people should never be given sleeping pills if it can be avoided, and if they do take Halcion, they should be cautioned about the possibility of dizziness or confusion. Medical supervision is always necessary.

If It Doesn't Work: It is unlikely that another sleeping pill will be much better. You should consider the possibility that your insomnia cannot be resolved with sleeping pills. A referral to a sleep disorder specialist might be considered. Above all, do not take extra pills if one doesn't help.

If It Does Work: Always try to skip some nights. Get into bed first and give yourself at least an hour before reaching for the pill. A night of insomnia once in a while is better than getting hooked on sleeping pills.

Cost: Generic triazolam is just as safe and effective as brand-name Halcion and cheaper.

Special Comments: Halcion is the shortest-acting and most powerful sleeping pill available. Because it is short acting, it is almost completely eliminated from the body by the next morning and therefore is unlikely to cause a hangover. It is medically safe and very effective. Some people take it on airplanes so they can sleep and prevent jet lag. The memory loss attributed to Halcion involves events that occur in the hours after the drug is taken. Halcion does not cause brain damage. It is important to avoid taking it every night without a break.

ESTAZOLAM

Brand Name: ProSom.

Used For: Insomnia.

Do Not Use If: You have a problem with drug or alcohol abuse unless your doctor is well informed of this.

Tests to Take First: None needed.

Tests to Take While You Are on It: None needed.

Usual Dose: Most people take a 1-mg or 2-mg tablet before going to bed. Elderly people may do best with 0.5 mg.

How Long Until It Works: You should fall asleep in about an hour or less after taking ProSom.

Common Side Effects: Some people feel sleepy the day after taking ProSom. If taken for too many nights in a row and then stopped, insomnia may be worse than before taking ProSom.

Less Common Side Effects: Some people feel anxious the day after ProSom has worn off and others feel dizzy.

What to Do About Side Effects: If you feel sleepy or dizzy the next day, try taking a lower dose of ProSom. Most important, sleeping pills like ProSom should not be taken every night for weeks in a row.

If It Doesn't Work: You will probably need to try a different sleeping pill, such as Ambien or trazodone.

If It Does Work: It is best not to use sleeping pills every night for longer than a week or two. Longer continuous use sometimes leads to tolerance, which means the drug stops working and you won't fall asleep even if you take it. Also, you may become dependent on a sleeping pill like ProSom, and then when you stop it your insomnia will be worse than it was in the first place.

Cost: Generic estazolam is as safe and effective as brand-name ProSom and cheaper.

Special Comments: For some reason, ProSom never caught on as a sleeping pill. This is unfortunate because in many ways it is the best of the benzodiazepine-type sleeping pills, which include Dalmane, Restoril, and Halcion. It has a good length of action so that most people do not feel sleepy the next day. It is safe and effective. Its lack of popularity is hard to understand, but it is now a moot point with the increasing popularity of Ambien and Lunesta as the sleeping pills of choice for most short-term insomnia problems.

ZOLPIDEM

Brand Names: Ambien, Ambien CR.

Used For: Insomnia.

Do Not Use If: You have a problem with drug abuse, particularly alcoholism. Some physicians will still be able to prescribe Ambien for you, but only in certain circumstances.

Tests to Take First: None needed.

Tests to Take While You Are on It: None needed.

Usual Dose: One 10-mg pill taken before bedtime. Elderly people may do better with a 5-mg pill instead. Ambien CR is usually effective with one 12.5-mg dose, with elderly people doing better on 6.25 mg.

How Long Until It Works: You should fall asleep in less than an hour after taking it.

Common Side Effects: Feeling sleepy the next day.

Less Common Side Effects: If you take it during the day and don't go to bed, you may forget things that happen to you after you take the pill. Diarrhea is an unusual side effect. There have been reports of people binge eating during the night after taking Ambien.

What to Do About Side Effects: Most people tolerate Ambien very well and have no problem with side effects. If you do feel drowsy or dizzy the next day, the lower dose (5 mg) may be a good idea. Binge eating during the night means the drug is not working properly and you should probably try a different approach to insomnia.

If It Doesn't Work: You may need to try a different medication, either trazodone or one of the older benzodiazepine sleeping pills like ProSom, Restoril, or Dalmane.

If It Does Work: In general, it is not a great idea to take sleeping pills every night for an indefinite period of time. After five to seven days of sleeping pill use, it is best to try to see if you can sleep without it. There is always a risk of becoming dependent on sleeping pills, including Ambien. However, Ambien has been shown to continue to work for long periods of time, and Ambien CR is approved by the FDA for "sleep maintenance," meaning longer use than just a week or two. Hence, for severe insomnia for which no other solutions have worked, it is possible to continue to use Ambien for prolonged periods of time.

Cost: Generic forms of Ambien and Ambien CR are not available, so the drug is expensive.

Special Comments: Strictly speaking, Ambien is not a benzodiazepine like Dalmane and Halcion. However, even though its chemical structure is different from the benzodiazepines, it still binds to the same brain receptors as these drugs. Hence, in many ways it is really the same kind of drug as Restoril or ProSom or Dalmane. Ambien has many attractive features as a sleeping pill. It does not last very long in the body and consequently most people do not feel sleepy the day after. There is also very little rebound effect so that patients do not feel anxious the next day and also do not find they have even worse sleep problems after stopping Ambien than they did before trying it. For the short-term treatment of insomnia, Ambien, along with Lunesta, has clearly become the preferred medication and should usually be prescribed instead of the older benzodiazepine drugs. For longer-term problems, it may still be useful, although many clinicians prefer trazodone for this situation. Ambien CR supposedly gives a "smoother" onset and length of action, but many people think it was developed only because Ambien is about to go off patent and there will be competition from generics. It is hard to see a reason to prescribe Ambien CR instead of regular Ambien, especially when Ambien goes generic and becomes less expensive.

ZALEPLON

Brand Name: Sonata.

Used For: Insomnia.

Do Not Use If: You have a problem with drug abuse, particularly alcoholism. Some physicians will still prescribe Sonata for you, but only in certain circumstances.

Tests to Take First: None needed.

Tests to Take While You Are on It: None needed.

Usual Dose: One 5-mg pill taken before bedtime is usually sufficient, but some people will require 10 mg. Elderly people may do better with a 5-mg pill.

How Long Until It Works: You should fall asleep in less than an hour after taking it.

Common Side Effects: Feeling sleepy the next day.

Less Common Side Effects: If you take it during the day and don't go to bed, you may forget things that happen to you after you take the pill. Diarrhea is an unusual side effect. There may be withdrawal effects after stopping Sonata if it has been taken for several weeks. These include insomnia, jitteriness, and agitation.

What to Do About Side Effects: Most people tolerate Sonata very well and have no problem with side effects. If you do feel drowsy or dizzy the next day, the lower dose (5 mg) may be a good idea.

If It Doesn't Work: You may need to try a different medication, such as Ambien, Lunesta, or trazodone, or one of the older benzodiazepine sleeping pills like ProSom, Restoril, or Dalmane.

If It Does Work: In general, it is not a great idea to take sleeping pills every night for an indefinite period of time. After five to seven days of sleeping pill use, it is best to try to see if you can sleep without it. There is always a risk of becoming dependent on sleeping pills, including Sonata. However, for severe insomnia for which no other solutions have worked, it is possible to continue to use Sonata for prolonged periods of time.

Cost: Generic forms of Sonata are not available, so the drug is expensive.

Special Comments: Strictly speaking, Sonata is not a benzodiazepine like Dalmane and Halcion. However, even though its chemical structure is different from the benzodiazepines, it still binds to the same brain receptors as these drugs. Hence, in many ways it is really the same kind of drug as Restoril or ProSom or Dalmane. Sonata has many attractive features as a sleeping pill. It does not last very long in the body, even shorter than Ambien, and consequently most people do not feel sleepy the day after taking Sonata. For unclear reasons, Sonata never caught on and is not often prescribed.

ESZOPICLONE

Brand Name: Lunesta.

Used For: Insomnia.

Do Not Use If: You have a problem with drug abuse, particularly alcoholism. Some physicians will still prescribe Lunesta for you, but only in certain circumstances.

Tests to Take First: None needed.

Tests to Take While You Are on It: None needed.

Usual Dose: 2–3 mg at bedtime is usually sufficient. Elderly people may do better with 1 mg.

How Long Until It Works: You should fall asleep in less than an hour after taking it.

Common Side Effects: Feeling sleepy the next day. Unpleasant taste in the mouth that lingers after the drug has been swallowed.

Less Common Side Effects: If you take it during the day and don't go to bed, you may forget things that happen to you after you take the pill.

What to Do About Side Effects: Most people tolerate Lunesta very well and have no problem with side effects. If you do feel drowsy or dizzy the next day, the lower dose (1 or 2 mg) may be a good idea. The unpleasant taste is annoying, but usually bearable and goes away in time. Some people find the taste is more bearable if Lunesta is taken with juice or milk instead of water.

If It Doesn't Work: You may need to try a different medication, either trazodone or Ambien, or one of the older benzodiazepine sleeping pills like ProSom, Restoril, or Dalmane.

If It Does Work: In general, it is not a great idea to take sleeping pills every night for an indefinite period of time, even though Lunesta is approved by the FDA for "sleep maintenance," meaning several months of continuous use. After five to seven days of sleeping pill use, it is best to try to see if you can sleep without it. There is always a risk of becoming dependent on sleeping pills, including Lunesta. Hence, for severe insomnia for which no other solutions have worked, it is possible to continue to use Lunesta for prolonged periods of time.

Cost: Generic forms of Lunesta are not available, so the drug is expensive.

Special Comments: Strictly speaking, Lunesta is not a benzodiazepine like Dalmane and Halcion. However, even though its chemical structure is different from the benzodiazepines, it still binds to the same brain receptors as these drugs. Hence, in many ways it is really the same kind of drug as Restoril or ProSom or Dalmane. Lunesta has many attractive features as a sleeping pill. It does not last very long in the body and consequently most people do not feel sleepy the day after. There is also very little rebound effect so that patients do not feel anxious the next day and also do not find they have even worse sleep problems after stopping Lunesta than they did before trying it. For the short-term treatment of insomnia, Lunesta and Ambien have clearly become the preferred medications and should usually be prescribed instead of the older benzodiazepine drugs. For longer-term problems, it may still be useful, although many clinicians prefer trazodone for this situation. The manufacturer of Lunesta has launched an aggressive "direct to consumer" advertising campaign and almost everyone has now seen the Lunesta butterfly on television. It is a good sleeping pill although not obviously better than Ambien, which will shortly become available in the less-expensive generic form.

Over-the-Counter Sleeping Pills

Brand Names: Excedrin PM, Miles Nervine, Nytol, Sleep-Eze, Sleepinal, Sominex, Unisom, Benadryl.

Used For: Insomnia.

Do Not Use If: You have an enlarged prostate gland, asthma, or glaucoma unless your doctor approves. Never take these drugs with alcohol.

Tests to Take First: None required.

Tests to Take While You Are on Them: None required.

Usual Dose: Read the label on the box or bottle. These sleeping pills do not require prescriptions.

How Long Until They Work: You should fall asleep within an hour.

Common Side Effects: Dizziness, disturbed coordination, stomachache, and thickening of the secretions normally found in your lungs.

Less Common Side Effects: Patients with narrow-angle glaucoma can get an attack after using some of these sleeping pills. Patients with an enlarged prostate gland or other problems with urination may find it very difficult to urinate. Confusion and disorientation.

What to Do About Side Effects: Never take more pills than recommended on the label, and do not use them more than one or two nights a month. If you experience dizziness or disturbed coordination, stop taking them immediately. Never give these to children without approval from your pediatrician.

If They Don't Work: Don't be surprised; my experience is that they frequently don't work. You may need to take a prescription sleeping pill like Ambien, Lunesta, or trazodone (Desyrel).

If They Do Work: If one of the over-the-counter sleeping pills does help you sleep, you should still use them sparingly. Your body will get used to them after a while and you will find that without them you won't be able to sleep at all. If you are taking them more than once or twice a month, call your doctor and get an evaluation.

Special Comments: These drugs represent one of the rare examples in this book of drugs for which a prescription is not required. Most of these sleeping pills contain the same chemical present in the antihistamine Benadryl (diphenhydramine). Antihistamines were developed to counteract allergic reactions, but many were quickly noted to have the annoying side effect of making the patient sleepy. That is why nonsedating antihistamines, like Claritin, were developed. This disadvantage was quickly turned into an advantage when drug companies realized they could sell these antihistamines as sleep aids without a prescription.

The fact that they do not require a prescription is their only advantage over prescription sleeping pills. Over-the-counter sleeping pills have side effects, frequently do not work, and are just as likely to become habit-forming as prescription sleeping pills. Once the body becomes used to the sleeping pill, it frequently refuses to sleep without it after it is discontinued. These sleeping pills should be taken infrequently. If you require more help to sleep, you should see a doctor anyway, and in most cases Ambien, Lunesta, trazodone (Desyrel), or a benzodiazepine sleeping pill is safer and more effective.

Prescription Antihistamines

Brand Names: Atarax (available only as the generic hydroxyzine), Vistaril (hydroxyzine), and others.

Used For: Treatment of allergies, insomnia.

Do Not Use If: You have just had an alcoholic beverage. If you have glaucoma, asthma, or an enlarged prostate, you should check with your doctor first.

Tests to Take First: None required.

Tests to Take While You Are on Them: None required.

Usual Dose: For Atarax and Vistaril, a 50-mg tablet or capsule is usually sufficient, but 100 mg is also sometimes prescribed.

How Long Until They Work: You should fall asleep within an hour.

Common Side Effects: Dry mouth, dizziness, disturbed coordination, and thickening of the secretions normally found in your lungs.

Less Common Side Effects: Asthma attacks in people who already have asthma, glaucoma attacks in people who have narrow-angle glaucoma, difficulty urinating in men with an enlarged prostate gland.

What to Do About Side Effects: They are usually very mild. If confusion or disorientation occurs, stop taking the medication and tell your doctor.

If They Don't Work: Do not be surprised. These are really not very good sleeping pills. They may make you drowsy enough to sleep on an occasional bad night, but do not rely on them to resolve serious insomnia. If a prescription antihistamine does not work and sleeping pills are clearly needed, you are probably better off taking a sleeping pill like Ambien, Lunesta, or trazodone (Desyrel).

If They Do Work: Prescription antihistamines, like over-the-counter sleeping pills, should be used sparingly, about one or two nights per month. Although they are medically safe, they can still be habit-forming. Your body will get so used to them that eventually they will be required for you to fall asleep. Then, if you decide to stop taking these drugs, you may experience worse insomnia than you did originally. If you find you need to take sleeping pills more than occasionally, tell your doctor to evaluate the problem thoroughly and consider referral to a sleep disorder expert.

Cost: Generic hydroxyzine is as safe and effective as brand-name Vistaril and cheaper.

Special Comments: The chemical ingredients of these prescription antihistamines are identical or almost identical to those of the over-the-counter sleeping pills. So why does one class require a prescription while the other can be obtained merely by walking into a supermarket or a drugstore? The reasons have more to do with drug company strategies than real differences in safety or effectiveness. Antihistamines are intended for the treatment of allergies. Many of them have as a side effect sleepiness, and therefore they are sold and prescribed as sleeping pills. As sleeping pills they are safe and sometimes effective. Taking them once in a while will not hurt, but if medication for sleep is required frequently, a sleeping pill like Ambien, Lunesta, or trazodone (Desyrel) is probably a better choice.

Sedative Antidepressants

Brand (generic) Names: Elavil (amitripyline), Desyrel (trazodone), Sinequan (doxepin).

Used For: Depression, insomnia.

Special Comments: These antidepressants are described in detail in Chapter 7. They all have the side effect of making a patient drowsy. Doses of these medications lower than those effective in treating depression are often prescribed to help people with insomnia. Trazodone is particularly good for this as it has very few side effects other than sedation. The usual dose for this purpose is about 50 mg one hour before bedtime. At this low dose, most of the side effects from the medications are minimal but the patient will still feel sleepy. There is some suggestion that these sedative antidepressants may be less habit-forming than the benzodiazepine sleeping pills, although this hypothesis requires further testing. I think they are useful in cases where some medication for insomnia is needed many nights in a row, for months or even years.

RAMELTEON

Brand Name: Rozerem.

Used For: Insomnia.

Do Not Use If: You are depressed or abuse alcohol.

Tests to Take First: None needed.

Tests to Take While You Are on It: None needed.

Usual Dose: One 8-mg pill taken before bedtime. It should not be taken with a high-fat meal.

How Long Until It Works: You should fall asleep in less than an hour after taking it.

Common Side Effects: Feeling depressed.

Less Common Side Effects: Worsening depression to the point of making someone feel suicidal.

What to Do About Side Effects: Rozerem is a brand-new drug. Therefore, it is hard to know if there are side effects that did not emerge during research studies that led to its approval by the FDA. Most people seem to tolerate Rozerem well and have no problem with side effects. However, there is a risk of getting depressed (or more depressed if you are already depressed), and this should be handled by stopping the drug and trying something else for insomnia.

If It Doesn't Work: You may need to try a different medication, either trazodone, Ambien, or Lunesta, or one of the older benzodiazepine sleeping pills like ProSom, Restoril, or Dalmane.

If It Does Work: In general, it is not a great idea to take sleeping pills every night for an indefinite period of time. After five to seven days of sleeping pill use, it is best to try to see if you can sleep without it. There is always a risk of becoming dependent on sleeping pills. However, Rozerem may be unique compared to most other sleeping pills in not causing dependency and not having withdrawal problems.

Cost: Generic forms of Rozerem are not available, so the drug is expensive.

Special Comments: It has always been known that melatonin, a naturally occurring hormone secreted by the pineal gland at night, makes people sleepy when taken in pill form. There is a receptor in the brain to which melatonin binds, and Rozerem is the first medication that binds to and stimulates that receptor, thus also making people sleepy. Unlike Ambien,

Sonata, Lunesta, and benzodiazepine sleeping pills, it does not bind to the benzodiazepine receptor and therefore does not seem to have problems like dependency and withdrawal. Because it is new, it is not yet possible to fully evaluate how well it works or how serious the depression side effect will be.

SUMMARY OF DRUGS USED TO
TREAT INSOMNIA

In almost all cases of insomnia, if there is no other solution than sleeping pills, Ambien, Lunesta, and trazodone (Desyrel) are the best choices. Rozerem may fall into this category as well, and sometimes Seroquel is the best in patients with other psychiatric illnesses. Over-the-counter sleeping pills and prescription antihistamines should be used only occasionally.

The following drugs should almost always be avoided in treating insomnia: Placidyl, Noludar, barbiturates (like Seconal and phenobarbital), Miltown, and Doriden.

Chapter 12

Drugs Used to Treat Drug Abuse

The very idea of giving drugs to stop people from abusing drugs may seem like a paradox. How can we tell an alcoholic or heroin addict that switching to a *different* drug will make him or her better and win the approval of his family, friends, and doctors?

Many people involved in the battle against drug abuse are vehemently opposed to prescribing any drug to drug abusers. They feel that only programs aimed at complete abstinence—the total drug-free state—make sense.

It is hard to ignore their point. For example, the best current treatment for alcoholism is Alcoholics Anonymous. AA attempts to induce alcoholics to give up drinking entirely; some view any form of drug therapy for alcoholism as simply another brand of drug dependence.

Although we may all agree that the best treatment for drug and alcohol abuse is to stop the habit entirely, most people with addiction problems find that stopping is more easily said than done. Rates of relapse after treatment for almost every form of drug abuse are very high. Think of all the cigarette smokers who are desperate to stop smoking, make it for a few weeks, and then relapse after the first stressful moment. We do not know how many alcoholics who go to AA remain abstinent for long periods, but there is good reason to believe that their relapse rate is also very high. And we have a very poor track record trying to convince heroin and cocaine users to stop cold turkey and remain drug free forever.

THE FEAR OF WITHDRAWAL

One of the biggest reasons addicts do not stop their habits is the fear of drug withdrawal. Addiction to cigarettes, alcohol, Adderall, OxyContin, heroin, or cocaine means that the body is physically dependent on the substance; take it away and there is a violent physical reaction. An alcoholic who suddenly stops drinking will become tremulous and may even develop delirium tremens (DTs), a syndrome that includes fever, seizures, and sometimes death. Cocaine and amphetamine addicts who stop may develop severe depression and a drug craving so powerful that they will do almost anything—including commit violent crimes—to get more drugs. Even sudden cessation of cigarette smoking is accompanied by an irritable, anxious, and depressed state that many find unbearable to the point that they must have another cigarette.

One aim of medication to treat drug addiction is reduction of the amount of withdrawal a person must undergo in stopping abuse of the drug. A person who can get through the acute phase of withdrawal, when drug craving is powerful and the physical symptoms unpleasant or even dangerous, has a good chance of remaining drug free forever. Antianxiety drugs, especially Librium (chlordiazepoxide), have been administered to alcoholics for almost thirty years to blunt withdrawal effects.

In most hospitals, it is considered dangerous *not* to give an alcoholic trying to detox some Librium for the first few days, because without it the patient might experience seizures or even die. Several years ago, the drug clonidine, best known as a treatment for high blood pressure, was found to reduce the withdrawal syndrome after discontinuation of heroin. The heroin addict given clonidine can stop "shooting up" and experience much less sweating, fever, and shaking than the addict not given clonidine.

Yet many addicts who get past the withdrawal period still relapse in time. Unfortunately, we do not yet know why. Animal studies, like those performed in the laboratories of Dr. Eric Nestler at the University of Texas in Dallas and Dr. Christina Alberini at the Mount Sinai School of Medicine in New York City, have shown that addiction to most substances changes the way genes in specific parts of the brain function. One important part of the brain in addiction, sometimes called the "reward system," involves a pathway from the ventral tegmental area to the nucleus accumbens. Manipulation of genes and proteins in this area of the brain in experimental animals reduces craving for addictive substances. This type of research holds great promise for developing new medications to treat addictions. Even after the addict loses the severe physical craving characteristic of the withdrawal period, which usually takes only a few weeks, an inner drive forces him or her to go back to the abused drug. There is now good evidence that at least in the case of alcoholics, some of this need for the drug is caused by a genetic defect. Strange as it may sound, some people apparently are born to be addicts, having inherited what scientists think is an abnormal gene. Different life stresses probably trigger the transformation of the person with the abnormal gene into an addict.

BLOCKING THE HIGH

We do not yet know how to repair such abnormal genes. Instead, several drugs have been developed that prevent addicts from receiving the full impact of their drug of choice or that make addicts sick when they take the abused drug. The idea here is that once an addict finds out that heroin won't produce a high, he or she will have little reason to continue taking it.

Antabuse was one of the first such drugs to be developed. If an alcoholic takes Antabuse and then drinks, he or she will become violently ill. One time is often enough to convince the alcoholic never to take another drink. The problem here, of course, is that the alcoholic has to agree to keep taking Antabuse. The effects of Antabuse last only about one day, so if the alcoholic simply refuses the pill for a couple of days, he or she can resume drinking without getting sick. Antabuse treatment requires a motivated alcoholic, the kind of person who might do just as well attending AA meetings and stopping drinking without drug treatment.

Naltrexone (ReVia) is a drug that blocks the effects of heroin and alcohol. It is relatively long acting, so the recovered heroin addict or alcoholic need take it only once a day. An injectable, long-acting form of naltrexone was recently approved for the treatment of alcoholism and needs to be administered only once a month. The anticonvulsant drug Topamax (topiramate) has shown promise in experimental studies for blocking the craving for alcohol. While the addict is on naltrexone, heroin has absolutely no effect. The alcoholic has a significantly reduced craving for alcohol. Both bupropion (Wellbutrin, Zyban) and varenicline (Chantix) block craving for nicotine and therefore help the cigarette smoker quit.

MIMICKING THE EFFECTS

In addition to decreasing withdrawal symptoms and blocking the effects of abused drugs, there exist medications that mimic the effects of abused drugs but do not produce the same serious health or social risks. The best known of these is methadone, a drug that mimics many of the effects of heroin. Because it is ingested orally instead of injected, methadone does not produce the same devastating physical diseases as heroin, such as infections of the heart and AIDS. Also, because methadone is given out under controlled conditions in clinics, it does not lead to crime and circumvents the drug pushers. Methadone treatment has been successful in treating about one-fourth of the nation's heroin addicts, but many people object to it as substitution of one addiction for another. More important, there are far too few methadone clinics in the United States to accommodate all of the country's heroin addicts. Recently, a drug called buprenorphine (Subutex, Suboxone) has been approved for treatment of opiate addiction, including heroin. It can be given in the doctor's office and then by prescription. It is particularly useful for treating addicition to opiate painkillers like oxycodone (OxyContin).

Not unlike methadone maintenance, although intended for use over a shorter period, are nicotine chewing gum, nicotine lozenges (Commit), nicotine nasal spray, and the nicotine patch. All contain nicotine, the addicting substance found in cigarettes. Cigarette smokers are asked to chew the gum several times daily, inhale the nasal spray, swallow the lozenge, or wear the patch, instead of smoking, to get their nicotine. Although nicotine itself is probably not great for health, chewing the gum or wearing the patch is far safer than inhaling the poison into the lungs. After chewing the gum or wearing the patch for several weeks, some smokers find they are gradually able to give up the nicotine substitutes without starting to smoke again. These nicotine substitutes are available without prescription.

TREATMENT OF AN UNDERLYING ILLNESS

There is a fourth way that medication may help an addict. We now have good evidence that some people who abuse drugs are attempting to treat an underlying psychiatric illness without going to the doctor. More women have anxiety attacks than men, but there are more male alcoholics. It is likely that some men with anxiety attacks go to the bar instead of going to the psychiatrist. Studies have shown that as many as one-third of patients undergoing alcohol detoxification had experienced panic attacks before they became alcoholics. Alcohol is a very powerful although very dangerous medication for anxiety attacks. Dr. Alexander Glassman of Columbia University has shown that smokers who find it the most difficult to stop smoking are more likely to have depression than smokers who successfully quit. The nicotine in cigarettes may act as a stimulant for some depressed people. Many, probably most, patients with schizophrenia smoke and have had a difficult time being admitted to hospitals with no-smoking policies. It is believed that nicotine acts as a stimulant to counteract some of the negative and cognitive symptoms of the illness itself and some of the cognitive and emotional blunting effects of drugs prescribed to treat schizophrenia.

Depression, schizophrenia, and anxiety disorders probably cause some of the cases of cocaine, alcohol, heroin, and cigarette addiction. Cocaine may give the chronically depressed patient a temporary lift, alcohol blocks panic attacks and reduces phobias, heroin blocks out almost all painful emotions, and cigarette smoking seems to have some relationship to depression and schizophrenia. Although I do not believe that more than a small fraction of cases of drug or alcohol abuse are directly the result of psychiatric illness, it is extremely important that addicts undergo a thorough psychiatric evaluation. If an underlying mental disorder is the root of the addiction problem, successful treatment of that disorder may also eliminate the need for the abused drug. In most cases, however, the patient will need separate treatments for the psychiatric disorder and the addiction. Psychiatrists have had some success in the use of antidepressant and antianxiety drugs to treat alcoholics, cocaine addicts, and even heroin addicts in whom a psychiatric condition was the real problem. They have even discovered patients with bipolar disorder (manic-depressive illness) whose abuse of alcohol or cocaine was an attempt to regulate moods either up or down. Such patients often stop abusing drugs after they are placed on lithium.

In cases of drug abuse, psychiatric medications must be prescribed by an experienced clinician, because some psychiatric drugs do not interact well with abused drugs. Antidepressants of the monoamine oxidase inhibitor class, for example, should never be given to people who continue to use cocaine. It is a serious mistake to prescribe a benzodiazepine-type antianxiety drug, for example, Xanax or Valium, on a long-term basis to an alcoholic patient without very careful monitoring. These drugs are often abused by alcoholics and, in some cases, merely add to their problems. Similarly, heroin addicts sometimes abuse antianxiety agents. Seroquel (quetiapine) is often prescribed to opiate addicts and alcoholics to treat anxiety and insomnia because it is less likely to be abused than benzodiazepines like Xanax, Valium, Ativan, and Klonopin. It is described in more detail in the chapter on drugs used to treat schizophrenia (antipsychotic drugs).

FOUR RULES FOR DRUG THERAPY

To summarize, there are four ways that medication may help an addict overcome addiction (Table 32):

1. By blocking withdrawal symptoms when the abused drug is stopped. This makes it easier to get through the first few weeks.

2. By blocking the effects of the abused drug or making those effects unpleasant. This reduces the addict's motivation to take the abused drug.

3. By mimicking the desired effects of an abused drug with a safer medication. The addict is induced to take a medication that has effects similar to those of the abused drug but has fewer adverse medical and social consequences.

4. By treating an underlying psychiatric disturbance that is the root of the drug abuse. Once the underlying depression or anxiety disorder is relieved, the addict may experience a reduced need to take the abused drug. However, treatment for the addiction is usually still necessary.

Table 32.

Drugs Used to Treat Drug Abuse

STRATEGY	ABUSED DRUG	TREATMENT DRUG
Block withdrawal	Alcohol	Librium, Valium, Ativan
	Heroin	Clonidine
Block effects of abused drug	Alcohol	Antabuse, naltrexone, acamprosate
	Heroin	Naltrexone
	Cigarettes	Bupropion, varenicline
Mimic effects of abused drug	Cigarettes	Nicotine gum, nicotine patch, nicotine nasal spray, nicotine lozenges
	Heroin and other opiates	Methadone, buprenorphine
Treat underlying psychiatric disorder	Alcohol, cigarettes, heroin, cocaine	Antidepressants, antianxiety medication, psychiatric medications; psychotherapy

CONVINCING THE ADDICT

Even if we accept that some patients with an addiction are properly treated with medication, there still remains the problem of convincing addicts that drug abuse is their problem. Psychiatrists miss this point many times. Doctors frequently forget to ask patients about drug and alcohol abuse. Some doctors, including psychiatrists, think that asking their patients about alcohol or drug abuse is insulting. As long as a person doesn't stagger into the office with alcohol on his or her breath, the doctor refuses to believe the patient has a drinking problem.

With physicians exercising this kind of denial, it is no wonder that many drug abusers with serious addiction problems fool themselves into thinking they are only recreational users. I now offer some simple guidelines to determine if you or someone you care about may have a drug abuse problem.

1. There is *never—absolutely never—a* recreational use for cocaine, heroin, amphetamines ("uppers" including Adderall), barbiturates ("downers"), OxyContin, Vicodin, Quaaludes, Talwin, or Dilaudid. Most of these drugs are illegal; others are sometimes prescribed by physicians. If you ever take any of these, even once, without a prescription from your doctor, then you have a drug abuse problem.

2. Cigarettes are as harmful as the former surgeon general Dr. Everett Koop said they are. Many people have quit smoking; the remaining smokers are likely to be people who have tried and simply cannot quit. They should see their doctor and try getting into a program that may include nicotine substitutes, bupropion (Wellbutrin, Zyban), and/or varenicline (Chantix).

3. Alcohol is tricky. There is, of course, a legitimate and legal recreational use for alcohol. Most people do not drink to excess because they do not find it pleasant. The average person feels relaxed and happy after a drink or two; more than that makes the person sleepy and then sick. Evidence now suggests that alcoholics tolerate much higher "doses" of alcohol before they feel these unpleasant effects. So an alcoholic can keep on drinking past the point at which the normal person's body says stop. This means that alcoholics may not recognize they are drinking too much at first. Later, they insist they are in complete control. Unfortunately, too many people believe this until it is too late. Alcoholics should join AA and see a physician who may prescribe naltrexone (either orally or in the long-acting injectable form) and/or acamprosate (Campral).

So here is a simple test. If you think you may have the slightest problem, do not have another alcoholic drink (including beer and wine) for one week.

No matter what. Don't make an excuse, like you have to go to a party or business meeting and it will look odd if you don't have a drink. If you cannot last one week without a drink, you have a drinking problem and should get help. If you do last a week, it does not mean you are home free, but you have demonstrated that you at least are no longer physically addicted. AA insists that an alcoholic who stops drinking is a "recovering" alcoholic, not an "ex-alcholic."

There are other warning signs of an alcohol problem:

- You drink to fall asleep at night.

- You drink alone.

- You drink because you feel you have to calm your nerves.

- You drink in the morning or the afternoon.

- You tell yourself you aren't going to have a drink but can't help yourself and have one anyway.

- You miss work because you are drunk or have a hangover.

- You have blackouts, that is, you forget everything that happened for several hours after getting drunk.

- Your body shakes several hours after your last drink (this is a component of withdrawal syndrome; your body is craving alcohol).

- Someone tells you that you have been drinking a lot.

- You lie to others about how much you drink or you hide bottles of alcohol so no one will know you are drinking.

- You have an automobile accident or get a speeding ticket while inebriated.

If you meet even one of these eleven criteria, you should consider the possibility that you have an alcohol abuse problem. Talk to your doctor. Join an AA chapter. Whatever you do, do not ignore the problem.

HOW TO PROCEED

Simply stopping use of the addicting drug is the preferred way to handle the problem. Even insurance companies, which usually resist paying for psychiatric care, are willing to pay for psychotherapies that specifically aim to stop addictions. Everyone knows that it costs far more to treat the medical and social complications of an addiction than to treat the addiction itself. So the first consideration is to try a drug-free treatment.

If therapy does not work, treatment with one of the drugs listed in this chapter, under the supervision of a qualified doctor, is worth trying. The following strategies are useful:

Alcohol. Be sure there is not an additional underlying psychiatric disturbance, for example, depression or panic disorder, which should be treated with the proper antidepressant or antianxiety drug. Librium or Ativan may be prescribed for a few days to block withdrawal symptoms. Chronic alcoholics may have to be admitted to the hospital for detoxification, because sudden discontinuation of alcohol can produce life-threatening withdrawal symptoms. Then, consider Antabuse treatment and naltrexone (ReVia or long-acting injectable) and acamprosate (Campral). Always join AA. Qualified addiction counselors are also extremely helpful and offer both individual and group therapy.

Cocaine. Be sure that there is not an additional underlying psychiatric disturbance, for example, depression or bipolar disorder, which should be treated with the proper antidepressant or mood-stabilizing drug. No medications are currently available that have been proved effective for cocaine use, so a drug treatment program is always needed.

Heroin and other opiates. Clonidine is sometimes given to block the withdrawal symptoms. Then naltrexone is administered to block the high from heroin. Alternatively, methadone or buprenorphine (Subutex, Suboxone) maintenance mimics the action of heroin without incurring most of the medical and social risks. Methadone-maintained patients can then be switched to clonidine for detoxification.

Buprenorphine-treated patients may be able to taper off the medication without relapse after a while. Buprenorphine is also helpful in treating people who abuse opiate painkillers (also known as opiate analgesics) such as oxycodone (OxyContin), Vicodin (combination of acetaminophen and oxycodone), and fentanyl.

Cigarettes. During the initial abstinence period, nicotine chewing substitutes, available without prescription, may be used to mimic the effects of cigarette smoking with far fewer health risks. Also, be sure that there is no underlying psychiatric disturbance, for example, depression or anxiety, which is increasing the need for cigarettes. Nicotine substitutes are usually discontinued after a few weeks to months. It is important to remember that nicotine substitutes work best when combined with behavioral therapy and prescribed medication (bupropion or varenicline) to stop smoking.

DRUGS USED TO TREAT DRUG ABUSE

Until more is learned about the causes of addiction, it will fail to be stopped in many cases. Combinations of therapy and medication have saved many people. The following information on the specific drugs used to treat drug abuse should be useful to addicts and to people who care about addicts.

ACAMPROSATE

Brand Name: Campral.

Used For: Alcohol abuse.

Do Not Use If: Caution must be exercised if you have very severe kidney disease.

Tests to Take First: None needed.

Tests to Take While You Are on It: None needed.

Usual Dose: Two 333-mg pills are taken three times a day.

How Long Until It Works: The effects are gradual, but after several weeks the patient should notice reduced craving for alcohol.

Common Side Effects: Side effects are uncommon, but the drug can make people feel anxious or moody, and nausea, diarrhea, and insomnia sometimes occur.

Less Common Side Effects: Severe depression and suicidal thinking have been reported, but this is very uncommon.

What to Do About Side Effects: Side effects are uncommon and most people tolerate Campral well.

If It Doesn't Work: Even if there is a relapse and the patient starts drinking again, it is worthwhile to stay on Campral. If multiple relapses occur or the patient does not experience any reduction in alcohol craving at all, it is probably time to stop the drug.

If It Does Work: Campral should be continued indefinitely. There is little known risk from long-term use of the drug, but alcohol abuse relapse is always a risk.

Cost: Generic forms of Campral are not available, so the drug is expensive.

Special Comments: Campral seems to work by decreasing the activity of the brain's most abundant neurotransmitter, glutamate. The question in treating alcoholism is how well does a drug work. A recent study showed that Campral is less effective than naltrexone, a treatment that has been available for alcohol abuse for several years. Many physicians are trying the combination of naltrexone and Campral, which appears to be safe, but it is unclear whether this increases the chance of successful cessation of alcohol abuse.

CHLORDIAZEPOXIDE

Brand Name: Librium.

Used For: Blocking the withdrawal symptoms after stopping alcohol. Note: Librium is one of the many drugs in the benzodiazepine class of antianxiety agents, which are described in detail in Chapter 8. Although Librium has traditionally been used by doctors to prevent serious alcohol withdrawal symptoms, like delirium tremens, any of the benzodiazepines can be used for this. Ativan is also frequently prescribed. When a patient is hospitalized for alcohol detoxification, benzodiazepines are frequently given by injection.

Do Not Use If: You are not serious about stopping drinking. Alcoholics are at very high risk of getting hooked on Librium. It should be given for only a few days to prevent serious withdrawal reactions like seizures and heart failure. Librium is not to be taken along with alcohol.

Tests to Take First: Your doctor will do many medical tests as part of the alcohol withdrawal process, including blood tests to determine how much damage alcohol has done to your liver. You will also be given the vitamins and minerals, like magnesium, thiamine, and folic acid, that alcohol usually depletes from the body.

Tests to Take While You Are on It: During alcohol withdrawal, it is important that your pulse, blood pressure, and temperature be checked frequently. Rapid pulse, high blood pressure, and fever are signs that serious and potentially life-threatening alcohol withdrawal reactions may be about to start.

Usual Dose: In some situations, it is best to have a brief admission to the hospital for alcohol detoxification. The first dose of Librium (50 or 100 mg) is sometimes given intramuscularly or intravenously (directly into the vein). Then, 50 or 100 mg is given by mouth every three hours to a maximum of 300 mg per day. The key is to keep agitation to a minimum.

How Long Until It Works: The treatment takes effect immediately. The patient should be relatively sedated and calm throughout detoxification.

Common Side Effects: There are no side effects to the use of Librium in alcohol detoxification. Too much Librium may make the patient too sleepy, but this is probably desirable.

Less Common Side Effects: There is a very small chance that such drugs as Librium, when given intravenously, will cause a temporary (a few minutes) decrease in breathing. Very rarely, the patient actually stops breathing. For this reason, of course, intravenous drugs are given only to patients in the hospital. A doctor or nurse is present when the dose is given, and if a breathing problem develops, a bag is placed over the patient's nose and mouth and air is pumped in by hand for a few minutes. This may sound frightening, but it is actually a very simple procedure (much less complicated than administration of anesthesia during surgery). After a few minutes, the patient starts breathing regularly again.

What to Do About Side Effects: If the patient is too sleepy, the dose of Librium is reduced or the interval between doses is extended to more than three hours.

If It Doesn't Work: This is very rare. If given properly, Librium and related benzodiazepines almost always block serious withdrawal symptoms of alcohol detoxification. Sometimes, however, seizures occur even with Librium protection; then, anticonvulsants, for example, Dilantin and phenobarbital, are given.

If It Does Work: The treatment usually lasts about three days. During this time, the dose is gradually decreased and the intervals between doses are increased. At the end of three days, Librium is stopped.

Cost: Generic chlordiazepoxide is cheaper and just as safe and effective as brand-name Librium.

Special Comments: Alcohol withdrawal is very serious. Unlike the situation that results when benzodiazepine use is stopped, patients can die during alcohol detoxification. Immediately after abrupt discontinuation of alcohol, patients can become agitated and develop fever, high blood pressure, and rapid pulse. Some hear voices (hallucinations) and have seizures. In delirium tremens (the DTs), the patient develops severe agitation and hallucinations and signs of hyperactivity of the nervous system. At one time, this medical emergency proved to be fatal in many cases. The use of drugs like Librium now makes this a very treatable condition. A long-term alcoholic ready to quit should be cared for by a physician knowledgeable about alcohol detoxification and withdrawal.

DISULFIRAM

Brand Name: Antabuse.

Used For: Motivating an alcoholic to stop drinking. Drinking while on Antabuse causes a severe and very unpleasant physical reaction.

Do Not Use If: You are not completely serious about stopping drinking and are not ready to begin an alcohol treatment program like AA; you have almost any serious medical problem, for example, heart disease, diabetes, epilepsy, kidney disease, liver disease, and thyroid disease; you are taking other medications, unless your doctor determines that these other drugs do not interact badly with Antabuse; you abuse any drugs besides alcohol, like barbiturates; you have had a drink in the last twelve hours.

Tests to Take First: A complete medical evaluation is necessary, including physical examination, blood tests, urine tests, and an electrocardiogram.

Tests to Take While You Are on It: None are automatically necessary, but your doctor may want to order various blood tests if there is any suspicion that Antabuse is causing side effects.

Usual Dose: First, you must not have ingested alcohol for at least twelve hours. This means alcohol in any form, including cough medicine, mouthwash, sauces, or even aftershave lotion splashed on your face or isopropyl alcohol rubbed on your back. Then, a dose of 500 mg is given every morning for one to two weeks. Antabuse can also be taken at night if you feel it makes you sleepy during the day. After two weeks, the dose is often cut back to 250 mg.

How Long Until It Works: Immediately. After the first dose of Antabuse, you should not ingest alcohol in any form, for example, sauces containing wines and desserts containing liqueurs. If you do, you will develop a violent physical reaction that includes severe nausea and vomiting, headache, flushing, dizziness, low blood pressure, and rapid heart rate. This can be dangerous, especially if you have a preexisting medical condition, such as heart disease. In many ways, patients on Antabuse must follow as strict a diet as that followed by patients taking monoamine oxidase inhibitors. Many alcoholics on Antabuse are tempted to try drinking because they don't believe they will actually have these reactions; they are very used to people trying to scare them about the dangers of drinking. Don't give in to the temptation to drink while on Antabuse. If you cannot stay away from drinking, do not take Antabuse.

Common Side Effects: There are no common side effects, but some of the less common side effects are serious.

Less Common Side Effects: Neuritis—inflammation of nerves causing pain and difficulty with vision; liver problems like hepatitis; skin rashes; drowsiness, headache, impotence, and a bad taste in the mouth—these usually go away after the first two weeks of treatment; psychosis.

What to Do About Side Effects: Neuritis, psychosis, and hepatitis are reason to stop the medication immediately. Antihistamines can be given for rashes. The side effects of drowsiness, headache, impotence, and bad taste usually go away on their own. Sometimes, reduction of the dose is necessary.

If It Doesn't Work: If you cannot stay away from drinking, do not take Antabuse. Antabuse works only for the motivated alcoholic who needs the extra impetus of a physical threat to keep from drinking. If you aren't ready to stop drinking completely, you should not take Antabuse. Try Alcoholics Anonymous and other alcohol treatment programs first.

If It Does Work: You may stay on Antabuse as long as you feel you need to. Some patients take it for months or even years. It is hoped that at some point you will feel that you have enough willpower to not drink without Antabuse.

Cost: Generic disulfiram is no longer available, so you will have to get brand-name Antabuse, which is costly.

Special Comments: Very few doctors prescribe Antabuse anymore. Most of us have learned that a highly motivated alcoholic will stop drinking without the threat of physical harm that Antabuse presents. On the other hand, less highly motivated alcoholics should not be given Antabuse, because the physical reaction is very extreme and sometimes dangerous. Nevertheless, the occasional alcoholic who decides that Antabuse will help his or her resolve should be allowed to try it. These people should carry a card in their wallet or wear a MedicAlert bracelet that identifies them as on Antabuse.

CLONIDINE

Brand Name: Catapres.

Used For: Blocking withdrawal symptoms after discontinuation of heroin or methadone.

Do Not Use If: You have heart disease, unless your doctor tells you it is okay.

Tests to Take First: Clonidine is most commonly used to lower blood pressure in patients with high blood pressure, so it is a good idea to have your blood pressure recorded before starting treatment.

Tests to Take While You Are on It: Blood pressure should be checked every day during heroin detoxification.

Usual Dose: To block withdrawal symptoms after discontinuation of heroin or methadone, the patient is usually started at 0.1 to 0.3 mg a day three times daily. After five days, the dose is reduced; the patient is treated for a total of one to two weeks.

How Long Until It Works: For heroin addicts who stop shooting up and go on clonidine in a one- or two-week detoxification program, many of the physical withdrawal symptoms—tremors, yawning, sweating, and rapid pulse—are blocked after the first few doses. The patient usually still has a psychological temptation to get heroin. Many heroin addicts are first placed on methadone and then switched to clonidine. Clonidine then blocks the symptoms of withdrawal from methadone, which are much the same as those of withdrawal from heroin.

Common Side Effects: Sedation, drowsiness, dry mouth, and light-headedness, the latter caused by the lowering of blood pressure.

Less Common Side Effects: Very few. Rarely, nausea and vomiting, skin rash, and a feeling of physical weakness.

What to Do About Side Effects: Some amount of sedation may not be so bad, especially for an addict trying to withdraw from heroin. Reducing the dose usually reverses sedation and low blood pressure.

If It Doesn't Work: If clonidine does not block withdrawal symptoms sufficiently and the patient feels he or she must have something, he or she is usually placed back on methadone.

If It Does Work: After one or two weeks, most heroin addicts no longer have withdrawal symptoms. Heroin addicts will probably need long-term psychological treatment to prevent relapse.

Cost: Generic clonidine is as safe and effective as brand-name Catapres and cheaper.

Special Comments: Clonidine has been prescribed for many years for treatment of high blood pressure. It also blocks the excess nervous system excitement that occurs when people suddenly stop using substances to which they are addicted. Clonidine is an established component in some detoxification programs for heroin addicts. It is a very safe treatment, although too great a reduction of blood pressure can produce the uncomfortable side effects of dizziness and light-headedness. Elderly people should use clonidine only under a physician's strict supervision, because these side effects can result in falls.

NALTREXONE

Brand Name: ReVia, Vivitrol (injectable extended-release formulation).

Used For: Blocking the high from heroin (oral form only), blocking craving for alcohol (both forms).

Do Not Use If: You are not serious about stopping use of heroin or alcohol or you have liver disease. Alcoholics who receive naltrexone, especially the extended-release form, must not be taking opiates like heroin, OxyContin, Vicodin, or morphine. In some cases of patients with liver disease, the physician may still prescribe naltrexone.

Tests to Take First: Blood tests for liver problems are recommended. Patients using oral naltrexone to treat heroin addiction should not start naltrexone until at least a week has passed since they used heroin; a blood or urine test is required to confirm the absence of heroin in the body.

Tests to Take While You Are on It: Blood tests to confirm that naltrexone is not hurting your liver should be done periodically.

Usual Dose: For patients using oral naltrexone to treat heroin addiction, treatment is not begun until the patient has been off heroin at least one week. This fact is often confirmed by obtaining a blood or urine test. For both heroin addicts and alcoholics, 50 mg can be given every day to block the high. Because naltrexone has a very long length of action, many patients being treated for alcohol addiction eventually take it only three times a week. One schedule, 100 mg on Monday and Wednesday and 150 mg on Friday, seems to offer sufficient blockage. Patients trying to stop alcohol use usually take 50 mg daily.

For patients with alcoholism using the injectable form (Vivitrol), an injection of 380 mg is given in the muscle of the arm or buttocks once every four weeks.

How Long Until It Works: For heroin detoxification, the effect is immediate. If, after taking naltrexone, a patient shoots up with heroin, he or she will not get high. This quickly discourages the patient from shooting up. For discontinuation of alcohol, the effect is more subtle. The patient should experience decreased craving for alcohol in conjunction with a comprehensive alcohol cessation program.

Common Side Effects: Nervousness, insomnia, low energy, headache, joint and muscle pain, nausea and vomiting, difficulty ejaculating, impotence, dizziness, diarrhea, constipation, rash, increased thirst, decreased appetite, and chills. Injectable naltrexone (Vivitrol) can cause redness or rash at the site of injection.

Less Common Side Effects: If a person is mistakenly prescribed naltrexone while still addicted to heroin, he or she will experience an acute withdrawal syndrome. In other words, naltrexone will suddenly block all of heroin's effect and the patient will be in the same boat as if he or she had suddenly stopped heroin. The withdrawal syndrome includes tremors, sweating, shaking, runny nose, tearing, and rapid pulse. Injectable naltrexone (Vivitrol) carries a very small risk of causing liver disease, although this seems most likely at higher doses than given to patients. Vivitrol was also associated in research studies with a very slightly elevated risk of depression and even suicidal thoughts compared to placebo. There is also a small risk of pneumonia and serious rash at the injection site from Vivitrol.

What to Do About Side Effects: The abrupt withdrawal syndrome induced by mistakenly prescribing naltrexone to someone still addicted to heroin can be treated with methadone or, in some cases, with clonidine. It is best to wait a week before trying naltrexone again. The common side effects are not dangerous and may subside in time on their own. In actual practice, few former heroin addicts or alcoholics are very bothered by the side effects of naltrexone. The nausea that often occurs with the first injection of Vivitrol usually passes quickly and does not occur with subsequent injections. For mild skin reactions at the injection site, applying heat can be helpful and it may be best to choose a different place for the next injection. However, if swelling and redness last more than four weeks or are severe, the doctor should be warned immediately. Similarly, if cough, shortness of breath, extreme fatigue, depression, or suicidal thoughts occur, tell your doctor right away.

If It Doesn't Work: Patients who cannot stop injecting heroin even though they are taking naltrexone to block the high should probably be placed on methadone. For patients with alcohol abuse, some doctors add acamprosate (Campral). Naltrexone will probably not work for alcoholism unless you are also in a treatment program like AA.

If It Does Work: Treatment can continue indefinitely, although liver problems can rarely occur that warrant stopping naltrexone. It is hoped that psychological treatments will work so that the patient can ultimately stop naltrexone without returning to heroin or alcohol abuse.

Cost: For users of oral natrexone, the generic drug is just as safe and effective as brand-name ReVia and less expensive. There is no generic form of Vivitrol, making it an expensive treatment.

Special Comments: Naltrexone treatment requires a motivated alcoholic or heroin addict who really wants to quit. It is easy to stop taking naltrexone at any time and start injecting heroin or drinking again. After about a week off naltrexone, the effects wear off and the addict is able to get high again. The effect of Vivitrol, however, lasts for four weeks after the injection. Naltrexone treatment works for patients with alcoholism but unfortunately is underused.

BUPRENORPHINE

Brand Names: Subutex, Suboxone (also contains naloxone).

Used For: Addiction to opiates (heroin or opiate painkillers like OxyContin or Vicodin).

Do Not Use If: Except for people who are very medically ill, almost all opiate addicts can take buprenorphine for detoxification and treatment of their addiction. Because Suboxone also contains naloxone, a drug that immediately blocks the effects of opiates, it should not be taken if you are still taking, or have recently taken, any type of opiate. Usually, Subutex is given first for "induction" (getting treatment started) and then in a few days the patient is switched to Suboxone for maintenance.

Tests to Take First: None needed.

Tests to Take While You Are on It: None needed.

Usual Dose: People who are currently using opiates (that is, have recently shot up heroin or taken an opiate painkiller) must stop the opiate, and induction of treatment is done with Subutex, which is pure buprenorphine. This is usually done in the doctor's office because some patients may still experience the signs of opiate withdrawal and need extra treatment. Induction with Subutex is generally started with between 2 and 8 mg taken under the tongue, depending on how much opiate the patient has been taking. Then,

8–16 mg are given every day for the next several days. At that point, the patient is switched to Suboxone, 12–16 mg a day under the tongue for maintenance. The dose of Suboxone can be raised slowly over the next few days to a maximum of 32 mg.

How Long Until It Works: It may take a few days for the craving for opiate to be gone.

Common Side Effects: Nausea, constipation, chills, and insomnia may occur in the first few days, more because of withdrawal from the opiate than from the drug itself. Sleepiness can also occur from both Subutex and Suboxone.

Less Common Side Effects: Withdrawal from opiates can cause severe symptoms. If the dose of Subutex is not enough to substitute for whatever you have been taking, withdrawal will occur, which includes severe agitation, sweating, insomnia, diarrhea, nausea and vomiting, increase in heart rate and blood pressure, and fever. There is a very small risk from buprenorphine of liver problems. If while on Suboxone you use heroin or an opiate painkiller, you may also precipitate withdrawal because of the naloxone component to the drug.

What to Do About Side Effects: The trick to using buprenorphine is to pick a dose that prevents withdrawal symptoms and then blocks the craving for opiates without getting too high a dose and causing sedation. As physicians have gotten more experience with buprenorphine, they are usually able to do that based on how much opiate you have been using prior to starting buprenorphine treatment. Sometimes, dosing adjustments are needed, either upward to fully block craving or downward to decrease sedation.

If It Doesn't Work: For heroin addicts who do not respond to buprenorphine, methadone is usually the next step. For other opiate addicts, there are few other choices at present.

If It Does Work: Buprenorphine is continued for as long as needed to protect against opiate abuse relapse. It is always given in conjunction with a complete treatment program that includes rehab and counseling.

Cost: Neither Subutex or Suboxone are available as generic drugs, so they are expensive.

Special Comments: The FDA recently approved buprenorphine for the treatment of opiate addiction. It seems most effective for pill addicts— people who abuse prescription opiate painkillers (analgesics), like OxyContin (oxycodone), Vicodin, fentanyl, or morphine—and somewhat less effective for treating heroin addiction. The advantage over methadone is that buprenorphine can be prescribed by a doctor in his or her office, unlike methadone, which can be administered only in a methadone clinic. Most states have restricted access to buprenorphine, making physicians take special training before they can prescribe it and limiting the number of patients on buprenorphine each doctor can have at any one time. The latter restrictions will probably be eased over time, making access to buprenorphine easier. The difference between Subutex and Suboxone is that Suboxone is a combination of buprenorphine and naloxone. If a patient tries to abuse Suboxone by raising the dose above 32 mg or taking other opiates along with it, the naloxone component will actually block the effect of buprenorphine or other opiates and cause withdrawal. Therefore, it is fairly difficult to abuse buprenorphine, which is the reason the FDA felt comfortable allowing doctors to prescribe it and patients to obtain it from regular pharmacies without the kind of supervision that is required for methadone maintenance. Many patients placed on opiate painkillers by physicians for real medical problems or who obtain them on their own from other sources, like the Internet, become addicted to them. For these people, buprenorphine is often a very helpful way to overcome the addiction.

NICOTINE SUBSTITUTES

Brand Names: Nicotine patch: Nicoderm, Habitrol, Prostep, Nicotrol; nicotine gum: Nicorette; and others.

Used For: Stopping cigarette smoking.

Do Not Use If: You are not committed to stopping smoking, are pregnant, have unstable heart disease.

Tests to Take First: None required.

Tests to Take While You Are on It: None required.

Usual Dose: The strength of the nicotine substitutes varies and the starting dose depends on how many cigarettes you smoke. The strongest patches have 15–22 mg in them. Over a period of several weeks to months, the dose is decreased. All of these forms of nicotine substitute are available without prescription (some cities and states have programs to give them free to cigarette smokers who want to quit). Just follow the directions on the package or ask your doctor for advice.

How Long Until It Works: Nicotine is released into the body immediately after the patch is applied, the spray is inhaled, the gum is chewed, or the lozenge is swallowed. This means that some reduction in craving for a cigarette is realized quickly. Nevertheless, smoking cessation may take weeks to months.

Common Side Effects: The various types of nicotine substitutes are very well tolerated. Skin irritation can occur with the patch.

Less Common Side Effects: Occasionally there can be dizziness, insomnia, nausea, and vivid dreams. Although it is not a good idea to smoke cigarettes while using a nicotine substitute, the combination does not seem to cause heart attacks as originally reported.

What to Do About Side Effects: Rotating the patch to different parts of the body on different days is usually effective in preventing skin irritation. The other side effects usually diminish on their own or by decreasing the dose or frequency that you take the substitute.

If It Doesn't Work: Quitting cigarettes is very hard to do and most people relapse a few times before finally getting off them. So the first rule if the nicotine substitute doesn't work is to try again and never lose hope. It is also a good idea to combine the patch with some form of behavioral therapy and consider one of the prescription medications (bupropion or varenicline) as well.

If It Does Work: Then you are a hero! The nicotine substitute is usually used regularly for at least several months, with the dose decreased over time. Then try to do without it.

Cost: Prices vary from pharmacy to pharmacy. They can be expensive and usually not covered by health insurance because no prescription is required. Some municipalities have programs in which nicotine substitutes are given out for free.

Special Comments: Although nicotine is not a healthy substance—it is the addicting part of cigarettes—it is nonetheless much better to use a nicotine substitute than to smoke. There are now lots of ways to take a nicotine substitute (patch, gum, lozenge, inhalant) and the choice is basically up to you. Many people do best using several forms. For example, some ex-smokers put a patch on in the morning and then chew nicotine gum each time they have a craving to smoke. Studies show that nicotine substitutes work best in conjunction with behavior therapy and the prescription medication bupropion. Also, although varenicline (Chantix) probably works better than bupropion for smoking cessation, it is not yet clear if it is safe to combine it with a nicotine substitute or bupropion, so this requires further research.

VARENICLINE

Brand Name: Chantix.

Used For: To stop cigarette smoking.

Do Not Use If: There are no known absolute reasons to avoid Chantix.

Tests to Take First: None needed.

Tests to Take While You Are on It: None needed.

Usual Dose: A single 0.5-mg tablet is taken on a full stomach with a full glass of water every morning for the first three days, then the 0.5-mg tablet is taken morning and night (always with a full glass of water and after a full meal). After four days of 0.5 mg twice a day, the dose is raised to 1 mg twice a day.

How Long Until It Works: After one week many smokers begin to feel less craving for cigarettes, although it can take longer than that to feel comfortable not smoking.

Common Side Effects: Nausea, insomnia, and vivid dreams.

Less Common Side Effects: No other side effects have yet been detected, but this is a brand-new drug.

What to Do About Side Effects: The common side effects are generally mild and go away on their own. If they persist, lowering the dose may help.

If It Doesn't Work: Give it at least twelve weeks. If there is no response, switch to the combination of bupropion and nicotine substitute. Whatever treatment you are using, it is always best to get behavior therapy as well.

If It Does Work: It is recommended that patients who respond by twelve weeks continue to take Chantix for another twelve weeks.

Cost: Generic forms of Chantix are not available, so the drug is expensive.

Special Comments: Chantix was approved by the FDA in 2006, so it is too early to have a full impression. Nevertheless, it was impressive in clinical research trials in which it outperformed bupropion (Zyban, Wellbutrin). Chantix is the first antismoking drug to work by stimulating the receptor in the brain to which nicotine itself binds. Most physicians will now consider it the first-line medication for cigarette smoking cessation, although it is more expensive than generic bupropion and it is unclear to what extent managed care pharmacies will cover it. I hope that further research will show that it is safe to use with nicotine substitutes and increase the success rate of Chantix even further.

BUPROPION 12-HOUR TABLETS

Brand Names: Budeprion SR, Budeprion XL, Wellbutrin, Wellbutrin SR, Wellbutrin XL, Zyban.

Used For: Cigarette smoking cessation, depression.

Usual Dose: To help stop smoking, a single 150-mg tablet of bupropion 12-hour tabs (Wellbutrin SR, Zyban) is taken in the morning for the first three days and then twice a day, usually separated by four to eight hours.

How Long Until It Works: It takes at least a week and usually several weeks until craving for a cigarette becomes manageable.

Common Side Effects: See description of bupropion in Chapter 7.

Less Common Side Effects: See description of bupropion in Chapter 7.

What to Do About Side Effects: See description of bupropion in Chapter 7.

If It Doesn't Work: Switching to varenicline (Chantix) is a good option.

If It Does Work: Keep taking it until you are sure you won't smoke. Sometimes this will mean several months or even years.

Cost: Generic buropion 12-hour tablets is just as safe and effective as Wellbutrin SR and Zyban (the same drug with different brand names) and less expensive.

Special Comments: Bupropion has already been described in detail in Chapter 7 because it is also used to treat depression, so please refer to that description for information about side effects. After it was marketed for this problem, it was discovered that it also helps cigarette smokers stop smoking, whether they are also depressed or not. Combined with nicotine substitutes and behavior therapy, success rates are fairly robust. Interestingly, patients who use bupropion to stop smoking often do not gain weight, a noted problem among those who quit. The manufacturer of brand-name Wellbutrin decided to call the drug Zyban for cigarette smoking cessation treatment, but it is exactly the same drug.

METHADONE

Brand Name: Methadose, Dolophine.

Used For: Substitution for heroin in long-term maintenance treatment. Methadone is also sometimes used for severe pain in patients with cancer and other serious medical problems.

Do Not Use If: You have serious respiratory (breathing) disease. Some people with thyroid, liver, and kidney disease, with Addison's disease, an enlarged prostate gland, or other serious medical problems also should not take methadone. Of course, they should not take heroin either, and there is almost no situation in which remaining on heroin is better than taking methadone.

Tests to Take First: A complete physical examination and routine blood tests should be done.

Tests to Take While You Are on It: At least once a year most patients on methadone are required to have a physical examination and routine blood tests.

Usual Dose: Dosage varies greatly and is controversial. Most patients are started at 20 mg a day. The dose is increased to the point that the patient has no withdrawal symptoms and no desire to take heroin. Some patients take as much as 80–100 mg per day in a single dose.

How Long Until It Works: After the first dose or two of methadone, the patient should feel little desire to take heroin.

Common Side Effects: Most side effects wear off in time. These include light-headedness, dizziness, sedation, nausea, vomiting, and sweating.

Less Common Side Effects: These occur mostly in people who also have other medical problems and include respiratory and heart problems.

What to Do About Side Effects: The more common side effects usually go away in time. Reducing the dose may help. Less common—and more serious—side effects almost always require reduction of the dose or even discontinuation of methadone.

If It Doesn't Work: It sometimes doesn't. Some heroin addicts drop out of methadone programs and return to heroin. A good number of these, however, will try again and, eventually, even after several attempts, successfully stop shooting up heroin. A more serious problem is the shortage of methadone clinics in large cities in the United States. Many heroin addicts cannot get into methadone treatment because of the long waiting lists.

If It Does Work: Being on methadone is always superior to injecting heroin. Some patients stay on methadone the rest of their lives. Many attempt to get off methadone, often by taking clonidine to block withdrawal symptoms (see earlier in this chapter) and then naltrexone to block the heroin high (see earlier in this chapter).

Cost: Methadone, when taken as part of a methadone maintenance program, is often paid for by the state. Some programs also take the Medicaid, Medicare, or private health insurance for reimbursement. Usually patients do not have to pay anything themselves.

Special Comments: By taking methadone every day, a heroin addict loses the need or desire to take heroin. Methadone is much safer than heroin; AIDS or heart infections cannot be contracted by drinking methadone, as they can by injecting heroin. Also, heroin obtained on the street is often secretly mixed with other substances, sometimes making injecting it fatal. Methadone is also safer for society: Heroin addicts must often engage in criminal activities to obtain heroin; methadone is legally available from special clinics and can be given free of charge to indigent patients. As methadone can also be abused and sold on the street, methadone clinics have strict regulations controlling the dispensing of methadone. By law, most methadone clinics offer counseling to their patients and always attempt to get them off all drugs. Methadone maintenance is often successful and certainly superior to heroin injection.

Part III

SPECIAL TOPICS ABOUT PSYCHIATRIC DRUGS

Chapter 13

Treating the Violent Patient

It is a popular notion, perpetuated by television and the movies, that people with psychiatric illnesses are violent and dangerous. For the most part, this view is absolutely false.

Certainly, the vast majority of patients with depression, bipolar depression, and anxiety disorder are no more violent, and probably less so, than anyone else. That is, as long as we mean violence toward others; patients with these diagnoses, of course, are prone to violence against themselves. There are a few psychiatric syndromes associated with violence toward others, although violence among psychiatric patients is not nearly as common as we are often led to believe.

Certain forms of schizophrenia may predispose people to violence. Patients with paranoid schizophrenia—those with schizophrenia who develop delusional ideas that people are out to harm them—may feel threatened and believe they need to defend themselves by violent means, as in this example:

Ralph, a twenty-two-year-old patient with chronic schizophrenia, decided to stop taking his antipsychotic medication one day. Three days later he began to feel that people on the street were talking about him. Then he became convinced that his next-door neighbor had been hired by the Mafia to kill him. He attempted to avoid the neighbor, but voices told him the neighbor was about to shoot him. One afternoon he saw the neighbor in the lobby of his apartment building. When the neighbor put his hand in his pocket, Ralph was sure he was reaching for a gun to shoot him. Ralph screamed and threw a small table in the lobby at the neighbor, then ran out the door into the street. He began screaming for police and throwing garbage cans at the door of the apartment building, hoping to hit his neighbor in case he ran out after him. Police were called and they immediately restrained Ralph and brought him to the emergency room. Ralph's violent behavior was motivated by fear, not a real or malicious desire to hurt anyone. Patients with schizophrenia do not routinely plot murders and are not vicious. They should not be shunned on the false belief that they are killers.

Direct injury to specific regions of the brain and some types of neurological illness can unleash violence, although this is not common. A form of epilepsy variously called temporal lobe epilepsy, psychomotor epilepsy, and partial complex seizures (the official name used by neurologists) is sometimes cited as a cause of violent behavior. Patients with this type of epilepsy are said to commit violent acts as part of an involuntary seizure. This behavior has never been well documented; if it occurs, it must be extremely rare. Most patients with temporal lobe epilepsy engage in purposeless behavior of a nonviolent nature during seizures.

The next example is of violent behavior that is the direct result of brain injury:

Donald was a hardworking electrician, devoted father of three children, and regular churchgoer until one fateful day when he tried to change a tire on his car. While he was kneeling to remove the lug nuts, the car suddenly fell off the jack, propelling the tip of the jack handle directly into Donald's head. He was knocked unconscious, bleeding severely, and was rushed by ambulance to the hospital. Miraculously, he survived the injury, but two days after regaining consciousness a marked disturbance in his behavior became apparent. The formerly mild-mannered Donald began swearing, screaming at people, and throwing things around the room. He violently attacked a nurse's aid. Eventually, he was transferred to the psychiatric unit for management of his violent behavior.

Another tragic form of violence associated with psychiatric illness is the rare case in which a new mother develops a psychotic postpartum depression. She has delusions that the baby is really a "devil" and hears voices that she must kill it to save the world. Fortunately, this is also a rare outcome. The vast majority of cases of postpartum depression do not follow this course, but it does highlight the importance of being vigilant and treating postpartum depression when it does occur.

Sometimes a psychiatric illness is used as an excuse to commit a violent crime. A person who can convince a judge or jury that he or she is "insane" by virtue of brain damage, drug abuse, or psychosis may not be held criminally responsible for his or her crimes. Obviously, this book is not the place to debate this point. I merely want to reiterate the point that psychiatric illness is rarely the cause of violence. Psychiatric patients have enough stigma with which to deal.

Drug abuse is probably the only psychiatric condition that regularly produces violence, for two reasons. First, addicts are so desperate to get drugs that they often commit acts of violence to obtain the money to buy drugs. Second, drugs like cocaine and amphetamines produce violent feelings in patients, and drugs like heroin and alcohol may unleash violent feelings that are already there but usually under control. Unlike patients with schizophrenia or manic bipolar disorder, who act on impulse in the occasional situations in which they become violent, a person driven crazy by cocaine may carefully plot a violent crime to get the money for drugs.

MEDICATIONS FOR VIOLENCE

In some instances, medications are needed to treat violent behavior when it is caused by a mental disturbance.

Agitated Schizophrenia or Manic Bipolar Disorder Patients

Antipsychotic medication or benzodiazepines like Ativan (lorazepam) should be given as soon as possible to the agitated patient with schizophrenia or the manic phase of bipolar disorder, by injection if the patient will not take the medicine by mouth. Many civil libertarians and patients' rights advocates have correctly questioned administration of antipsychotic drugs to patients against their will. Almost everybody agrees, however, that in the face of a dangerously violent situation, medication should be given immediately. It is not doing the patient any favor to let him or her continue being violent. Patients with schizophrenia or in the manic phase of bipolar disorder occasionally become violent when they feel threatened, and this is almost always a treatable condition. All the drugs used are described in detail in Chapter 10.

Brain-Damaged Patients

In the acute, emergency situation, the antipsychotic drugs are appropriate to stop violent behavior in a patient with brain damage.

If it is determined that the violence is actually part of a seizure, anticonvulsant medication is given. For longer-term management of chronic violent eruptions in patients with brain damage, especially in cases in which antipsychotic medications do not work sufficiently to control violence, many other drugs have been tried. These include anticonvulsants (Tegretol and Dilantin), lithium, and propranolol. Propranolol (Inderal) can be especially valuable. Its use in treating violence was pioneered by Dr. Stuart Yudofsky of Baylor College of Medicine. Propranolol is usually given to treat such medical conditions as high blood pressure, angina, and migraine headaches. It has been observed that propranolol, often in very high doses (more than 320 mg and as high as 1,000 mg a day), reduces violent behavior in brain-damaged patients. It can be given in combination with antipsychotic drugs like Risperdal, Geodon, Seroquel, or Zyprexa. Blood pressure and pulse must be carefully monitored because propranolol lowers both.

Psychotic Postpartum Depression

When a new mother develops a postpartum depression with psychotic symptoms (delusions and/or hallucinations), she should be given both an antidepressant (described in Chapter 7) and an antipsychotic medication (described in Chapter 10). It is often necessary to hospitalize such a patient, although this is not ideal as it separates the mother from her baby. Nevertheless, if there is any concern of violence toward herself or her baby, hospitalization is obviously the safest option.

Drug Abusers

The situation of the drug abuser is very difficult because drugs that produce violence often interact badly with drugs used to control violence. Cocaine, amphetamines, and angel dust (phencyclidine, PCP) can induce a violent state. This can be treated with antipsychotic drugs but should be done in an emergency room under careful medical supervision. The best treatment for violence in a drug abuser is physical restraint until the effects of the abused drug have worn off.

A few tips to family members: If your son, daughter, husband, wife, or other relative has a psychiatric problem and becomes violent, you should almost always call the police or an ambulance. It is very easy to say the wrong thing to psychotic patients and make them even more frightened and confused. Psychosis, by its very nature, makes people difficult to reason with and resistant to logic. In a psychotic state, frightened patients can be unbelievably strong; they truly believe that their life is threatened and that everybody, even their closest relatives, are the enemy. As difficult as it may be, it is best to get help quickly.

Also, do not let your love for your relative stand in the way of quick and effective treatment. Violent patients can hurt people and can themselves be hurt. It is best to allow trained people to restrain and quickly medicate a violent patient. There will be plenty of time, after the acute situation is resolved, to decide calmly on a proper course of treatment.

Finally, even in a person with a clear-cut diagnosis of schizophrenia or other mental disorder, always suspect alcohol or drug abuse if violence suddenly becomes a problem. Patients with schizophrenia or in the manic phase of bipolar disorder tolerate alcohol, cocaine, and heroin especially badly and are very prone to lose control when intoxicated.

Most violence does not involve psychiatric patients and should be taken care of by police and courts, not psychiatrists. However, when a psychiatric patient is out of control, a rapid response with physical restraint and medication is both humane and effective.

Chapter 14

Family, Environment, and Genetics

A mother came to see me about her thirty-five-year-old daughter. For about two years I had been treating her daughter with lithium for bipolar disorder. Recently, the daughter had developed a mild depression despite the lithium treatment, and I had prescribed an antidepressant as well. The mother was very concerned.

"Does this mean she is getting worse and lithium won't help anymore?" she asked me.

"No," I answered. "It is very common for lithium-treated patients to develop occasional breakthrough depressions. If treated quickly enough, these depressions usually resolve without any serious consequences. I do not think it means the lithium has stopped working."

"That's good to know. Is there anything we, my husband and I, should be doing? I mean, we never know whether to leave her alone when she gets depressed or urge her to go out and do things. Sometimes it's very frustrating when all she wants to do is stay in bed. And should we say anything about her weight? She's gained a lot since you put her on lithium."

These are all very common questions from family members of patients with psychiatric illness. Here was my answer:

"The most important thing is not to get angry at your daughter and make her feel you blame her for her problems. You have been very supportive in the past, and I think part of the reason she has done so well is the way you have treated her with respect and encouragement. When people get depressed, it's natural that they don't feel like doing things, and sometimes they really can't. So I wouldn't go overboard pushing her. Try to help her do the things that are essential and leave it at that. When the depression is over, she will pick up on her own. The weight gain troubles me too. It is a side effect of lithium, and also, depressed patients sometimes overeat. Right now I wouldn't make a big deal about it, but when her depression resolves, I definitely think we should encourage her to go on a diet and start an exercise program."

Then the mother asked me the question that is probably on the mind of every parent of a patient with psychiatric illness.

"Doctor, how did she get to be this way in the first place? Do you think it is because I had to go back to work when she was two? I think we always had good babysitters, but I wasn't home all day. My husband might have been a little gruff with the children in those days. He is really a good father, but you know how it is. He was just starting his business when our daughter was born, and at first it didn't go so well. Maybe he wasn't, you know, emotional enough with her. Could that do it?"

This kind of question breaks my heart. People have been brainwashed into believing that parents are responsible for mental illness. So mothers and fathers carry a tremendous burden of guilt and shame when their children require psychiatric care.

I explained what we know about the roots of mental illness. "We really do not know what causes any psychiatric illness. That's what the research is aimed at right now. There are a few things you should know. First, if working mothers and less than the most gushingly emotional fathers were the cause of mental illness, about half the world's population would be seeing psychiatrists right now. From what I have heard from you and your daughter, you were as good parents as most and the things you mentioned are not the cause of mental illness. It is possible that an abnormal gene causes some forms of psychiatric illness and there is some evidence for that with the specific problem your daughter has. But for all we know, it might be a virus, a toxin in the air, or just bad luck. I think bad parents can make mental illnesses worse and good parents can help make them a lot better, but parents don't cause schizophrenia, bipolar illness, serious depression, or panic attacks."

Did the mother feel relieved by my answer? Only partially. She felt better to know that I don't blame her and that scientists do not believe that bad parenting causes psychiatric illness. But do most of her friends and acquaintances know that? Or will she feel blamed by the people with whom she ordinarily comes into contact?

Furthermore, I could not give her a definite answer. I could not say, "Your daughter's illness is the result of a childhood viral infection that affected her brain." People are most reassured when they know the cause of an illness. Vague answers—the only kind that can honestly be given in psychiatry—are only partially helpful.

GENES AND MENTAL ILLNESS

Do genes cause psychiatric illness? There is good reason to think so, at least in part. The first step in determining whether a particular disease, psychiatric or otherwise, is inherited is to see whether it runs in families. In so-called family history studies, a group of patients with a disorder is selected along with a group of people without the disorder. The latter group is called the "normal" controls ("comparison" group is a better term for them—the people in this group are "normal" only insofar as they don't have the psychiatric illness under study). Then the history of psychiatric illnesses in first-degree relatives of the patients and of the comparison subjects is ascertained, either by asking the patients and comparison subjects about their families or, even better, by interviewing family members directly.

Through these studies, it was determined that such psychiatric disorders as schizophrenia, bipolar disorder, serious (major) depression, panic disorder, obsessive-compulsive disorder, and alcoholism clearly run in families. These disorders occurred in more relatives of patients than in relatives of comparison subjects.

Nevertheless, this tells us only that if a parent has a psychiatric condition there is a greater likelihood that his or her children will have it also. Is that because an abnormal gene is passed down or because the children learn to adopt the parent's behavior? Is it nature (genes) or nurture (the experience of being raised by a parent with a psychiatric condition)?

One way to try and tease this apart is to look at psychiatric conditions in twins. Identical twins (scientists call them monozygotic) have the same genes; fraternal twins (called dizygotic) share as many of the same genes as do ordinary brothers and sisters. In other words, monozygotic twins are genetically identical, and dizygotic twins are genetically similar.

If a disease is truly genetic, if one identical twin has it then the other twin should also have it, because they have the same genes. On the other hand, if one fraternal twin has the disease, the other fraternal twin need not also have it, because they may not have both inherited the abnormal gene. Scientists say that if a disease is genetic, the concordance rate should be higher for monozygotic twins than for dizygotic twins.

Excellent places to study twins are in Japan, Israel, Iceland, and the Scandinavian countries, where very complete health records, including twin registries, are maintained and groups of people have tended to stay in the same communities for generations. The United States is a particularly difficult country in which to do these studies because we keep awful health records and people move around so much that it is often very difficult to locate generations of relatives of a person with a particular disorder. Nevertheless, some of the most elegant twin studies of psychiatric illness have been done by Dr. Kenneth Kendler of the Medical College of Virginia. By studying the inheritance of psychiatric conditions in twins, it has been shown that schizophrenia, bipolar disorder, and panic disorder are probably, at least in part, genetic illnesses. I say in part because genes do not explain all cases of these disorders. In fact, about 60 percent of the risk for schizophrenia and about 30 percent of the risk for anxiety disorders and depression seems to come from inheriting a gene or several genes that predispose to those illnesses. The remaining risk comes from experiencing stressful life events, particularly during childhood, or environmental factors such as viral infection during pregnancy.

Now there exist even more powerful scientific methods for determining whether a disease is genetic. These methods involve molecular biology, a field that opened up with the discovery of the structure of DNA, the genetic molecule, in 1953 by James Watson and Francis Crick. Molecular biology is a very complex field. Basically, scientists can now take DNA and RNA from blood cells or from postmortem brain tissue, chop it up in test tubes, and find out whether people with a particular illness have a similar genetic pattern. By doing this, it is possible to determine on which of the twenty-three human chromosomes an abnormal gene for a given disorder resides and in some cases find a specific gene that increases risk for a specific psychiatric illness.

Using molecular biology, scientists localized the gene for the neuropsychiatric disorder Huntington's disease to chromosome 4. They have also found that the cause in a small number of people of Alzheimer's disease is inheritance of one or more of several genes.

There is now also evidence that some other psychiatric illnesses may be associated with abnormal genes. One group, studying Amish families, found evidence that bipolar disorder may be associated with chromosome 11, although follow-up studies have failed to confirm this finding. Another group, working in Israel, linked bipolar illness to the X chromosome, one of the two chromosomes that determine sex. It is possible, indeed very likely, that both groups are correct and that there are different genetic routes to bipolar illness. Significant progress has been made in finding genes for schizophrenia, although it is now clear that mutations must occur in several genes in order for a person actually to be at risk for this illness. A mutation that changes a gene for a receptor in the brain's serotonin system, called the serotonin transporter protein, clearly increases the risk to get depression and probably an anxiety disorder. A mutation in the gene for a chemical in the brain called monoamine oxidase (the antidepressants called monoamine oxidase inhibitors or MAOIs block this enzyme) may increase the risk in children and adults for antisocial behavior.

All of this work, which has occurred with remarkable speed, has the field of psychiatry at a high pitch of excitement. Molecular biology is now one of the top priorities of the National Institute of Mental Health's research program. There is good reason to expect that within the next decade, genes responsible for specific mental illnesses will be located.

Once a gene is located, it is still a long road before it is known what the abnormal gene does. It may make an abnormal substance that produces the illness, or it may be unable to make a necessary substance that normal genes make. For example, the gene for the protein neuregulin seems to be one of at least ten genes that can increase the risk for schizophrenia, but scientists are not entirely sure about all the things that neuregulin does in the brain, and it is clear that the neuregulin by itself is not the only culprit but must interact with abnormalities in several other genes, some still not discovered, before risk of schizophrenia is increased. Knowing that a specific gene or genes are involved in a disorder leads to obvious attempts to treat genetic mental illness either by blocking the action of abnormal genes or by giving patients necessary substances that abnormal genes fail to produce. We are a long way from being able to do this. In this regard, psychiatry is no different from most of the rest of medicine. We have known exactly what the mutation in a specific gene is that causes sickle-cell anemia for almost half a century, but that knowledge has not yet helped us treat or cure the disease.

Genetics clearly will not provide all the answers. Even in those conditions that we are pretty certain have a genetic basis, like schizophrenia, we sometimes find that only one member of an identical twin pair is affected. How did the other member escape the illness? One possibility is that he or she does have the abnormal gene but for some reason it is not expressed. Another possibility is that to get the disease, there must be a combination of abnormal genes and other factors. These other factors could be viruses, poisons, or stress. Obviously, we have a long way to go before we know how all these factors come together to produce an illness.

BLAMING GENES FOR EVERYTHING

With all the emphasis on genes and biology in psychiatric research, some people wonder if family and environment are ever factors in psychiatric illness.

In some situations, it may truly be harmful to blame everything on biology. A good example occurred to me after reading a very sad story in the newspaper.

A mother and father were suing the local school system for negligence. Their teenage son had recently committed suicide. The parents claimed that the school should have known their son was depressed and gotten help for him. I wondered if the parents believed that the school personnel should have known their child better than they did. Didn't they notice that their son was depressed? Should families be entirely "off the hook" for psychiatric problems?

I can only offer my own opinion. The major psychiatric illnesses like schizophrenia, bipolar disorder, major depression, panic disorder, alcoholism, and obsessive-compulsive disorder probably have genetic roots. Without abnormal genes I do not think it is possible to develop these conditions.

But stress, including a poor home environment while growing up, can influence the degree to which these abnormal genes are expressed. And this must vary from illness to illness. Schizophrenia is probably among the least influenced by stress. Warm, supportive treatment will make the life of a patient with schizophrenia easier, but I do not think it can prevent or cure the illness. The same seems to be true of bipolar illness. On the other hand, a good childhood with relatively little stress may prevent a person with a gene for alcoholism from becoming an alcoholic. A striking example is the serotonin transporter gene that I mentioned earlier. A milestone study performed in New Zealand showed that a mutation in that gene makes people more susceptible to stressful life events causing depression and suicide. This is a classical example of gene and environment interacting to cause a genetic disease. With that knowledge, scientists like Dr. Daniel Weinberger of the National Institute of Mental Health have been able to show using sophisticated brain-imaging techniques that the very same mutation in the gene for the serotonin transporter protein also alters the way specific parts of the human brain respond to stressful stimuli. Clearly, this information brings us closer to understanding what causes depression and makes depressed people commit suicide. Unfortunately, there is a still a lot of work to do because the research indicates that the serotonin transporter gene is probably only one of several genes that must be mutated before someone becomes depressed.

Certainly, the burden remains on family members to recognize a psychiatric problem promptly so that it can be treated. Depression may not be preventable, but suicide almost always is if the depressed patient receives prompt and humane care.

Parents should not feel guilty or ashamed if their children develop psychiatric problems. They should not believe they are bad parents or made horrible mistakes; however, they are responsible for getting their children help and for giving them as much support and encouragement as possible. Until the exact causes of mental illness are known and the cures are found, family members will continue to be the psychiatrist's most powerful allies in treatment.

Chapter 15

Weight Loss and Weight Gain

While reading through the side effects caused by psychiatric drugs, you may have noticed that one side effect crops up unusually often—weight gain. This is a plague for psychiatric patients and their doctors. Often, it seems that just when everyone is happy with the way a drug is working and the patient is ready to resume life, someone notices that the patient is gaining weight.

At first, it may not appear to be a major problem. During the acute part of a psychiatric illness, many patients lose their appetite, stop eating, and lose weight. So the first few pounds gained may seem like a breakthrough, a simple return of the ability to get exercise combined with a healthy appetite and eating habits.

Soon, however, the patient realizes that she is continuing to gain weight without seeming to eat all that much extra. Often, doctors fail to realize this weight gain as a side effect of the drug and mistakenly tell the patient that the cause of the problem is simply that she must be eating more. "Stop eating cake and cookies," the doctor pompously insists, "and the weight will disappear."

So the patient stops eating dessert, but the weight gain continues. Soon, the patient believes the treatment is worse than the disease and contemplates stopping the medication. Everyone accuses the patient of being a glutton. The patient feels so criticized that she indeed stops the medication without informing her physician. A month later, relapse occurs.

DRUGS CAUSE WEIGHT GAIN

The fact is that many psychiatric drugs—including some antidepressants, lithium and Depakote, and most drugs for psychosis—cause weight gain. We really do not understand why. Indeed, we understand a lot less about obesity in general than we once thought.

Physicians, nutritionists, and scientists used to insist that how much a person weighed was almost entirely a function of how much he ate and how much he exercised, with an emphasis on the former. The more calories consumed, the more weight gained. Vigorous exercise burns calories and eliminates a few pounds but not enough to offset a high caloric intake. So overweight people were told it was all up to them: Diet and exercise or your fatness is your fault.

Things are not so simple. Evidence now exists suggesting that weight is in part determined by metabolic rate, the rate at which the body burns calories and uses exercise. Each person apparently has a specific set point for weight, something akin to body temperature. A regulator, probably located in the part of the brain called the hypothalamus, controls how fast the body uses calories in almost the same way that body temperature is maintained at 98.6°.

Another factor seems to be the sensitivity of cells in the body to the hormone insulin. In so-called type I diabetes, the kind that usually begins in childhood, the pancreas does not make enough insulin, blood sugar (glucose) levels skyrocket, and the patient must take insulin to survive. Type II diabetes, which usually begins in adulthood, seems to be triggered by being obese. However, the underlying problem is usually an insensitivity of cells in the body to insulin, rather than actual insulin deficiency. This is called insulin resistance and itself may lead to obesity. Studies have now shown that two drugs that cause a great deal of weight gain, the antipsychotic medications clozapine (Clozaril) and Zyprexa (olanzapine), cause insulin resistance even before the patient becomes obese. Here again, the drugs are causing a metabolic abnormality that is not related to diet and exercise. This also explains why patients on clozapine and Zyprexa are so prone to developing diabetes. Other weight gain–inducing medications may also cause insulin resistance, although research studies have not yet been completed to confirm this.

Overeating absolutely causes weight gain. Decreasing calories causes weight loss. Below a certain point, however, scientists now believe, the hypothalamus will not permit any further burning of calories. Once a certain weight is reached through dieting, the body's metabolism slows and further weight loss becomes impossible. The only way to overcome this appears to be through absolute starvation, which is why patients with illnesses like anorexia nervosa can reduce their weight to the point that they come close to death.

Psychiatric drugs may cause weight gain by artificially slowing the metabolic rate. They may do this by tricking the hypothalamus into somehow changing its set point, or by causing insulin resistance, or they may affect the way fat cells throughout the body burn fat. All of this is speculation. What is clear is that many psychiatric drugs produce weight gain, even if the patient does not eat a lot.

Because so many psychiatric drugs have this unfortunate side effect, it is easier to list the drugs that do *not* cause weight gain (Table 33).

Keeping in mind the large number of drugs reviewed in this book, it is immediately obvious that the list of psychiatric drugs that do not produce weight gain is comparatively small. Patients taking cyclic antidepressants (for example, Tofranil, Elavil, Norpramin, Pertofrane), monoamine oxidase inhibitor antidepressants (for example, Parnate and Nardil), serotonin reuptake inhibitors and other newer antidepressants (especially Remeron, Paxil, and Effexor XR but also Prozac and Zoloft and probably Celexa, Lexapro, and Cymbalta too), antipsychotic drugs (especially clozapine and

---

Table 33.

Psychiatric Drugs That Do Not Cause Weight Gain

Antidepressant Drugs
Wellbutrin (bupropion)

Antipsychotic Drugs
Moban (molindone)
Geodon (ziprasidone)
Abilify (aripiprazole)

Drugs for Bipolar Affective Disorder
Tegretol (carbamazepine)
Lamictal (lamotrigine)

Drugs for Anxiety
All benzodiazepines (for example, Valium, Librium, Ativan, and Xanax)
BuSpar (buspirone)
Luvox (fluvoxamine)

Zyprexa but also Seroquel and Risperdal), and mood stabilizers (lithium and Depakote) may all gain weight. An interesting drug is the anticonvulsant (that is, a drug used to treat epilepsy) Topamax (topiramate). This drug was tried for bipolar disorder and failed (it may have utility in helping alcoholic patients), but it turned out to be one of the few medications that cause weight loss. Patients often lose five to ten pounds in the first few weeks of taking Topamax and do not regain the weight. Unfortunately, the drug is sedating and sometimes adversely affects memory (some have called it "dopeamax"), so many patients cannot tolerate it. Nevertheless, adding Topamax is one strategy for helping patients on psychiatric drugs lose weight. Another medication used for weight loss is Meridia (sibutramine). This drug has the same neurotransmitter properties as Effexor XR (venlafaxine) and Cymbalta (duloxetine), but for some reason it didn't work out as an antidepressant. It can promote a mild weight loss and is also sometimes added to other drugs when they cause weight gain. An experimental treatment for weight gain caused by clozapine is Glucophage (metformin). Glucophage is currently used to treat type II diabetes because it increases insulin sensitivity. It is too early in the research to know how well this works. Taking amphetamines or other stimulants is definitely not a good idea, however. Weight loss from stimulants lasts only a few weeks and then most people regain all the weight.

COMMONLY ASKED QUESTIONS

Is the weight gain always severe? No. It varies tremendously from patient to patient. Some people gain only a few pounds, which is usually acceptable. Other patients, however, gain ten, twenty, or even more pounds.

Is dieting while on psychiatric drugs useless? No. Staying on a diet often limits the amount of weight gained. It just is not fair to blame a patient who gains weight on a psychiatric drug for not dieting enough. Some of the weight gain may not be preventable, even with strict caloric reduction.

Does weight gain continue as long as the drug is continued? No. After a few months, it usually stops and weight levels off.

Can any of the drugs that do not produce weight gain on the list be used to help with dieting and weight loss programs? As mentioned above, Topamax and Meridia are sometimes added and promote weight loss, although there are interactions between them and some psychiatric drugs that limit their use. Amphetamines like Dexedrine were once widely prescribed for the sole purpose of weight loss. It is true that they speed up metabolism and curb appetite and, if taken regularly, cause weight loss at first. But the effect is very transitory and most people quickly gain back what they lose, probably because the hypothalamic set point is reset to slow the metabolic rate. Furthermore, the patient who uses amphetamines for weight loss quickly becomes addicted and cannot stop the drug without suffering withdrawal depression. Consequently, amphetamines should not be prescribed for weight loss. On rare occasions, described in more detail in Chapter 7, they are useful as antidepressants. They are also prescribed for attention-deficit/hyperactivity disorder.

When Prozac was first tested as an antidepressant, many depressed patients were observed to lose some weight. Sometimes this loss was substantial, five to ten pounds. Rumors quickly spread that Prozac would be effective and safe as a weight-reducing pill for overweight people. Although the company that makes Prozac did not contribute in any way to the spread of these rumors, there is no doubt that some physicians initially prescribed Prozac to nondepressed patients to help them lose weight. As it turns out, most patients do not lose very much weight from Prozac and the little they do lose is usually regained in a few months.

It is now clear that after long-term exposure (that is, several months), many patients gain weight on the SSRI antidepressants like Prozac, Zoloft, and Paxil. Even worse are the new antipsychotic drugs like clozapine and olanzapine, which almost always produce substantial weight gain.

The other drugs on the list are more or less neutral when it comes to weight gain and loss. Tegretol does not cause weight gain the way lithium and Depakote often do, but it usually does not induce weight loss either. Benzodiazepine antianxiety drugs and BuSpar also do not affect weight one way or the other.

Are any psychiatric drugs useful for treating anorexia nervosa?
Anorexia nervosa is an illness affecting mainly young women in which the patient develops a fixed idea that she is overweight. No matter how thin she becomes, she still looks in the mirror and sees herself as fat. The patient stops eating and abuses water pills (diuretics) and laxatives to try to lose more weight. Often, she becomes an exercise fanatic and makes herself vomit after meals, which are both attempts to lose weight. The illness can be fatal, as the sad case of the popular rock star Karen Carpenter made clear to the world.

Many psychiatric drugs have been used to treat anorexia nervosa. Some clinicians have observed the high rate of depression in people with anorexia and tried antidepressants. Others have likened patients' insistence that they are fat when in fact they are wasting away to a psychotic delusion and prescribed antipsychotics. There is little evidence that antidepressants or antipsychotics work in anorexia nervosa. In fact, a recent study conducted by Dr. B. Timothy Walsh of Columbia University showed that antidepressants in fact do not work for anorexia nervosa. Patients with anorexia nervosa are often extremely anxious, and for this reason antianxiety drugs are sometimes used.

Can any of the drugs be used to treat bulimia? Like anorexia nervosa, bulimia is an eating disorder that affects primarily young women. Recent reports indicate that college students are especially prone to developing bulimia, although many experts suspect that this hypothesis is more the result of who is surveyed than the true prevalence of bulimia. The primary feature of bulimia is binge eating. People with bulimia seem periodically to develop uncontrollable urges to eat as much as they possibly can, often consuming jars of peanut butter, gallons of ice cream, and boxes of cookies at a single sitting. Many make themselves vomit immediately after bingeing, so only a portion of bulimics actually gain weight. Some patients go through periods of bulimia and anorexia nervosa in cycles.

There is now evidence that antidepressants, such as Zoloft and Prozac, are effective in the treatment of bulimia. Studies also suggest that Topamax may be effective. This seems particularly true if medication is combined with nutritional counseling and cognitive and behavioral psychotherapy.

Is weight gain important enough to warrant switching drugs or even stopping a psychiatric drug? Sometimes. Being overweight is unpleasant and bad for your health. Sometimes, a small weight gain is a reasonable price to pay for freedom from a debilitating psychiatric illness. Like any side effect, a balance must always be struck between the harm a drug does and the benefit it provides. Some people gain a lot of weight from psychiatric drugs and this may mean that switching to a different drug is in order. For example, some depressed patients who gain too much weight from drugs like Paxil or Effexor XR can be switched to Wellbutrin (bupropion) and maintain the depression-free state while losing the drug-induced weight gain. Others, however, relapse into depression with this switch. Keep in mind that there are rules for switching from one drug to another that must always be observed. You must wait for two weeks after stopping Nardil before trying Paxil, for example.

When a psychiatric drug is stopped, will the weight be lost? Any weight gained because of a psychiatric drug is usually lost once the drug is stopped. It may take a few months, however, to return to baseline weight.

Are there medical disorders that produce both weight gain and psychiatric illness? There are several, but probably the most important is an underactive thyroid. This condition, called hypothyroidism, results in weight gain, lethargy, fatigue, hair loss, intolerance to cold, and constipation, among other symptoms. It is increasingly recognized that some very subtle forms of hypothyroidism can be associated with chronic depression. For this reason, psychiatrists sometimes order blood tests of thyroid function when treating patients with psychiatric illness. Also, if a depressed patient fails to respond to the usual antidepressant drug therapy, more extensive thyroid tests are recommended because hidden thyroid problems may be the reason.

Lithium, the primary drug used for patients with bipolar disorder, causes both hypothyroidism and weight gain. Sometimes, but not always, lithium causes weight gain by bringing about a decrease in thyroid gland function. Therefore, it is important to undergo thyroid tests every six months to a year while on lithium. If hypothyroidism is the problem, then adding thyroid hormone to lithium can lead to some weight reduction.

Are there medical conditions that cause weight loss and psychiatric illness? Yes, and many of these are serious. Many forms of cancer, for example, produce weight loss and depression. Another illness that can do this is AIDS. As depression itself results in a reduced appetite, it is very common for depressed patients to report weight loss; the vast majority do not have serious underlying medical problems. Any patient with depression and weight loss should, however, be evaluated by a medical doctor to rule out the possibility of an underlying medical problem. Often, the doctor can do this simply by taking a good medical history and ordering routine blood and urine tests, but sometimes a more in-depth medical workup is needed.

Chapter 16

Sex and Psychiatric Drugs

Psychiatrists are supposed to be the doctors to whom people can tell anything and everything without feeling embarrassed. Maybe that is true, but it is surprising how reluctant people are to reveal to their doctor that a psychiatric drug is producing a side effect that interferes with sex and sexual function.

Today, most medical schools teach young doctors to obtain a sexual history from every patient they see. Medical students are told it is their responsibility to bring this subject up, not the patient's. Most people are reluctant to reveal they have a sexual problem or to ask questions about how illness or medications may affect their sex lives.

Unfortunately, many doctors—psychiatrists included—are also embarrassed to discuss sexual issues. Elderly patients are especially likely to leave the doctor's office without discussing sexual concerns or difficulties because even physicians maintain the ridiculous myth that old people do not have sex.

SEX AND PSYCHIATRIC ILLNESS

Many psychiatric illnesses have a profound effect on sexual functioning. One of my professors used to insist that "if a depressed person still has a good sex drive, you know he isn't too far gone." As general rules, depressed patients usually lose their interest in sex at least to some degree, anxious patients have a sex drive but cannot calm down long enough to have sex, and manic patients want to have sex all day long.

For diagnostic purposes, then, a psychiatrist should also ask at least a few basic questions about a new patient's sex life. Here is a typical discussion about sex I might have during the evaluation of a thirty-five-year-old married man complaining of depression:

"You've told me so far that you have lost your appetite and have felt blue most of the time for the last six weeks or so. You also do not have interest in a lot of things you used to enjoy. How about your interest in sex?"

"Forget it," the patient replies emphatically. "We haven't had sex in six months."

"You mean you and your wife haven't had sex at all in the last six months?"

"That's right, if you could call what we have sex."

"Is the problem that you have lost your interest in having sex—your sex drive is low—or that you and your wife are having trouble with your relationship?"

"I'm not interested."

Obviously, everything doesn't quite fit together with this story. "You told me you have been feeling depressed for about a month and a half, but you haven't had sex with your wife for six months. What was the problem before you started feeling depressed?"

Now I get the story. "She's never home, so how can we have sex?" my patient explained. "And when she does come home from work in the middle of the night, she is usually exausted—who wouldn't be, with a work schedule like that?—and falls asleep."

After some more discussion, I was able to figure out that the patient really had maintained his sex drive. He still thought about sex and often became aroused. The problem here had to do with his relationship with his wife. Although he was clearly depressed, loss of libido (sex drive) was not one of his symptoms, as it often is with depressed patients.

This man's sexual difficulty required counseling and therapy, not antidepressant medication. Other times, however, a loss of interest in sex is a direct result of depression.

Patients with anxiety disorders, for example, generalized anxiety disorder, may be so nervous that they can't take their minds off their troubles long enough to enjoy sex. These patients may suffer from impotence or difficulty with vaginal lubrication. Anxiety disorder may make it difficult to relax enough during sex to maintain an erection or have an orgasm.

A cardinal symptom of mania, on the other hand, is increased sex drive. Manic patients often speak incessantly about sex, sometimes at inappropriate times or places. They become sexually irresponsible, often forgetting about the risks of pregnancy or sexually transmitted diseases. Although psychiatrists are not interested in spoiling someone's good time, the increased sex drive of manic patients usually leads to unfortunate consequences and requires treatment.

DRUGS AFFECT SEX

Treatments, however, sometimes produce more sexual impairment than the original illness. A number of psychiatric drugs, particularly the antidepressants, can produce sexual side effects (Table 34).

Antidepressants such as Prozac, Paxil, Zoloft, Luvox, Celexa, Lexapro, Cymbalta, and Effexor XR (see Chapter 7) are noteworthy in this respect. These drugs are used for patients with many forms of depression and anxiety disorder. Patients with depression typically lose their sex drive while anxiety disorders often make it hard for patients to relax enough to enjoy sex.

About four weeks after beginning treatment with one of these drugs, the patient with depression or anxiety disorder typically feels more energetic

Table 34.

Sexual Side Effects of Psychiatric Drugs

SYMPTOM	DRUGS
Delayed orgasm	Many antidepressants, especially monoamine oxidase inhibitors (for example, Nardil, Parnate), SSRIs and SNRIs, (for example Prozac, Paxil, Lexapro, Effexor), and Anafranil
Priapism (prolonged erection)	Trazodone (Desyrel)
Retrograde ejaculation (ejaculation into bladder)	Many antidepressants and antipsychotics (for example, Mellaril)
Hypersexuality	Any antidepressant that produces manic behavior, including Nardil, Parnate, and Prozac

and hopeful, stops worrying, and begins to anticipate events with pleasure, including sex.

About one month after this good feeling, however, the patient often (about 70 percent of the time in my experience) notices a problem. Both men and women find that the length of time needed to achieve an orgasm lengthens. Men are usually not concerned at first. They are able to maintain erections for long periods and view this effect as good. But then the frustration sets in.

Unfortunately, patients are often embarrassed to discuss such subjects as orgasms with the doctor, so they suffer. They sometimes think there is something wrong with them and do not realize that delayed orgasm is a fairly common side effect of many antidepressants. If it goes on too long, the patient finds sex too frustrating and begins to lose interest. It also occurs with use of other antidepressants, including the cyclic antidepressants like Tofranil and Elavil and monoamine oxidase inhibitors like Nardil.

Antidepressants, then, do not usually cause impotence or decreased sexual desire. If anything, they increase sex drive by relieving depression; however, they may cause delayed orgasm. It is important to discuss this problem with the doctor, because several solutions are possible. First, it is important to know that delayed orgasm occasionally goes away with time, so sometimes realizing it is a side effect and waiting for it to go away is the best solution. Second, reducing the dose of the drug may help. If these remedies do not work, a counteracting medication can be added. Wellbutrin (bupropion) is the only drug so far shown by research studies to counteract the sexual side effects of other antidepressants. Finally, it may be wise to switch to one of the three antidepressants that do not cause sexual side effects: Wellbutrin, Remeron, or Serzone (although the latter has other problems). The mood stabilizer Lamictal does not cause sexual side effects and sometimes is effective by itself for patients with depression who do not have bipolar disorder.

Retrograde ejaculation is another sexual side effect that occasionally occurs with psychiatric drugs. The male ejaculation goes the wrong way, back into the bladder instead of out of the penis. Report this effect to the doctor immediately. Usually, dose reduction or switching to another drug is required.

Patients who take benzodiazepine antianxiety drugs (like Xanax and Klonopin) for prolonged periods occasionally complain of reduced sex drive. Very occasionally, men on lithium complain of difficulty maintaining an erection.

One final rare, but potentially dangerous, side effect should be mentioned. Some men taking the antidepressant drug Desyrel (trazodone) develop prolonged erection, a condition called priapism. It is estimated to occur in only one in one thousand to one in ten thousand men who take Desyrel. This can be an emergency because an erection lasting more than an hour may result in serious damage to the penis. Men who take Desyrel should be warned about this side effect and should call the physician immediately if they have a sustained erection for no apparent reason.

DRUGS TO IMPROVE SEX

What about the use of psychiatric drugs to improve sexual function? Many people find that alcohol, marijuana, cocaine, amyl nitrite, Quaaludes, and other "recreational" drugs make sex more intense or more enjoyable. Are there prescription drugs that also do this?

This is a tricky area because the potential for abuse is obvious. Of course, a depressed patient who takes an antidepressant will realize improved sexual performance and desire once the depression abates. However, this is not treatment of a sexual problem but rather treatment of a sexual impairment caused by underlying depression.

In some situations, extreme anxiety surrounding sex can be treated with antianxiety agents. Some patients, for a variety of reasons, develop intense anxiety about sex. This may stem from unconscious prohibitions about sex learned in childhood or from performance anxiety and fear of failure. It may stem from negative feelings about the sexual partner that the patient is unable to recognize and deal with. Most of these call for psychotherapy; medications are generally unwarranted, but short-term prescription of small doses of benzodiazepine antianxiety drugs like Valium or Xanax may be helpful. It is important not to prescribe these too liberally or the patient may come to feel that he or she cannot have sex without them. It thus can become a psychological dependency.

Psychiatrists, psychologists, and psychoanalysts are often portrayed as being preoccupied with sex. Some people think that everything they say to the psychiatrist will be interpreted with respect to sex. Therefore, they resist openly discussing sexual problems and sexual side effects. Let me emphasize the two main points of this chapter: First, the doctor must obtain a sexual history as part of the initial psychiatric evaluation, and second, any possible sexual side effects of psychiatric drugs must be brought to light.

Chapter 17

Treating the Elderly

Too many doctors are frightened and refuse to prescribe psychiatric drugs for elderly patients, and thus many elderly patients with psychiatric illness remain untreated.

This problem has been made worse by media attention to overprescription of psychiatric drugs to patients in nursing homes and recent warnings that antipsychotic drugs increase the risk of dying among elderly patients with dementia (such as Alzheimer's disease). It is true that many nursing home patients are given drugs without proper medical supervision, often resulting in serious side effects. There also exists the prevailing misconception that it is somehow normal for older people to feel depressed and anxious. After all, younger people reason, it is depressing to grow old, so what is there to treat with medication?

It is important to set the record straight on these issues. First, it is not dangerous to prescribe psychiatric drugs to elderly people who have treatable mental disorders. Certain skills and knowledge are required, but treatment should not be avoided just because someone is over sixty-five.

Second, what goes on in some nursing homes is bad medicine and should be corrected. The appropriate solution, however, is better medical care, not abandonment of psychiatric treatment for the elderly.

Third, depression, psychosis, and anxiety disorder are absolutely never normal, no matter how old someone is. This does not mean that psychiatric drugs always cure these disorders, but some form of treatment should always be considered. Most elderly people do not become depressed, although the incidence of depression does rise in the elderly.

RULES FOR TREATING THE ELDERLY

There are three important features to stress in treating elderly people with psychiatric drugs:

1. The diagnosis of psychiatric illness may be complicated.

2. There may be preexisting/coexisting medical problems that pose particular challenges.

3. Elderly people are very sensitive to all drugs and may experience more side effects than younger people.

These points require further explanation.

Diagnosis

Whenever an elderly person develops a psychiatric symptom, the first consideration must be whether a physical medical problem exists. With age, the chance of developing medical problems increases, as does the possibility that a new psychiatric problem is really a symptom of medical disease. All people over age sixty-five who complain of depression, loss of interest, decreased appetite, constipation, change in sleep habits, or anxiety, or who exhibit abnormal behavior (for example, hallucinations and delusions) need a complete medical and neurological workup.

The list of medical problems that can cause psychiatric symptoms in the elderly is very long and includes all forms of cancer, hormonal disturbances, heart problems, unrecognized strokes, and Alzheimer's dementia. Note these examples:

Mrs. C., an eighty-year-old widow, complained to her married children on several occasions that she frequently felt dizzy and light-headed. Sometimes she experienced a fluttering in her chest and broke out in a sweat. Her internist examined her, drew some routine blood tests, and performed an electrocardiogram. All the tests were normal, so Mrs. C. was told it was her "nerves" and sent home with a prescription for a tranquilizer.

Fortunately, one of her daughters felt a second opinion was in order and referred her to another physician, who performed a twenty-four-hour monitor test of her heart. This revealed a serious, but intermittent, irregularity in Mrs. C.'s heart rhythm. A simple electrocardiogram, which monitors heart rate for only a few minutes, can easily miss this kind of problem. Mrs. C. required a pacemaker, which solved her problem. Tranquilizers were clearly the wrong treatment.

Mr. B., a sixty-six-year-old retired shop owner, complained of trouble sleeping and seemed listless and bored. His wife noted that he had been picking at his food for several weeks and often seemed distracted. His family doctor found nothing wrong, so Mr. B. was referred to a psychiatrist. Here is how the beginning of the consultation went:

"How are you feeling today, Mr. B.?"

"I'm okay, I guess. About the same as before."

"Your wife says that you have not seemed yourself lately. Have you noticed that yourself?"

"Yeah, maybe for about a month or so."

"When exactly did it start?"

"Oh, maybe a month ago, September I guess."

The problem was that it was February and a "month ago" would have been January. The psychiatrist then gently tested Mr. B.'s memory by asking him questions about what he had done the day before, what he had eaten for breakfast, and where his children were living. Mr. B. seemed confused and could not answer most of the questions. As he tried to answer, he became visibly upset, then clammed up and seemed disinterested in the rest of the interview.

Further testing revealed that Mr. B. was suffering from Alzheimer's dementia, not depression. This devastating illness is the most common form of dementia and results in progressive loss of memory and other intellectual functions. There is no cure, but drugs called cholinesterase inhibitors—Aricept (donepezil), Exelon (rivastigmine), and Razadyne (galantamine)—and Namenda (memantine) can slow the progression of the disease. Research has indicated the strong possibility of a genetic basis to the disorder. Frequently, demented patients are first thought to be depressed or psychotic. Antidepressants and other psychiatric drugs often make the memory ability of patients with dementia even worse, so the diagnosis is particularly important.

On the other hand, everyone was convinced that Mrs. G. was suffering from dementia because at age seventy-one, she started to forget things and act confused. She talked very little, looked glum, and seemed disinterested. A psychiatrist noted, however, that Mrs. G. did well on memory tests but seemed to have trouble concentrating. Careful questioning revealed that she also had crying spells, loss of appetite, and insomnia, and felt that she had raised her children so badly that now they were all suffering. In fact, Mrs. G.'s children were happy and well adjusted. Mrs. G. was suffering from major depression. What seemed like a memory problem was really the result of poor concentration, a common symptom of depression. Mrs. G. was treated with an antidepressant and made a full recovery.

Research into depression in the elderly has revealed that it may take a form distinct from depression in younger people. The concept of "vascular depression" has been pioneered by Dr. Ranga Krishnan of Duke University and Dr. George Alexopoulos of Cornell University. It is found in elderly people who have their first episode of depression after age sixty-five and who have had a history of diseases involving the blood vessels, such as high blood pressure, transient ischemic attacks (TIAs), or stroke. These patients seem more apathetic than sad and usually do not have a family history of depression. MRI scans show small abnormalities scattered throughout the deep regions of the brain, particularly in the front. Antidepressants seem less likely to work in patients with vascular depression, and sometimess electroconvulsive therapy is the only thing that works.

A final case is that of Mr. R., a vigorous eighty-year-old man who had walked five miles and spent at least one hour daily in his garden until he began complaining that the neighbors were stealing his gardening tools. He refused to walk his usual five miles because he became convinced that his wife was having an affair while he was gone. Finally, he accused his grandson of hiding his glasses on purpose to confuse him. These clear signs of paranoid delusions often occur in elderly patients with Alzheimer's disease, but the curious thing about Mr. R. is that his memory seemed fine. Paranoid delusions also occur in patients with major depression, but Mr. R. had no other symptoms consistent with depression. Paranoid delusions are also a component of schizophrenia, but this disorder rarely manifests for the first time in someone of Mr. R.'s age. A neurological examination revealed a number of abnormalities that turned out to be secondary to a brain tumor. Fortunately, the tumor was benign, and with the proper treatment, Mr. R.'s paranoid delusions disappeared completely.

Another problem in deciding what is and is not a psychiatric illness in the elderly is the effect of the various drugs they frequently must take for medical problems. Many common medications, like those prescribed to treat high blood pressure, can produce serious psychiatric symptoms. As elderly people are more likely to take medications, development of a psychiatric symptom should be carefully analyzed with respect to initiation of a new drug for a medical problem.

All of this is not to say that a diagnosis of psychiatric illness in an elderly person is impossible. It merely reinforces the need for careful attention to many factors, especially the possibility of underlying medical illness.

Preexisting/Coexisting Medical Problems

Medical problems can make psychiatric drug treatment of the elderly tricky. Although a medical problem may not be the cause of an elderly person's psychiatric symptoms, an elderly person is more likely than a younger person to have some medical problem that will interfere with a psychiatric drug. For example, heart conditions that make the use of cyclic antidepressants like Tofranil and Elavil more risky are relatively rare in young adults but become more common with age. Some psychiatric drugs, like monoamine oxidase inhibitors, clozapine, and Zyprexa, may cause problems in patients with diabetes, which also is more common in elderly people. Most cyclic antidepressants and many antipsychotic drugs (like Thorazine and Mellaril) can result in a serious medical problem in an older man with an enlarged

Table 35.

Some Drugs That Are Comparatively Safe for Elderly Patients

ILLNESS	DRUG	ADVANTAGE
Depression	Nortriptyline[a]	May not lower blood pressure as much as other cyclic antidepressants
	Prozac, Paxil, Zoloft, Celexa, Lexapro[a]	Do not affect blood pressure, heart rate, bowel function, or urinary function
	Effexor XR, Remeron	Few interactions with other drugs
Psychosis	Risperdal, Zyprexa, Seroquel, Geodon	Minimal sedation, no EPS
Anxiety	Xanax, Ativan	May be more easily metabolized by elderly people than Klonopin Valium, Librium, or Tranxene

[a]See Chapter 7.

prostate. Hence, medical problems—and the drugs used to treat them—may interfere with the use of psychiatric drugs.

Again, this does not mean that psychiatrists should hesitate to treat the depressed or anxious elderly patient. It does mean that the psychiatrist and the medical doctor treating an elderly patient should work together to find the safest treatment plan.

There is now a controversy about whether the newer antidepressants like Prozac, Paxil, and Zoloft are as effective for elderly people with serious depression as the old cyclic antidepressants like nortriptyline (Pamelor). A few studies have suggested that the older drugs are slightly more effective; others find the SSRIs (Paxil, Zoloft, Celexa, Lexapro, and Prozac) to be just as effective. Because the newer SSRI antidepressants, along with newer drugs like Effexor XR, Remeron, and Cymbalta, are so much safer than the cyclics in terms of effects on the heart and other organs, most clinicians will recommend them first to elderly patients with depression. If they do not work, however, the cyclics, particularly nortriptyline, will be considered.

Increased Sensitivity to Side Effects

Many psychiatric drugs produce a drop in blood pressure when the patient stands up quickly. This is particularly serious in elderly patients, who can experience significant decreases in blood pressure when taking some antidepressants and antipsychotic drugs. This decrease in pressure may cause dizziness and light-headedness and result in serious falls. Some psychiatric drugs also cause drowsiness. Depakote is more likely to cause a decrease in platelets and anemia in older than younger people, and the elderly are more likely to have a drop in sodium level when on SSRI and SNRI antidepressants. Again, elderly people are more sensitive than younger people to this side effect. In general, elderly people are more sensitive to drugs of any kind because the capacity to metabolize (break down) drugs declines with age. A younger person given a drug rapidly breaks it down, but in elderly people, the drug may hang around in the body for a longer period.

Special mention should be made of the recent finding that antipsychotic drugs increase the mortality risk in elderly people with dementia. The leading cause of nursing home placement for people with dementia is behavioral disturbance, not memory loss. Behavioral problems in elderly patients with dementia are serious and can include severe agitation, paranoid delusions, hallucinations, and even violent behavior. Many drugs have been tried to help with these problems, including clonidine, propranolol, anticonvulsants (Depakote and Tegretol), BuSpar, and benzodiazepines. Some work, but often their side effects are difficult to manage. The drugs that work the best are the antipsychotic medications given in very low doses. Risperdal, Haldol, Trilafon, Zyprexa, and Seroquel are popular choices. Often they can be given for a short period of time and then stopped without a return of the problem. The recent finding of increased death rates, usually from heart problems or infections, came from carefully looking over data from clinical trials of these drugs that were mostly completed years ago. None of these studies were specifically designed to investigate this particular problem, and the risk is small, only a few percentage points. Nevertheless, more elderly people died while on an antipsychotic drug than while on a placebo in these studies, causing the FDA to force drug companies to issue special warnings to physicians. Some physicians are skeptical about this finding, and others wonder what they are supposed to do to treat the agitated or psychotic elderly patient. There is no easy answer, but sometimes with the approval of the family there is no choice but to administer antipsychotic drugs to elderly people and monitor them carefully.

With very few exceptions, elderly people should always be given lower doses of medication and should be evaluated for side effects more frequently than younger people. Some medications may be safer than others for elderly people, as shown in Table 35. In general, for any drug, it is prudent to start the elderly patient with half the dose that a younger person would start with. Lower doses may actually work well in elderly patients. If it is recommended that blood levels be obtained for a drug for safety reasons, for example, lithium blood levels, these should be obtained about twice as often in elderly people as in younger people.

One of the most tragic situations is the elderly person left to suffer with psychiatric illness. A major problem here at present is the terrible Medicare rule that limits people over sixty-five to the barest minimum of outpatient psychiatric care. An older person essentially has to become so sick with a psychiatric problem that he or she needs hospitalization before Medicare will pay for treatment. When Medicare does pay, reimbursement rates are very low, even though taking care of an elderly person with psychiatric illness is usually more time-consuming than caring for a young patient.

Elderly people can and should be treated for psychiatric illness with medications. Careful diagnosis, skillful prescription, good communication between psychiatrist and primary care physican and with family members, and vigilance for potentially serious side effects are required. In other words, it takes good medical practice.

Chapter 18

Psychiatric Drugs and Pregnancy

Scientists, especially those who work for drug companies, have expended many years and great effort in engineering drugs with the special properties necessary to cross from the blood into the brain. After all, unless a drug can gain access to the brain, it probably will not be much help in treating a psychiatric problem.

Unfortunately, many of the properties that enable a drug to cross the blood-brain barrier also enable the drug to cross the placenta and enter the fetus. Since the 1950s and thalidomide, we have become acutely aware of the potential dangers to the fetus of a pregnant woman who takes medications. We also know that alcohol, cigarettes, and cocaine are bad for the unborn baby. Recent research has suggested that depression and anxiety disorder in a pregnant woman may also be deleterious to the fetus and cause lifelong problems for the offspring.

In the evaluation of the potential harm a psychiatric drug may do to a fetus, special problems arise. These drugs affect the brain and it is hard to determine right away if a newborn infant has subtle brain damage because its mother took psychiatric medications during pregnancy. Infants exposed to psychiatric drugs in utero will not show lower intelligence, learning disabilities, hyperactivity, or any of a number of behavioral problems for years.

A problem in sorting out to what degree illness during pregnancy affects the fetus is also complex because of the nature-versus-nurture issue. Because most psychiatric illnesses have a genetic component, the fact that a women who is depressed during pregnancy has a child who grows up to have depression could mean that she has passed along a gene for depression or that depression during pregnancy changes the chemical environment sufficiently to affect the fetus's brain as it is developing. It turns out that both things are true. We should not let fathers off the hook, by the way. One series of studies has shown that the older the father at the time of conception, the more likely the offspring to develop schizophrenia. That is, there is a risk to being involved with old sperm.

Drug companies and medical textbooks usually offer the following vague advice: When contemplating use of a psychiatric drug in a pregnant woman, the benefits of the treatment must be weighed against the risks to the fetus. I cannot think of a more useless sentence. Without evidence one way or the other, what can actually be weighed? Who decides when treating a psychiatric illness in a pregnant woman if it is worth risking even the most remote possibility of harm to the fetus? In this age of rampant malpractice suits, psychiatrists are going to be very reluctant to make such a decision. Can a pregnant woman with severe depression or panic attacks or psychosis be expected to decide and make a well-informed decision? Should we involve the lawyers?

WHAT WE DO KNOW

Let me first go over the few things we do know with some certainty about psychiatric illness and psychiatric drugs during pregnancy.

Contrary to previous beliefs, pregnancy is not a time when psychiatric illness is relatively quiet. Psychosis, depression, mania, and anxiety attacks all occur during pregnancy, usually in women who have had these problems before.

A big problem in figuring out if psychiatric drugs increase the risk of birth defects is that birth defects themselves are very uncommon. If a particular birth defect occurs in one out of ten thousand live births, for example, then it is hard to know if two out of ten thousand that occur in women taking a drug is a significant increase or just chance (in fact, using statistics themselves, it is not significant, but no one would want to be that second parent who would blame herself for taking the drug or that doctor who prescribed them). Furthermore, studies tend to contradict themselves. One study may say a particular drug is safe during pregnancy and then a few years later another finds a problem. A good example of this is antidepressants and pregnancy. A number of studies, mostly involving newer serotonin reuptake inhibitor antidepressants like Prozac, Paxil, Zoloft, Celexa, and Lexapro, seemed to indicate that they were safe during pregnancy. Psychiatrists began to prescribe them to very depressed pregnant women. More recently, however, studies have been published suggesting a small risk of a condition called pulmonary hypertension in babies born to mothers who had taken antidepressants during pregnancy. Pulmonary hypertension is often fatal, so even a small risk is unacceptable. Now, most psychiatrists refuse to prescribe antidepressants to pregnant women, with good reason.

Another problem in evaluating whether psychiatric drugs cause problems when taken during pregnancy is that it is impossible to perform formal studies of this problem. We cannot deliberately give some women with a psychiatric illness a specific drug and some a placebo as we would normally do in nonpregnant patients to evaluate if a drug works. In fact, almost all studies of psychiatric medications specifically exclude pregnant women. Therefore, the only way we know if drugs are harmful to the fetus is to poll women who took them, usually relying on reports of their doctors when a problem occurred. Because good outcomes are usually not reported, the deleterious effects of drugs during pregnancy might be exaggerated.

Even getting pregnant may be affected by psychiatric drugs. Certainly, losing sex drive or not being able to have an erection, both side effects of some psychiatric drugs, will make it hard to have a pregnancy.

SOME RECOMMENDATIONS

I recommend the following guidelines to women on psychiatric drugs who want to get pregnant:

1. It is best to try to get off the drug before you try to conceive. The first step is to taper off the medication; most psychiatric drugs should never be stopped abruptly. Then stay off the medication for several weeks before trying to get pregnant to ensure that the body has completely eliminated the drug. During that time, use birth control measures.

2. Most psychiatric illnesses do not return immediately upon discontinuation of the drug, so there is a safety zone between your last pill and the time you get pregnant.

3. Although the most critical time for fetal development is the first trimester, and the brain is almost completely formed by the end of the second trimester, this does not mean that it is okay to take psychiatric drugs

late in pregnancy. In fact, babies born to mothers who take benzodiazepine antianxiety drugs like Xanax and Klonopin close to delivery may have babies that are sluggish from the effects of the drugs. Babies born to mothers who take antidepressants associated with withdrawal problems when discontinued, like Paxil and Effexor XR, will themselves have withdrawal problems.

4. If a serious psychiatric disturbance develops during pregnancy, psychotherapy should be considered first. For those conditions that have evidence-based psychotherapies, like cognitive behavioral therapy for any of the anxiety disorders and cognitive behavioral therapy or interpersonal psychotherapy for depression, it is best to employ them before considering medication. If these don't work, or the woman has a condition like mania or psychosis as part of schizophrenia, medication should be considered only if the problem is severe and the patient cannot wait until delivery for treatment. It is a lot to ask a person to live with mania, severe depression, panic attacks, or hallucinations and delusions for six months. Furthermore, some of these illnesses can themselves potentially be dangerous to a fetus. If a depressed woman cannot eat and loses weight, the fetus may be malnourished. If a psychotic woman abuses alcohol or cocaine or becomes paranoid and refuses routine medical care, the consequences can be serious for the newborn baby. Many women have taken antidepressants, antipsychotic drugs, and benzodiazepine antianxiety drugs during pregnancy and delivered normal babies. Originally, it was believed that use during pregnancy of the antianxiety drugs like Valium and Librium caused cleft lip or cleft palate in the infant, but this has recently been disputed. One would think that by now if any of these drugs did produce serious birth defects, we would know about it, although it is possible that subtle defects have been missed. The best advice is, if a psychiatric disturbance is so severe that the mother's and/or the fetus's life and health are jeopardized, it is reasonable to prescribe medication in small doses after the first trimester.

5. If psychiatric medication is prescribed, it should be one of the drugs that have been on the market for several years. In other words, avoid drugs that have only recently been released. There is no theoretical reason to think that these drugs would be more harmful to a fetus than other drugs in their classes, but it is certain that fewer pregnant women have used them and therefore there is a greater chance that they cause birth defects we do not yet know about. For example, Lamictal (lamotrigine), a medication used for patients with bipolar disorder (and for epilepsy as well), was first thought to be safe for pregnant women to take, but after only a few years on the market there were reports that it causes fetal malformations, just like the other anticonvulsant medications.

6. For bipolar patients, lithium appears to be safe for the fetus. As pregnancy progresses, the lithium blood level declines and an increase in lithium dose is usually required to maintain mood stabilization. Tegretol, Depakote, and Lamictal should not be given to pregnant women. Older antipsychotic medications, like Trilafon, are said to be safe during pregnancy. Although they have many side effect disadvantages compared to the newer "ayptical" antipsychotic drugs like Risperdal and Zyprexa, the latter have not been around long enough to know if they are really safe for pregnant women. Therefore, I recommend Trilafon if antipsychotic medication is needed for a woman with mania, schizophrenia, or psychotic depression during pregnancy.

7. As in the case of the antipsychotic drugs, older antidepressants may be the best choices if depression during pregnancy does not respond to psychotherapy. Nortriptyline is often selected in those cases. Despite the bad press it has received, electroconvulsive (shock) treatment is probably the safest way to treat depression in a pregnant woman. It causes seizure activity in the brain much like the activity that occurs during epileptic seizures, and we know that women with epilepsy have normal babies. Although it is usually hard to convince patients and their families of this, it may be true that shock treatment is safer than antidepressant medication for a depressed pregnant woman.

8. If anxiety disorder absolutely must be treated during pregnancy, benzodiazepine antianxiety drugs like Klonopin and Valium can be used, but low doses should be given and they should be tapered and discontinued if at all possible before delivery.

9. Drugs of abuse, like alcohol and heroin, are clearly bad for pregnant women and the fetus, so medications to treat these addictions are warranted if necessary. Unfortunately, we do not know if naltrexone or acamprosate (Campral) are safe during pregnancy, and most physicians will elect to stop them and hope that AA is sufficient to keep the pregnant woman from drinking. Methadone is usually continued for heroin addicts during pregnancy as a safer alternative to heroin.

The following case history may illustrate these recommendations best:
Joan had serious emotional disturbances as a teenager and young adult. At age seventeen she experienced her first serious depression and began psychotherapy. She went to college but took six years to graduate because of two more severe episodes of depression, one of which required hospitalization. After graduation, she had a manic episode and again required hospitalization. Unfortunately, she was not placed on lithium until she had two

more manic episodes and a depression that resulted in a serious suicide attempt.

When at age twenty-four Joan was finally placed on lithium, her life was in disarray. She had never held a job for any length of time, had lost many of her friends during her episodes of highs and lows, and never had a serious romantic relationship. Over the next ten years, because of her courage and intelligence, she went to graduate school, got a job, reestablished friendships, met a man, and got married. Now, at age thirty-four, she is happily married and successful. She also is stable on lithium with ten years of no mood swings. Understandably, she wants to get pregnant, but should she risk a severe depression or manic episode to have a child? Although her husband is very understanding and loves her, he has never seen her in the middle of a high or low. Joan wonders how it will affect her relationship with her husband if she becomes ill. Will she lose all the ground she has gained in her career over the last ten years if she needs a hospitalization once taken off lithium and appears unstable to her bosses?

It would be a tragedy for Joan to deny herself the opportunity of having a child in these circumstances. Naturally, no one can predict what will happen. It is possible that she will become depressed or manic once off lithium. Given the stigma attached to mental illness, it is also possible that her husband, friends, and coworkers will have a negative attitude toward her if she becomes psychiatrically ill. The alternative, however, is to voluntarily give up the chance of having a baby.

I would tell Joan and her husband that although there is no absolute guarantee that lithium won't harm her baby, the consensus is that it should be continued during pregnancy. I would coordinate her care with her obstetrician, looking carefully for any sign of new side effects from lithium, getting ultrasound examinations at appropriate intervals, and checking the lithium level at least monthly and adjusting the dose of lithium according to the blood test results. If Joan developed depression during her pregnancy, I would recommend a trial of cognitive behavioral therapy or interpersonal psychotherapy and try to avoid giving her antidepressant medication. Because of the high risk of postpartum depression in women with bipolar disorder, once the baby is born I would give Joan two options: (1) start antidepressant medication immediately because this has been shown in one study to prevent postpartum depression and does not appear to affect the newborn or (2) watch carefully for any signs of depression and treat immediately if they occur with antidepressant medication. With Joan's permission, I would alert both her obstetrician (whom she will see at least once after delivering the baby) and her child's pediatrician (whom she will probably see many times in the year following delivery) of her psychiatric history and the need to watch for signs of depression.

There are many situations, psychiatric and otherwise, when couples are well advised to forgo having children. But, whenever possible, we should not further stigmatize psychiatric patients by making this an absolute rule for everyone who needs psychiatric medication. For many of us, having children is the best thing we can do to improve our mental health.

Chapter 19

AIDS: Dealing with Psychiatric Problems

Patients suffering from many different medical diseases can develop psychiatric problems. Sometimes, as I have stressed many times in this book, a hidden medical illness is actually the *cause* of a psychiatric symptom like depressed mood, panic attacks, or hallucinations.

All of this is true with respect to AIDS—acquired immune deficiency syndrome. AIDS is known to be caused by HIV (human immunodeficiency virus), which slowly destroys the infected patient's immunological system. Stripped of its natural defenses, the body becomes susceptible to a host of serious infections and tumors. Ten years ago, most people with HIV infection went on to develop AIDS and die. The situation is vastly different now. Modern antiviral medications, including drugs called protease inhibitors, have turned HIV infection from an inevitably fatal condition to a chronic one with which most people live for years. The cocktail of drugs that people with AIDS take is called "highly active antiretroviral therapy" or HAART. People still die from AIDS, particularly in our inner cities and in third world countries where good medical care is insufficiently available. Many AIDS patients develop a second infection with the hepatitis C virus. Although this too can be treated with a drug called alpha interferon, the combination of AIDS and hepatitis C has made liver disease a major cause of death for AIDS patients. Nevertheless, the prognosis is much, much better for AIDS patients today.

At the beginning of the AIDS epidemic, there was much talk about "high-risk groups"—specific groups of people who seemed most likely to be infected by HIV. We now know that anyone who engages in *high-risk behavior* can be infected with HIV. The most common behaviors are unprotected sex (without using a condom) and intravenous drug use. Although drugs like the protease inhibitors can prolong the life of someone with AIDS, the only way to avoid infection with HIV is to avoid unprotected sex and intravenous drug use.

Psychiatrists and their mental health professional colleagues have therefore become very involved in the AIDS epidemic because they are the experts in behavioral change. The National Institutes of Health is spending millions of dollars annually to fund research aimed at learning how to change behavior and stop the spread of HIV. Studies show that providing clean needles to drug addicts helps reduce the spread of AIDS, but for reasons I consider totally misguided many states refuse to legalize needle exchange programs.

It might seem logical that the person infected with HIV, knowing the high likelihood that he or she will develop AIDS, would become highly anxious or depressed. So far, studies are contradictory about whether AIDS patients have higher risks for psychiatric illness than the general population. The emotional reaction to learning that one is infected with HIV seems to follow a pattern: The person who thinks she or he may be infected usually feels very anxious undergoing the HIV blood test and awaiting the results. If the results are positive—the person is indeed infected—depression and suicidal thoughts can occur: "I'll kill myself before I get sick." "I'll never let myself suffer and die a slow, painful death." "I'd rather be dead than have anybody know I have AIDS."

As far as we can tell, however, these reactions are temporary. Within two weeks of hearing the test results, patients with HIV infection seem to begin making peace with themselves. They recognize that it may be years before any medical symptoms develop from the infection and that scientists throughout the world are working to find a cure. HIV-infected patients often develop hope and optimism at this point, channeling negative thoughts and energy into work, family, and various altruistic efforts. In fact, in my own research work with people infected with HIV, I have been consistently impressed with their fortitude, courage, and resilience.

During the period in which the HIV-infected patient remains medically asymptomatic, which thanks to HAART can last a lifetime, he or she may develop psychiatric symptoms at about the same rate as an uninfected person. The treatment of these patients, however, may not be the same.

Patients with HIV infection have an immune system that is precarious at best. Many drugs—prescribed and not prescribed—can affect the immune system. The last thing we want to do is give patients antidepressant or antianxiety drugs that might harm their immune system.

On the other hand, we do not wish to leave HIV-infected patients to suffer with anxiety disorder or depression. We want them to lead normal lives while awaiting the scientific breakthrough that will cure them. Fortunately, almost all medications used in psychiatry to treat HIV-positive patients have been shown not to have adverse effects on the immune system.

Of course, just as in noninffected individuals, whenever possible I think that a person with HIV infection who becomes depressed or develops anxiety disorder should be treated with brief nonpharmacological methods. Support groups, counseling, interpersonal psychotherapy, and cognitive behavioral therapy are all good choices. If these are going to work for the depressed or anxious patient, they should do so in a few weeks.

If medication is needed to treat depression or anxiety disorder, I recommend starting with low doses. Because the virus gets into the brain, HIV-positive patients are often more sensitive to antidepressant drug side effects. They are more prone, for example, to develop agitation and insomnia from SSRI and SNRI antidepressants like Celexa, Paxil, Zoloft, and Effexor XR than are uninfected depressed patients. This increased sensitivity is complicated by the fact that many HIV-positive patients continue to abuse substances, also making them more sensitive to antidepressant side effects. Many of the drugs that are part of HAART regimens cause weight gain and increases in cholesterol and triglyceride levels so that psychiatric drugs like Paxil, Remeron, Zyprexa, and Seroquel that cause weight gain themselves can be an added problem. Finally, there is the problem of poor adherence. Patients with HIV infection have to take a lot of different drugs for their illness and can become forgetful or resentful about taking them, just as anyone with any chronic disease can. It is very important to query HIV-positive patients about whether in fact they are taking their medications and, if they are not, to try to understand why not and to help them develop better adherence.

Psychoneuroimmunologists believe that treating depression and anxiety disorder may actually improve immune function. Some research, especially that led by Dr. Dwight Evans of the University of Pennsylvania, has shown that stress and depression may themselves harm the immune system; therefore, it might be expected that reversing these psychiatric conditions will lead to improvement. It is therefore very important to recommend that depression and anxiety disorder be treated in patients with HIV infection.

A complicating factor in treating HIV-positive patients with psychiatric drugs is that some of the drugs used in HAART regimens interact with drugs prescribed for depression, anxiety, and psychosis, potentially causing serious drug reactions. For this reason, some physicians are afraid to treat psychiatric illness in HIV-positive patients. This is unfortunate, because it is not difficult to learn about the potential drug interactions and to avoid them by

Table 36.

Some Recommended Psychiatric Drugs for Patients with HIV or AIDS

Depression
Patients who are medically asymptomatic—Celexa, Remeron, Effexor XR
Patients with serious medical symptoms—Ritalin or Provigil

Anxiety
Low doses of Xanax, Klonopin, or Ativan

Psychosis
Low doses of Risperdal, Geodon, or Trilafon

picking the right drugs. Many of my recommended psychiatric drug choices for HIV-positive patients are guided by avoiding drug-drug interactions with anti-HIV medications.

A complicating part of HIV infection is AIDS-related dementia. The patient's mental faculties are slowed, memory is reduced, and powers of reasoning are weakened. It is extremely important to stress that this is usually a late event in most patients, although more subtle signs of cognitive deficits may occur earlier in the illness. Sometimes, the stimulant medications like Ritalin (methylphenidate) or Provigil can be helpful in these situations. It is particulary important to get patients with any sign of cognitive problems to stop abusing alcohol and other drugs.

Because of problems like dementia, brain infections, and brain tumors that sometimes occur in patients with HIV infection, it is important to coordinate psychiatric care with primary care physicians and other specialists to be sure that a new psychiatric illness is not the effect of one of these problems.

As mentioned earlier, many patients with HIV infection are co-infected with hepatitis C virus. The treatment for hepatitis C is a combination of drugs called alpha interferon and ribavirin. Alpha interferon causes depression in about half of patients who take it. Fortunately, this depression can usually be treated successfully with antidepressant medication. In fact, a research team at Emory University led by Dr. Charles Nemeroff showed that antidepressants prevent depression in patients with melanoma who are also treated with alpha interferon.

We obviously want to treat the HIV-infected patient with psychiatric problems with medications that produce the smallest number of side effects. Here are some recommendations (see also Table 36).

DEPRESSION

Anticholinergic antidepressants such as Tofranil (imipramine), Elavil (amitriptyline), Sinequan (doxepin), and Pamelor (nortriptyline) should be avoided. A full list of these drugs is provided in Table 12 in Chapter 7. The new antidepressant Wellbutrin (bupropion) is usually avoided because it is sometimes too activating for HIV-positive patients. Good choices are Celexa (citalopram), Remeron (mirtazapine), and Effexor XR. All three are relatively devoid of interactions with other medications. Celexa and Remeron are both available as inexpensive generic medications. Remeron is particularly good if the patient suffers from nausea, insomnia, and weight loss.

To treat depression in HIV-positive patients who are very lethargic and who have cognitive problems, many clinicians now recommend psychostimulants such as Ritalin (methylphenidate) and Provigil (modafinil) and amphetamines (Dexedrine, Adderall XR). Surprisingly, these drugs produce few side effects, although weight loss may be a problem. The main problem with stimulants, as discussed in more detail in Chapter 7, is that except possibly for Provigil they are addicting and this can be a particular problem in the patient who also suffers from a drug addiction problem.

ANXIETY

A review of Chapter 8 might be useful at this point to understand the many different forms of anxiety disorder. For generalized anxiety symptoms, I recommend cognitive behavioral therapy first. If this doesn't work, the same antidpressants that are recommended for depression in the section above—except for stimulants, which usually make anxiety worse—are usually the next step. Low doses of the benzodiazepine drugs—Xanax (alprazolam), Ativan (lorazepam), and Klonopin (clonazepam)—are also useful but can cause sleepiness and worsen cognitive problems and are also sometimes abused by patients with a history of drug abuse. Some clinicians prefer to prescribe trazodone (Desyrel) for insomnia and Seroquel (quetiapine) for anxiety and agitation, both in low doses, for patients with HIV infection. To my mind, it is cruel to deny an anxious patient with HIV infection safe and effective treatment.

PSYCHOSIS

Psychotic symptoms like hallucinations and delusions (see Chapter 10) are fairly uncommon in patients with HIV infection or AIDS unless they had these problems before becoming infected or were destined to develop them anyway. They also can result from drug abuse and from brain infections or tumors. Such patients should be treated with antipsychotic medications. Zyprexa and Seroquel are effective but also are sedating and cause weight gain and therefore are problematic for many patients who are already gaining weight because of HAART drugs. Low-dose Risperdal or Trilafon (perphenazine) also work, although patients with HIV infection are particularly prone to the so-called extrapyramidal symptoms such as muscle stiffness (dystonia), Parkinsonism (tremor and rigidity), and restlessness (akathisia) that these drugs can cause.

It must be stressed that these are only recommendations. Individual circumstances vary widely. The best advice is to try nondrug treatment first, but never permit the HIV-infected patient to suffer with psychiatric symptoms when medication might help. Always remember the possibility of brain infection and observe the patient very carefully for drug-induced side effects.

Most important, the psychiatric treatment of an HIV-infected patient should be coordinated with the other doctors involved in his or her care. Psychiatric symptoms should never be passed off as the "expected" or "understandable" reaction to life-threatening illness. It is bad medicine to ignore the emotional suffering of patients with HIV infection or any other serious illness.

Chapter 20

Adult Attention-Deficit/ Hyperactivity Disorder

Much has been written in the lay press about attention-deficit/hyperactivity disorder (ADHD) in children. The number of prescriptions for medications used to treat ADHD has skyrocketed, resulting in an outcry, almost entirely from nonpsychiatrists, of inappropriate prescription. Some have claimed that the drug companies have nefariously created a market for a disorder that doesn't really exist in order to sell their drugs. Indeed, the market for drugs like Concerta and Ritalin (methylphenidate), Focalin (desmethylphenidate), amphetamine (Adderall XR and Vyvanse), Strattera (atomoxetine), and Provigil (modafinil) is extremely lucrative. Psychiatrists and pediatricians, on the other hand, know that ADHD is a very real illness that responds remarkably well to medication. A recent study sponsored by the National Institute of Mental Health showed that methylphenidate worked better than behavioral therapy for children with ADHD. These children, much more often boys than girls, are fidgety, emotional, cannot concentrate, and do worse in school than would be predicted from standardized intelligence tests. Medications can produce dramatic results in helping them, with surprisingly few side effects. The truth between the naysayers and promoters of ADHD as a diagnosis and medication as a treatment for it probably rests in the middle. I believe that ADHD is overdiagnosed to some extent—there are not nearly enough child psychiatrists in the United States to see all of the children with possible ADHD to make sure that the diagnosis is correct. Effective behavioral therapies likely will be developed eventually. It is a big mistake, however, to deny a child with properly diagnosed ADHD medication because without it his or her life will be one of misbehavior, academic frustration, and poor social interactions.

Sometimes, even without treatment, ADHD goes away on its own after several years. Many other times, however, it persists into adulthood and then the adult psychiatrist is presented with the issue of adult ADHD. Many of the drugs that work for children with ADHD also work for adults, and three of these drugs, Strattera (atomoxetine), Adderall XR (amphetamine), and Focalin (dexmethylphenidate), have been approved by the FDA for the treatment of adult ADHD. Adults with ADHD, besides having the same academic and social problems as children with ADHD, also seem to be more prone to smoke cigarettes and abuse alcohol and other drugs. On the other hand, many of the drugs prescribed for ADHD can themselves be abused. This has been a particular problem on college campuses with respect to Ritalin for many years and has recently also become a huge problem with the amphetamine preparation Adderall. Also, in addition to increasing heart rate and blood pressure, causing insomnia and weight loss, and sometimes causing psychotic symptoms, the stimulant medications used for ADHD (methylphenidate and amphetamines) may cause heart disease if taken for a long time. The latter problem led to a debate within the FDA, well covered by newspapers, about whether to issue a special warning to doctors. In the end, the FDA decided not to do this, but the risk remains.

Because many of the drugs used to treat ADHD in adults are also used to boost the effects of antidepressants, they are all covered in more detail in Chapter 7 on treating depression. Here, I will give my own "hierarchy"—that is, order in which I prescribe drugs—for treating ADHD.

1. **Psychotherapy.** Although there is as yet no psychotherapy for ADHD that has been accepted as having sufficient research evidence to be broadly recommended, nevertheless several are in experimental phases. For example, Dr. Mary Solanto of Mount Sinai School of Medicine in New York City has a grant from the National Institute of Mental Health to study a brief psychotherapeutic intervention that holds promise for ADHD in adults. So first see if there is such a program in your area.

2. **Bupropion 12-hour tablets (Wellbutrin SR).** Although I admit that the research evidence for bupropion working for adult ADHD is weak, it sometimes works and is safe for long-term use. As long as the patient does not have a history of seizures or bulimia, there is little risk from bupropion, it doesn't cause sexual side effects or weight gain, and it is not abused. It is also available in generic form, making it less expensive than the other drugs for ADHD.

3. **Strattera (atomoxetine).** Strattera has actions in the brain similar to the antidepressants Effexor XR and Cymbalta. It is not abused but can cause constipation, nausea, and dry mouth. Some patients also complain of sexual problems. However, there is a good research database for its use in adult ADHD.

4. **Provigil (modafinil).** Provigil is available for treating narcolepsy and conditions that cause excessive daytime sleepiness, like multiple sclerosis and shift work. A number of studies show that it works in ADHD, although the FDA is still debating whether to approve it for this use. Nevertheless, physicians are allowed to prescribe it for ADHD. It has relatively few adverse side effects other than insomnia if it is taken too close to bedtime. It does not cause sexual problems or weight loss and is said to be less likely to be abused than stimulants, although I am skeptical that it has no abuse potential. It should not be used by patients taking birth control pills, as it will render them less protective against pregnancy.

5. **Long-acting version of Ritalin (methylphenidate).** Ritalin is the original drug used to treat ADHD. It is now available in generic form, but its main drawback is its short length of action in the body (short half-life). This means it has to be taken several times a day and there are often periods in between doses when the patient feels especially sluggish. The longer-acting forms that can be taken once a day include Concerta, Metadate, Ritalin LA, and Focalin (which is a slight chemical variant of other forms of methylphenidate). These are more expensive than regular methylphenidate but have the advantage of once daily dosing. All of them can be abused and in adults can cause inomnia, agitation, weight loss, and anxiety. If dosed correctly, however, they are almost always effective for adult ADHD.

6. **Amphetamine (Adderall, Adderall XR, and Vyvanse).** Although Adderall is referred to as "mixed amphetamine" salts, it is still amphetamine, meaning that in adults it is easily abused and can cause insomnia, agitation, anxiety, and sometimes psychotic symptoms like seeing things or becoming paranoid. Adderall XR is the once-a-day version. Physicians like to prescribe it because it is almost always effective, but my reluctance stems mainly from side effects and the fact that abuse of Adderall is becoming a major problem, especially among young adults and college students. Vyvanse was just approved when this edition was nearly completed. It is a "pro-drug" for amphetamine and, therefore, will work only if it is swallowed. Drug abusers will not be able to snort it or inject it. It is hoped that this will limit abuse of Vyvanse.

Not all patients are willing to try one drug after another until they find one that works, so I always describe this hierarchy to them and give them choices. It is true that this list goes from least likely to work to most likely to work—with the exception of Strattera and Provigil, which are probably a toss-up—but I try to encourage patients at least to start at level three before going to a stimulant. The most important thing, however, is to make sure the diagnosis is correct. ADHD rarely begins in adulthood. Adults who claim they got it for the first time and never had any signs when younger are usually suffering from a different condition (like hypomania or mania), looking for an "edge" at school or work, or drug abusers.

Chapter 21

Generic Versus Brand: What's in a Name?

Despite the fact that millions of Americans take some form of medication every day, most haven't the slightest idea how all these drugs get on the market. Many of us simply take it on faith that the government makes sure that medication is safe and effective before doctors are allowed to prescribe it.

One of the biggest areas of confusion for doctors and patients alike is whether to take brand-name or generic drugs. Every drug usually has three names: (1) the formal chemical name useful almost exclusively to scientists; (2) the generic name, a shortened version of the chemical name; and (3) the brand name, the name given to the drug by the company that wants to market it.

As an example, let's take the antianxiety drug Xanax. The scientific name for Xanax is (8-Chloro-1-methyl-6-phenyl-4H-s-triazolo [4,3-α] [1,4] benzodiazepine)—not something that rapidly falls off the tongue! When the compound was first discovered and thought to be potentially useful, it was given the generic name alprazolam. A drug company then assigned the name Xanax. A drug can have many brand names if different companies obtain the right to market it, but it can have only one generic name and one chemical name.

For example, the antidepressant paroxetine, which is available as a generic drug, has two brand names, Paxil and Pexeva, but both are still paroxetine. Sometimes the same company will give a drug two different names if it wants to pursue different purposes for the drug. The generic drug bupropion is called Wellbutrin for depression and Zyban for cigarette smoking by the same company.

DEVELOPING A NEW DRUG

Once a person, usually working for a drug company, discovers a compound that he thinks may be useful in treating a medical condition, he (actually, usually the company he works for) usually applies for a patent to ensure exclusive rights over the compound. Relatively few drugs are discovered by scientists working in medical school laboratories or in their own basements.

A patent on a drug is good for twenty years, but usually many years pass before a new drug is ever prescribed to an actual patient. Once the patent is issued, the company must run the drug through exhaustive tests according to the regulations of the U.S. Food and Drug Administration. First, there must be tests on animals that indicate that the drug is not likely to cause serious harm to humans. If mice or rats develop cancer or liver failure from the new drug, it is probably the end of the road.

If nothing terrible happens to the animals, the drug company submits an application to the FDA for permission to test the drug in humans. There are three mandated phases of this testing. In phase 1, patients and normal volunteers are given the drug to establish its safety, the best doses, and its usefulness in specific medical problems. In phase 2, several hundred patients are entered into controlled trials of the drug. In a controlled trial, some patients receive the active drug under study and others are given an inactive placebo. Phase 2 testing must determine whether the drug works better than a placebo to treat the targeted condition. Placebo is rarely used anymore in tests of any drugs except psychiatric drugs because in most other diseases there are medications that are established to work. Therefore, the FDA mandates that a new drug must be at least as good as, if not better than, the existing drug. Patients with pneumonia don't get better if given a sugar pill (that is, a placebo), so a new antibiotic has to be tested against an established one. It would obviously be unethical to give someone with bacterial pneumonia a placebo. In psychiatry, however, patients do respond to placebo, probably because the extra attention given patients in research studies makes some people with depression or anxiety disorder get better without real medication. Thus, the FDA mandates that psychiatric drugs must be tested to be sure they are better than placebo. Finally, phase 3 usually involves thousands of patients in controlled trials and must result in data that prove the drug is safe and effective. In some of these studies a third "arm" is added, which is an established drug. For example, a drug being tested for schizophrenia might be compared to placebo and to an established antipsychotic drug such as risperidone. There is currently a lot of controversy about the use of placebo in research studies in psychiatry, and although the FDA insists on it before they will approve a drug for marketing, many medical school and hospital human research approval committees will not allow it. When all three phases are completed, the company submits a new drug application (NDA) to the FDA, which must include all of the results from the three phases. If a company decides not to go ahead with an NDA, it is not legally obligated to submit its data to the FDA. The recent public outcry that companies may be hiding data that show their drugs are unsafe has led to the creation of registries where these data are made publicly available.

It takes an average of almost three years between submission of an NDA and FDA approval to market a new drug. As many as two-thirds of the NDAs are returned to the drug company by the FDA with requests for more information or even more studies on patients.

During all of this time, the clock on the patent is ticking. When a drug is finally approved by the FDA, it gets five years of "exclusivity." This is similar to patent protection and prohibits a generic company from making a cheap version. The difference between patent protection and exclusivity is that a patent begins whenever the company gets one for a drug, often years before it is approved. Exclusivity begins immediately upon FDA approval. The twenty-year patent can therefore expire before exclusivity begins, during exclusivity, or after exclusivity depending on where in the process of development the patent was obtained. If a company tests its drug for children, it gets six extra months of exclusivity. If it gets a new indication for an already approved drug, it gets three years of exclusivity but only for that new indication.

Let us take the example of a drug that first gets appoval to treat depression. The drug has three years of patent protection left (seventeen years have gone by in the development phase since the company first obtained a patent) but gets a full five years of exclusivity upon approval. These are not added up; the company has five years until generic companies can kick in. However, before the five years are up, the company does some studies to see if the drug works for depression in children. Whether the result is positive or negative, simply by doing the studies the drug can get an extra six months of exclusivity. Therefore, at the end of five and half years for this drug, generic forms can start to appear. If, in the meantime, the company does studies with the same drug for patients with panic disorder and gets FDA approval for this indication, it gets three years during which time generic companies can make the drug and advertise it for depression but cannot advertise it for panic disorder. This is complicated, but it basically means that drug companies have many things to figure out in order to try and delay generic competition as long as possible. Companies spend millions of dollars getting through the regulatory process, so if they are lucky enough to get FDA approval for a new drug, they want to make a profit quickly before the patent or exclusivity runs out.

Until the patent or exclusivity does run out, only the drug company that received permission from the FDA can market the new drug.

For the first few years, then, most new drugs are marketed only under one brand name. At the time of this writing, for example, the antidepressant drug escitalopram is available only under the brand name Lexapro. If a doctor prescribes escitalopram to a patient, the patient is automatically given the Lexapro brand.

With the lack of competition and the need for drug companies to recover the expenses incurred in developing the drug, it is clear why companies charge a lot for their brand-name drugs. Doctors rarely have any idea how much the drugs they prescribe actually cost, so they are not much help in keeping the cost to the patient for medications at a minimum. For that reason I have indicated which drugs are available as generics, because these are almost always cheaper than brand-name drugs. Managed care companies often charge higher co-pays for brand-name drugs if a generic is available.

Once a patent or exclusivity for a drug expires, the situation changes dramatically. Now, any drug company that meets FDA standards can manufacture and market the drug. For example, because it was such a successful drug, it was inevitable that in 1993, when the patent for Xanax expired, drug companies were ready to manufacture and sell generic alprazolam. Profits to a drug company plummet once its brand-name drug loses patent or exclusivity protection. Prozac, for example, went from making billions of dollars to making almost nothing for its manufacturer within months of the introduction of generic fluoxetine.

At the end of a patent's life, therefore, the generic drug becomes available. Now there is competition among companies and the price of the drug usually, but not always, falls. The generic drug companies have an important advantage over the brand-name companies that makes it possible for them to charge less for the drug: The generic companies did not spend millions of dollars developing the drug and therefore do not have to recover those expenses.

ARE GENERICS AS GOOD?

So it is almost always the case that the generic drug is cheaper than the brand-name drug. But are generic drugs as good as brand-name drugs? The

FDA is adamant about answering this question with an emphatic yes, and I fully argree. There are, of course, dissenters.

The brand-name drug companies obviously want doctors and patients to believe that generic drugs are inferior. One of their main arguments is the FDA rule that says a generic drug can be anywhere from 20 percent less potent to 20 percent more potent than the same dose of the brand-name drug. If we take as the standard 100 mg of a brand-name drug, a 100-mg tablet of the generic drug must be equivalent in activity to between 80 and 120 mg of the brand-name drug.

In actual fact, say generic drug manufacturers and the FDA, generic drugs are much closer in strength to brand-name drugs. Furthermore, they insist, there are very few reported situations in which a patient has experienced trouble after switching from the brand-name drug to a generic medication. Because the FDA insists that generic drugs have exactly the same ingredients and are manufactured in exactly the same way as brand-name drugs, they are really the same thing.

Not so, say the brand-name drug manufacturers. They are quick to cite examples of patients well stabilized on a brand-name drug who became sick or developed new side effects when switched to a generic drug. They also claim that generic drugs are associated with more allergic reactions and do not taste as good as brand-name drugs. Scandals a number of years ago in the generic pharmaceutical industry involving submitting false data to the Food and Drug Administration are cited as evidence that generic drugs are not reliable.

Doctors usually start prescribing a medication when it is still patented and therefore get to know it by its brand name. They are visited regularly by representatives of drug companies, who encourage prescription of their company's brand-name drugs. Generic drug companies do not have the money for reps and do not spend money on advertisements in medical journals. So physicians usually become accustomed to writing prescriptions using brand names. In most states, however, unless the doctor has a very good reason for insisting on the brand-name drug, the generic is automatically given.

The brand-name drug companies also lobby doctors to prescribe their drugs by pointing out that they use part of their profits to pay scientists and equip laboratories so that new drugs can be discovered. At this point, the bulk of new drug development in the United States takes place at the brand-name drug companies; without them, there is no question that new drug development would virtually grind to a halt, and diseases for which cures might be found would remain untreated.

All of this explains why brand-name companies think your doctor should always prescribe a brand-name drug and why insurance companies, state governments, and generic drug companies would like your doctor to prescribe less expensive generic drugs. What is better for you?

I have two recommendations:

1. When your doctor writes a prescription, ask if there is any medical reason why you shouldn't take the generic instead of the brand-name drug. Many times, the doctor will acknowledge there is no good reason and write the generic name.

2. Do not be worried about switching from a brand-name drug to a generic in the middle of a treatment period. Do not be alarmed that the generic drug looks different from the brand-name drug; federal law mandates that the packaging and outer layer of generic drugs have to look different from brand-name drugs. Remember that on the inside, where it counts, generic and brand-name drugs are identical.

There is absolutely no reason why you should not take the price of treatment into consideration, and generic drugs, when they are available, are almost always cheaper. So by all means, ask your doctor if you can take the generic and make him or her provide a logical reason if you are told no. The reason may be correct, but it's your dollar that is at stake. Don't hesitate to shop around to different pharmacies and to go online to sites like drugstore.com to find out the relative prices of drugs.

Chapter 22

Can We Trust Drug Companies?

It is said that the American public ranks drug companies lower than tobacco companies and the news media in terms of trustworthiness. This is about as severe an indictment as an industry can get, and it is not getting better. In fact, recent headlines about our ability to be sure that drug companies are truthful with us are indeed disturbing. In particular, we fear that the pharmaceutical industry withholds negative safety data about its products, drives up the costs of drugs unnecessarily, and pays to influence physicians to prescribe their drugs.

I am not about to defend the pharmaceutical industry, but I would like to address these claims and what they mean to a person with psychiatric illness who is about to be prescribed a medication. How do you know that it is safe and that your doctor is picking it because it is the best drug for you and not because the company has repeatedly paid for lavish dinners or brainwashed him or her at so-called continuing medical education (CME) courses?

I will begin by describing some of the positive things you need to know about the pharmaceutical industry.

The pharmaceutical industry is the most heavily regulated industry in this country. There is nothing similar in intensity to the Food and Drug Administration for the automobile, insurance, home-building, or clothing industries. The FDA makes drug companies go through a rigorous process of testing before a drug is permitted to be prescribed and turns down many drugs, either because they are concerned about safety or do not think that effectiveness has been proved. The vast majority of drugs approved by the FDA have had good safety records. It is the few exceptions to this rule, like Redux and Vioxx, that make the headlines.

Pharmaceutical companies fund about 60 percent of postgraduate medical education (that is, for doctors who have already finished medical school). As managed care has proliferated and government spending on biomedical research and medical training dwindled, academic medical centers, including our teaching hospitals and medical schools, have no money to spend on teaching doctors so they stay current with medical advances. In some states and for most hospitals, doctors must earn a certain number of CME credits every year in order to maintain their licenses and privileges. These can be obtained by attending courses and lectures or reading articles in journals and then taking a test to be sure the information has been absorbed. The pharmaceutical industry pays for much of this either directly or by funneling the money through professional organizations, medical schools, or an ever-growing number of CME companies. Often, a course or lecture will be advertised as "supported by an unrestricted educational grant" from whatever drug company. This is supposed to mean that the drug company has had nothing to do with the content of the course and merely provided funds to pay for speakers' travel expenses and fees and other expenses. Many other businesses that profit from health care generally refuse to help fund postgraduate medical education, including generic drug manufacturers, managed care companies, and nursing homes. Without the brand-name pharmaceutical industry there would be a crisis in educating physicians in the United States. Paying for medical education is one reason drug companies charge so much for their products.

Drug companies are, with very few exceptions, our only source of new medications. The United States is the world leader in drug discovery, making the pharmaceutical industry one of the few for which we maintain an important international status. Drug companies attract some of the best scientific talent and spend billions of dollars attempting to develop better and safer ways to treat human disease. Most molecules discovered by drug company scientists that initially look promising never make it through all the stages of testing, either because they make an animal sick or prove to have side effects or lack effectiveness when tested in humans. It takes about ten years—sometimes more—to develop a new drug all the way from discovery in a test tube to final testing in people with the target disease and approval by the FDA. Each time the company goes through this process, it risks millions of dollars in the hope that one out of about a hundred times they will get something that works and will be approved. As explained in the previous chapter, companies often have only a few years to recoup money they have spent developing a drug before generic drug companies, which spend nothing on drug development, enter the picture. This kind of research is another reason for the high cost of drugs.

So at this point, we are heavily dependent on the pharmaceutical industry for medical education and new drug discovery and we are reliant on the FDA to ensure that what we take is both effective and safe. There are obviously problems in this system and here are some of them.

The FDA is, like many federal agencies, woefully underfunded and understaffed. FDA scientists and administrators in my opinion do heroic work trying to sort out what is safe and effective from what is not and push back on drug companies that try to pressure them to make hasty or incorrect decisions. But there is just not enough staff to spend the time needed to be entirely sure that what gets approved won't cause problems down the line.

The FDA is subject to the usual politics that plague all regulatory agencies. When a member of Congress has an ill relative for whom a new medication being tested might be useful, the FDA is accused of being too slow and legislation is introduced to speed up the process. When an adverse effect of an already approved drug crops up and makes the newspapers, Congress demands resignations and advocates legislation to tighten the process. While it is true that the FDA is not perfect, its track record in protecting us from ineffective or unsafe drugs is excellent. One way the FDA has responded to political pressure is by increasing the number of the dreaded "black box warnings" placed in the prescribing information or "label" of drugs. Every medication comes with prescribing information with exact language mandated by FDA that describes the drug's mechanism of action, indications, adverse side effects, interactions with other drugs, safety in pregnancy, dosing, and other important facts. This is known as the drug's label and is what appears about each drug in the popular *Physicians' Desk Reference.* When the FDA thinks that a drug does something especially dangerous but that the drug should still be allowed to be prescribed, it orders the company to place at the very beginning of the label a warning about the problem in bold black letters within a black box. Drug companies dread this because it makes doctors nervous about prescribing the drug and therefore hurts sales. Black box warnings are useful if there really is a problem with a drug about which physicians should pay particular attention. But many of us fear that public pressure from the media, interest groups, and legislators have made a skittish FDA overdo the black box warning application. Self-righteous public officials are unhelpful. If they were really concerned about making the FDA even more foolproof than it already is, they would give it a more realistic budget.

No matter how hard we try to put a firewall between drug companies and speakers at medical education events, there is no question that paying for them gives the company a stake, and therefore influence, in what gets taught to doctors. The pharmaceutical industry recently adopted a set of self-imposed rules that are supposed to end the lavish gifts, trips, and dinners that doctors used to receive as part of their medical "education." Still, they do pay for most CME courses, and even when the money is funneled through a supposedly un-biased agency, the money still talks. CME companies that are supposed to en-sure that there is a separation between the providers of funds and the providers of knowledge need pharmaceutical industry money to survive. Are they going to allow speakers to heavily criticize products of the company paying for the medical education course? Every year, the American Psychiatric Association (APA) tries harder and harder to ensure that its industry-sponsored courses at its annual meeting are unbiased, something called "fair balance." Money from the drug company goes to the APA, which then uses it to pay the speakers' honoraria and expenses. Monitors sit in on the courses and make sure that speakers include information about competing products. Speakers must elab-orately disclose all of their financial ties to drug companies. Yet despite all of these safeguards, the APA collects a hefty fee from the drug companies for each course and needs the money in order to afford the annual meeting. Com-panies pay to advertise their courses in journals and newsletters that psychia-trists receive. It is rare that speakers bash the drugs made by the sponsoring company. Psychotherapy is usually mentioned as an afterthought when dis-cussing the treatment of a particular illness. In addition to this kind of edu-cation, drug company representatives still call on doctors in their offices to pitch their products and still pay for pizza lunches for medical students and residents, who appreciate the free food. There is no question that the phar-maceutical industry influences which drugs are prescribed. Advertising their products is an even bigger factor in the cost of prescription medication than paying for medical education or developing new drugs.

Like it or not, drug companies are businesses that must show a profit in or-der to survive. They are not nonprofit or charitable organizations. They have stockholders who demand a return on their investment. In the capitalist society that we have chosen, a drug company that loses money goes out of business and people lose their jobs. I believe that the vast majority of people who work for drug companies, from reps to scientists to business executives, are honest peo-ple who want to help patients get better. Furthermore, if a new drug really is harmful, lawsuits can be very costly, so there is a clear incentive to avoid mak-ing mistakes and marketing unsafe products. Nevertheless, human nature dic-tates that there is a strong incentive on the part of every employee of a drug company to get drugs to market and then make them sell. We can see the problem in the recall of Vioxx, the nonsteroidal anti-inflammatory drug that was touted at first as very safe and effective and then, only years after being on the market, turned out to increase the risk for heart disease. It appears that data indicating this might be a problem existed before the drug was ever marketed.

How did the FDA miss that? Did the drug company that makes Vioxx deliberately hide those data? While I believe that "deliberately" is too harsh a word in cases like this, it is easy to see the strong (and as a shrink I would say at least partly unconscious) motivation to avoid making public very bad news about a very profitable drug. I recall a drug for depression that turned out not to work and therefore no application to market it was submitted to FDA. Unfortunately, the realization that it was ineffective did not come until millions of dollars had been spent in development. Many of the people who worked on that drug, most of whom could not have known that the drug was not going to make it, lost their jobs. When a new model of car is introduced and bombs out financially, we are used to seeing pople get fired. But it is disconcerting to realize that the same thing can happen at a drug company. It makes us wonder what incentives there are for pharmaceutical industry employees to go out of their way to point out shortcoming with their companys' products.

Benjamin Franklin invented the decision-making method of drawing a line down the center of a piece of paper and putting pros on one side and cons on the other. When we do this in evaluating the drug industry, my sense is that it is a draw. The FDA does great work, but no system works perfectly. Drug companies spend lots of money educating doctors and developing new drugs, but their motivation is not simply altruistic. When it comes to psychiatric drugs, the problems are even more complex and potentially explosive.

Recently, the FDA placed a black box warning on all antidepressants, informing us of the potential risk for suicidal thoughts among children given these drugs. Once again, this information came to light only years after these drugs were marketed and after millions of children had taken them. Since none of the studies were actually designed to test suicidal or antisuicidal effects of antidepressants, and given that there were no actual suicides among the thousands of children in the studies examined, some psychiatrists and scientists felt that the black box warning was excessive and premature. They also point to the fact that there has been no increase in the suicide rate among children since the introduction of antidepressants, that the risk for suicide among untreated depressed children is higher than the risk of suicidal thoughts among treated children, and that some studies suggest that since the introduction of the new antidepressants (the SSRIs and SNRIs) in the 1990s, the suicide rate has been dropping in the Western world. Others say that the drug companies hid the information that antidepressants can increase the risk of suicides and have contributed to newspaper articles that understandably strike fear in the hearts of doctors and patients alike. One of the interesting things leading up to this black box warning was an FDA hearing at which family members of children who had commited suicide while taking an antidepressant were invited to testify. Needless to say, bereaved parents were understandably angry and gave highly emotional speeches about the evils of antidepressant medication. Those presenting opposite opinions were roundly booed. The FDA responded with a black box warning. Although there has been no decrease in antidepressant prescriptions to children by child psychiatrists, pediatricians have markedly decreased their prescription rates.

All of this made me think back to my days as a budding pediatrician before I switched to psychiatry. When a child with cancer getting chemotherapy died, bereaved parents were sometimes angry and accused the medication of killing their child. Sometimes they may even have been correct—to treat an otherwise fatal cancer, powerful and potentially dangerous medication is needed that sometimes has a bad result. I wondered whether if the FDA decided to hold hearings on the use of chemotherapy for children with cancer, it would invite the parents of children who died to testify. My bet is that they would not be asked for their opinions. Although their anger is understandable, the FDA would undoubtedly decide that the evaluation of chemotherapy for the treatment of pediatric cancer is a complicated scientific issue and ask only scientists and oncologists to opine. But when it comes to psychiatry, everyone is considered an expert.

There is no easy answer to the question, "Can we trust the drug companies?" I think it is always reasonable to question your doctor about the reasons he or she has picked a particular drug for you to take. Ask about its safety record as well. Tell the doctor if you experience any adverse side effects. Look the drug up on the Internet to see if there is anything noteworthy about it. And, perhaps most important of all, urge your legislators to vote for more funds to the NIH so that scientists who are not drug company employees can participate more in drug discovery, to medical schools and teaching hospitals so that they stop relying so much on drug companies for medical education, and to the FDA so that it can improve its surveillance of new medications.

Chapter 23

How Psychiatric Drugs Work

It is not at all necessary to know how psychiatric drugs work in order to take them safely and benefit from them. Some people would just as soon be spared the biological details, and I advise them to skip this last chapter.

But the way the brain works is really one of the most fascinating aspects of science and also one of the great scientific frontiers ahead of us. It has billions of individual nerve cells. In fact, there are more nerve cells in one human brain than there are people who have ever lived on Earth. If we took the brain of a single person and stretched the cells out in a straight line, the line would go to the moon and back. We are now in the midst of a neuroscience revolution in which more top scientists and laboratories and more funds than ever before are directed at research to learn how the brain functions. Every week our journals, and sometimes our popular newspapers, magazines, and television news reports, are crammed with exciting new discoveries about the scientific basis for human behavior.

So if you have a lively scientific curiosity, you might want to read on. Furthermore, many patients find it helpful to know a little of the specifics of drug action to understand what the drugs are actually doing to them and what benefits and risks they can expect. It gives everything grounding in nuts-and-bolts facts.

Although the brain is indeed nearly impossibly complex to understand, no one has to be a scientist to understand the basics of brain function and the way psychiatric drugs work. To explain the important features, it is first necessary to describe a little bit about how the human brain looks and works.

A LITTLE ABOUT THE BRAIN

In the broadest sense, any drug that affects the brain can be called a psychiatric drug. Alcohol and marijuana were among the first such drugs discovered, both obviously having profound effects on the brain and emotions. A wide variety of medications prescribed for nonpsychiatric conditions similarly have effects on the brain, although physicians are often unaware of this. Such commonly prescribed drugs as propranolol, used in the treatment of high blood pressure and angina; cimetidine, used for ulcers; and prednisone, used to treat many different diseases involving the immune system, all can produce marked changes in mood and behavior.

The ability of a drug to have an effect on mood and behavior is dependent on its ability to move from the digestive tract into the blood and then into the brain. The first step is relatively easy and scientists have known for many years exactly how to prepare orally administered medications so that they eventually are absorbed into the bloodstream. The second step, crossing from blood into brain, is problematic. Brain scientists often talk about a drug's ability to cross the blood-brain barrier. Perhaps appropriately, out of self-protection, the human central nervous system has evolved in such a way that many substances are blocked from getting into the brain, as if a wall stands between blood vessels and brain tissue. In general, drugs that are very fat soluble (technically called lipophilic), not bound to protein, and electrically uncharged have the best chance of getting into the brain. Furthermore, often the concentrations of drug necessary to have an appreciable effect on the brain are much larger than those needed to affect another organ of the body. For example, in relatively low doses, the once commonly prescribed antidepressant drug imipramine (Tofranil) dries mucous membranes in the body, causing dry mouth; however, doses of the drug as much as ten times higher than the mouth-drying dose may be needed to get an antidepressant effect. This is probably because of the difficulty drugs have in getting into the brain. Making drugs that safely affect mental processes is clearly a difficult task.

Once in the brain, a drug faces the most intricate, complex, and mysterious organ of the body. Nothing in the universe comes close to the human brain in complexity. Sometimes, psychiatric researchers complain that whoever designed the brain did so just to frustrate their attempts to understand it. Like other parts of the body, the brain is a collection of cells, the most important of which for our purposes are the neurons. Neurons send out long filaments, or branches, called axons and dendrites, that entangle each other in an endlessly complex web of connections and interconnections. A dendrite from one neuron may communicate with an axon, dendrite, or cell body of another neuron. But at each point of communication, there is an empty space between the two neurons, called the synapse. Brain cells essentially communicate by sending electrical signals, sometimes called action potentials. When a signal reaches the end of one neuron—just before the synapse—it causes the cell to secrete a chemical messenger into the synapse. This chemical messenger, called a neurotransmitter, floats across the synapse and binds to a receptor on the surface of the cell on the other side, the postsynaptic neuron. The binding of the neurotransmitter to the receptor on the other cell initiates a chemical process in that cell that either excites it and makes it continue to transmit the electrical signal or inhibits it and stops further transmission of the electrical impulse. Whether the process is excitatory or inhibitory depends on a number of complicated factors, including the kind of neurotransmitter involved. Once the neurotransmitter has done its job, it either is degraded by enzymes or is reabsorbed into the cell that originally secreted it (the presynaptic neuron). The most important components of this system are the pre- and postsynaptic neurons, the synapse, the neurotransmitter, the receptor on the surface of the postsynaptic neuron, and the degrading enzymes (Figure 2).

This process may seem simple and you may wonder at this point why I marveled earlier at the complexity of the brain. But consider the following. There are at least one hundred billion synapses in the human brain. There are about thirty different known neurotransmitters, but at the rate new ones are being discovered, some speculate that there are probably hundreds. Many neurons make or respond to two or more neurotransmitters. Although psychiatric drugs have traditionally focused on four neurotransmitters— acetylcholine, dopamine, noradrenaline (also called norepinephrine), and serotonin—two others are actually more abundant, glutamate and GABA (gamma-aminobutyric acid). Drugs now under development typically target these two. There is even a receptor in the brain for marijuana (actually, at least two), called the cannabanoid receptor, and marijuanalike neurotransmitters that occur naturally in the brain. Because marijuana makes people hungry, a drug that blocks the cannabanoid receptor, called remonibant, is currently being developed to treat obesity. Finally, a host of cofactors, such as calcium and chloride ions, have an effect on the strength of neurotransmitter responses.

Scientists are also beginning to learn that many things can affect the sensitivity of the postsynaptic neuron's receptors for neurotransmitters. Starve these receptors of neurotransmitter for a while and they become supersensitive to the chemical's effect the next time. Or the postsynaptic neuron may actually produce new receptors. It is quickly becoming apparent that the process by which receptor binding of a neurotransmitter leads to excitation or inhibition of the neuron depends on a very complicated chain of chemical

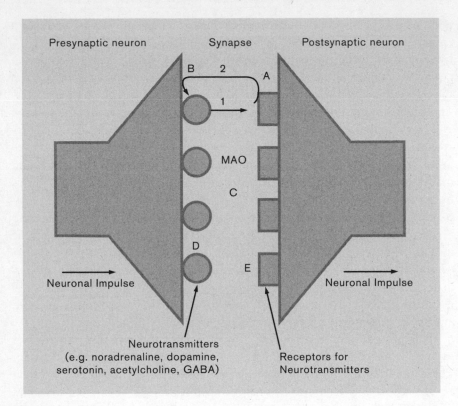

Figure 2.

reactions. In many cases, it involves chemicals called second messengers that work within the postsynaptic cell once it has bound the neurotransmitter on its surface. In fact, scientists now believe that we may understand only the tip of the iceberg about how neurotransmitters work. Once bound to its receptor, there is a cascade of events that must occur before a neurotransmitter has an effect. Ultimately, the process involves activating genes that may have been silent or at least slumbering. This results in increased production of proteins. The regulation of genes in the brain may be the ultimate way we develop psychiatric illness, the environment affects our behavior and personalities, and both psychotherapies and psychiatric medications work.

Most psychiatric drugs first exert their effects at the level of the synapse and therefore affect neurotransmitter binding to receptors in one way or another. For example, most of the drugs used to treat psychotic illnesses like schizophrenia attach to postsynaptic receptors that normally bind the neurotransmitter dopamine. By doing so, these antipsychotic drugs prevent dopamine from getting to the receptor and therefore stop nerve cell activity that depends on dopamine to maintain signal transmission.

The antidepressants, on the other hand, mainly block the reabsorption or reuptake of the neurotransmitters noradrenaline and serotonin into the presynaptic neuron after they have bound to the postsynaptic receptor. This prolongs the life of the neurotransmitter in the synapse and allows it to reattach to the receptor, thus increasing neurotransmission. The SSRI antidepressants (Prozac, Paxil, Zoloft, Celexa, Lexapro, and Luvox) potently block the reuptake of serotonin. The SNRIs Effexor XR and Cymbalta block the reuptake of both serotonin and noradrenaline. The antidepressant Remeron (mirtazapine) stimulates neurons to pump more serotonin and noradrenaline into the synapse. Antidepressant now under development are called "triple reuptake blockers" because they block reuptake of serotonin, noradrenaline, and dopamine. Other kinds of antidepressants, the monoamine oxidase inhibitors, reduce the amount of one of the degrading enzymes in the synapse, again increasing the life of the neurotransmitter in the synapse.

The benzodiazepine antianxiety drugs, for example, Xanax, Klonopin, and Valium, increase the activity of the inhibitory neurotransmitter GABA that is released by the presynaptic cell. This has the effect of reducing neuronal transmission and probably explains why these drugs, as well as the sleeping pills Ambien and Lunesta, reduce anxiety and make people sleepy.

Most drugs used in the treatment of Alzheimer's disease—donepezil (Aricept), rivastigmine (Exelon), and galantamine (Razadyne)—work by inhibiting an enzyme that breaks down the neurotransmitter acetylcholine, one of the first to be lost in this devastating disease. One new drug for Alzheimer's disease, memantine (Namenda), works by blocking the neurotransmitter glutamate. So does the mood stabilizer Lamictal (lamotrigine), used in treating bipolar disorder. In excess, glutamate has destructive effects on the brain, but if it is deficient it may cause cognitive problems. The latter effect explains why drugs to increase glutamate are being tested as a means of improving cognition for patients with schizophrenia. On the other hand, memantine and other drugs that block glutamate, like riluzole, may someday be marketed as antianxiety and antidepressant drugs.

HOW THE DRUGS WORK

At first, scientists believed that psychiatric drugs exerted their effects mostly by increasing or decreasing the amount of neurotransmitter available in the synapse. By increasing the amount of serotonin available, for example, it was reasoned that cyclic antidepressants improved neural transmission and cured depression. For a variety of reasons, it now seems pretty clear that this explanation is too simple. Instead, researchers are now focusing more and more on the effects of psychiatric drugs on receptors for neurotransmitters and on the events that occur inside the neuron after a neurotransmitter is bound to a receptor. Exciting new findings suggest, for example, that lithium may exert its complex effects for patients with bipolar disorder by working on one of these second messenger systems.

Almost immediately after the introduction of medication into psychiatric practice, major scientific effort was expended to determine if the actions of these drugs on the brain could tell us anything at all about the cause of psychiatric disease. This may sound a little like the tail wagging the dog, and indeed that is an apt analogy. The usual procedure in medicine is first to find out what causes an illness and then develop a drug for it. For example, once it was known that some forms of pneumonia are caused by bacteria, scientists developed antibiotics to kill the bacteria and cure the pneumonia. In psychiatry, however, the procedure has—until very recently—been exactly the opposite. The first step has almost always been the accidental discovery of a drug, usually through the astute and persistent work of a careful observer. Next, some knowledge of what the drug does is gained, and finally an attempt is made to relate drug action to cause of disease.

To use the example of the antipsychotic drugs, these were discovered mostly by anesthesiologists who first used them to anesthetize surgical patients and observed their calming effect. Then they were shown to have a specific effect in relieving certain psychotic symptoms, like hallucinations and delusions, commonly seen in patients with schizophrenia. Next, the discovery was made that these drugs block the dopamine receptor. Could that mean that a part of schizophrenia is the direct result of an excess of dopamine? This also led to the reiterative process of developing one new drug after the next that blocked dopamine. Even the newer antipsychotic drugs, despite being called "atypical," block dopamine.

Similarly, could the cause of depression be related to an insufficiency of the neurotransmitters serotonin and noradrenaline? Or could anxiety be caused by too little GABA? The obvious solution seemed to be to keep on developing drugs that increase those neurotransmitters.

We do not yet have answers to these questions, although as mentioned earlier, it already seems certain that simple theories based on too much or too little neurotransmitter will not be adequate to explain such complex, common, and variable illnesses as depression, anxiety disorder, and schizophrenia. But psychopharmacology has certainly turned attention to the real possibility that many of these illnesses are caused at least in part by alterations in the way genes in the brain function. This has had three main effects on research and our understanding of psychiatric illness. First, it has given us new leads into how psychiatric illness is inherited. Several genes have already been discovered that increase the risk for anxiety disorders, depression, and schizophrenia, and more will be found in the near future. Second, it explains how stressful life events and other environmental factors affect the brain and interact with genes to cause psychiatric illness. Finally, it has provided a rational way to develop new medications (and new psychotherapies) for psychiatric illness. The capacity to make images of the brain and its activity using sophisticated technology like functional MRI, magnetic resonance spectroscopy (MRS), PET, and SPECT and the recent major breakthroughs in molecular genetics will certainly help us find out what is wrong in the brains and the genes of people with psychiatric illness. For now, we must be content with the knowledge that psychiatric drugs are often of great benefit and the promise that research will someday tell us why.

WHAT RESEARCH WILL TELL US

We are experiencing an exciting and productive time in brain science research. Almost every day scientific journals and mass media announce a significant new breakthrough in our understanding of how the mind works.

These new findings will undoubtedly have a great impact on the way patients with psychiatric illness are treated, but the effect will probably not be seen for at least another decade. Right now, scientists are using new technologies to figure out how the brain actually works.

One of the most significant advances in recent years is the capacity to image the living, intact brain. Scientists studying psychiatric disease have long been hampered by the inaccessibility of the brain. Other organs of the body can be seen quite well with ordinary X-rays or can be biopsied so that tissue can be studied directly. Blood tests reveal a great deal about the function of such organs as the kidneys, liver, and heart. There is, however, little chance to obtain pieces of brain tissue from a living person, and the previously described blood-brain barrier means that little information about brain chemicals can be learned through blood tests.

Recently, and in rapid progression, new methods of seeing the brain have been developed. The first of these, called computerized axial tomography, or CAT scanning, reveals brain structures in great detail, allowing examination of small structures of the brain without harming the patient. Next, an even more sophisticated way of looking at the fine details of brain structure was developed, this time using no radiation. Magnetic resonance imaging (MRI) depends on the creation of magnetic fields and gives highly refined pictures of the brain. A related technique, magnetic resonance spectroscopy (MRS), permits measurement of the concentration of a variety of brain chemicals, including some neurotransmitters. Perhaps most exciting of all are the techniques called functional MRI (fMRI), positron emission tomography (PET), and its close relative, single-photon emission computed tomography (SPECT). These methods not only reveal brain structure but also show the degree of activity in various parts of the brain and allow visualization of brain chemicals and their receptors. For the first time, scientists can label drugs and chemicals with tiny, safe amounts of radioactivity, inject them into a person's bloodstream, and see exactly where in the brain they go and to what they bind.

Imaging techniques are already being used to describe abnormalities in the brains of patients with various psychiatric diseases, including panic disorder, depression, obsessive-compulsive disorder, and schizophrenia. They have taught us something about the receptors for antipsychotic and benzodiazepine antianxiety medications. And they have shown us the patterns of tissue destruction in Alzheimer's dementia and AIDS.

Another very exciting area in psychiatric research involves the powerful new tools of molecular geneticists. It was only a little over fifty years ago that Watson and Crick first described the structure of the genetic molecule deoxyribonucleic acid (DNA) and began a scientific revolution. At that time, it was probably unthinkable to most people that psychiatric disease would ever be found to have a genetic basis that could be linked to abnormalities on human chromosomes. Yet at least six neuropsychiatric disorders have now been linked to abnormal genes: schizophrenia, depression, attention-deficit/hyperactivity disorder, Huntington's disease, Alzheimer's disease, and bipolar disorder. Once discovered, knowledge about abnormal genes can lead to a complete understanding of the cause of an illness and ultimately to its cure. It has also helped us understand more about the ways environmental factors and inherited changes in genes cause brain disorders.

Molecular genetics and brain-imaging techniques are two dramatic examples of powerful research technologies being applied to the study of psychiatric illness. But other new approaches to psychiatric research, although not always so dramatic, also promise to provide important information that will change our treatment strategies. I have stressed the differences of opinion that have traditionally existed in psychiatry between pharmacologically and psychotherapeutically oriented practitioners. More recently, scientists have developed methods for studying psychotherapies under rigorous, controlled conditions. They can compare drug therapies directly to psychotherapies for specific conditions. This has already been done in large studies of depression, attention-deficit/hyperactivity disorder, post-traumatic stress disorder, social phobia, obsessive-compulsive disorder, and panic disorder.

The result is a more scientific understanding of the indications and limits of both kinds of treatment. We can expect that in the near future, doctors will have scientific information upon which to base treatment decisions, rather than relying on dogma or tradition.

NEW DRUGS ON THE HORIZON

It is hard to predict which new classes of drugs will turn out to be most important, but here are a few glimpses at the future.

For schizophrenia, many new drugs will focus on improving what scientists now believe to be the core symptoms of the illness, cognitive deficits. These drugs will increase the activity of neurotransmitters like glutamate and acetylcholine in the brain. Dr. Robert Friedman of the University of Colorado in Denver has already shown in pilot studies that a drug that stimulates one of the nicotine receptors in the brain, receptors that bind acetylcholine, improves the performance of patients with schizophrenia on neuropsychological tests. Other drugs may repair the coating on axons called myelin that is believed to be damaged in schizophrenia.

For depression and anxiety disorders, besides drugs that simultaneously increase the activity of three neurotransmitters believed to be involved in the illnesses, serotonin, noradrenaline (norephineprine), and dopamine, new drugs will try to increase the connectivity of brain cells and even stimulate the production of new brain cells. Extensive research has now shown that in animals, exposure to chronic stress causes neurons to retract their dendrites and lose connections with other neurons. Brain growth factors, called neurotropins, may be a future wave of antidepressant and antianxiety drugs. Also, drugs that reduce glutamate and increase GABA activity may hold promise in depression and anxiety disorders. As mentioned above, three drugs already available for other purposes that decrease glutamate activity have shown promise in preliminary studies. These are lamotrigine (Lamictal), used for bipolar disorder and epilepsy; riluzole, used to treat amyotrophic lateral sclerosis (ALS or Lou Gehrig's disease); and memantine (Namenda), used to treat Alzheimer's disease. A drug called indiplon that stimulates the GABA receptor is now being considered for approval by the FDA as a new sleeping pill.

Less activating and addictive drugs are in the pipeline for ADHD. Drugs that eat away amyloid plaques are being developed for Alzheimer's disease. Drugs that target gene changes caused by cocaine, heroin, and alcohol may someday be used to treat addictive disorders. For all of these disorders, the relationships between drugs and psychotherapies will be more intensively studied and will sometimes show that psychotherapy is better than drugs, sometimes that drugs are better than psychotherapy, and sometimes that a combination of the two is the best strategy of all.

Perhaps of greater importance, we now appear to be approaching an era in which psychiatric disease is less stigmatized, and scientists who study mental illness can receive support and funding—albeit dangerously decreasing—for their work. For the first time, private citizens, foundations, and special interest groups are focusing on the problems of the mentally ill and raising money for psychiatric research. Phil Satow of the JED Foundation, Jerilyn Ross and Alies Muskin of the Anxiety Disorders Association of America, and Steve and Connie Lieber and Dr. Herbert Pardes of NARSAD are but three examples of dedicated private philanthropies. Rather than blaming parents for causing mental illness, it is now understood that much psychiatric illness is the unavoidable result of abnormalities of brain function. Patients with the devastating diseases of schizophrenia or Alzheimer's dementia are now felt as worthy of our help and understanding as patients with multiple sclerosis or diabetes.

A Final Note

It is perfectly reasonable to expect that before much longer we will finally know what causes some psychiatric diseases and therefore have more specific remedies. In the meantime, we already have many treatments that are extremely effective and others that can at least help to reduce the suffering and social disturbance of psychiatric illness. In the preceding chapters, I have tried to be completely honest about the limitations of medications for emotional disturbances, even as I attempted to convey the great excitement shared by many psychiatrists about our ability to make a real difference in treating mental illness. It will always be impossible to describe every possible situation because in psychiatry, more than any other medical specialty, individual differences are of paramount importance. But the more the patient understands about psychiatric illness and treatment, the better he or she will be able to participate with the doctor in making good decisions.

If there is any overriding principle to this book, it is simply that the object of psychiatric treatment should always be to make the patient better. That may sound ridiculously obvious but in fact it will be challenged by many. Some feel the object of treatment is to make the patient understand more about himself or herself, to be better able to deal with complex emotions like anger and envy, or to follow societal rules and regulations better. I am not going to argue these points, because that would require another book. But I will bluntly assert that the object of psychiatric drug treatment has nothing to do with self-understanding or self-realization; it is a medical procedure intended to relieve symptoms and sometimes even cure disease. Thus, a patient can always ask himself or herself a simple question when evaluating the usefulness and success of a drug treatment: Do I feel significantly better now than before I started taking the medicine?

In historic Williamsburg, Virginia, stands the oldest continuously operating hospital in the United States dedicated to the care of patients with mental illness. The history of this Public Hospital serves as a metaphor for the changing attitudes toward mental health care in this country.

In the colonial period and through the early nineteenth century, the hospital resembled a prison. Rooms were tiny and had formidable bars on the windows. Patients, or inmates, as they were called, rarely left their rooms. There was no attempt at treatment. The patients were approached like criminals and kept in cells to protect society from their supposed irrational acts.

But through the years it was noticed that some of these "inmates" actually got better. Often, they were able to leave the hospital and return to their former lives. Some subsequently worked and raised families. By about 1830, attitudes had changed, and for the first time the patients in the Public Hospital were regarded as suffering from potentially treatable illness.

Doctors began to visit the patients regularly. Rooms were made larger, cleaner, and less prisonlike. The bars were replaced by fine wire mesh, which still kept patients from escaping but was less intimidating. Patients were let out of the rooms and every effort was made to rehabilitate them and return them to society as soon as possible. This was an era of great hope that with proper care and kindness, patients with mental illness could get better and leave the hospital.

This era too came to an end. Despite their best efforts, the physicians and other staff increasingly became discouraged by the number of patients who did not get better. As the hospital became a more humane place for the mentally ill, it also became a more popular place. The nation's population increased dramatically through the nineteenth century, and with that increase came larger numbers of chronically ill patients who could never leave the hospital. By the end of the nineteenth century, the Public Hospital again became a place dedicated mainly to chronic institutionalization rather than to treatment of patients with psychiatric disease. When the hospital burned down in the first half of the twentieth century, most of the optimism that mental illness was treatable had waned.

Clearly, we are now in a new age of hope. The reasons for the loss of optimism at the end of the nineteenth century are evident. Despite their best and noblest efforts, the doctors of that era had no idea what caused mental illness and no scientific basis for its treatment. Patients with time-limited illness like some forms of depression got better on their own; patients with chronic illnesses like schizophrenia remained ill. The ability to differentiate among different diseases was rudimentary.

Today we have sharpened our diagnostic skills and introduced powerful scientific methods to the study of the brain and its dysfunction. Scientific journals are replete with new and exciting findings that will lead the way to improved treatments. If the Public Hospital in Williamsburg were today a functioning hospital instead of a museum, it might look like any other general hospital, with doctors, nurses, social workers, X-ray machines, and laboratories. And it would be full of the belief that a combination of compassion and science will show us the way to relieving the pain and suffering of mental illness.

Glossary of Terms

ACETYLCHOLINE. A neurotransmitter in the brain that is destroyed in Alzheimer's disease.

ACUTE STRESS DISORDER (ASD). The symptoms seen during the first month after exposure to a life-treatening traumatic event. Sometimes leads into post-traumatic stress disorder.

AGRANULOCYTOSIS. A sudden decrease in a type of white blood cell needed to fight infection. This can occur in patients who take clozapine and is a medical emergency.

ANHEDONIA. Loss of interest in life, often experienced by depressed patients.

ANOREXIA. Loss of appetite.

ANOREXIA NERVOSA. An illness in which the patient has a fixed idea that she is fat and therefore must starve herself to lose weight. In addition to self-imposed starvation, patients with anorexia nervosa often abuse water pills (diuretics) and laxatives, induce vomiting, and become fanatical about exercise. The illness is potentially fatal.

ANTICHOLINERGIC. Generally refers to a set of side effects caused by many psychiatric drugs. The major anticholinergic side effects are dry mouth, constipation, difficulty urinating, and blurry vision. Many antidepressants and antipsychotic drugs cause anticholinergic side effects.

ATTENTION-DEFICIT/HYPERACTIVITY DISORDER (ADHD). An illness in children (usually boys) and adults characterized by short attention span, emotional lability, fidgeting, and difficulty with academic, social, and work performance.

ATYPICAL ANTIPSYCHOTICS. Drugs used to treat schizophrenia and bipolar disorder. They differ from older antipsychotics by being less potent dopamine blockers and more potent serotonin blockers. They have fewer neurological side effects than the older drugs.

ATYPICAL DEPRESSION. A form of depression in which the patient can usually be temporarily cheered up if something good happens. Often associated with overeating and oversleeping. Generally responds best to the newer antidepressants.

BENZODIAZEPINES. Medications used in the treatment of anxiety and insomnia that bind to the benzodiazepine receptor in the brain and increase the action of the neurotransmitter GABA. Examples are Xanax, Klonopin, Valium, and Ativan. Related drugs used to treat insomnia that are not chemically benzodiazepines but bind to the benzodiazepine receptor include Ambien, Lunesta, and Sonata.

BIPOLAR DISORDER. Illness in which the patient alternates between states of depression and states of hypomania or mania. A patient with four or more depressions and/or manic episodes in a year is said to have rapid cycling bipolar illness. Formerly called manic-depressive illness.

BLOOD-BRAIN BARRIER. A wall-like separation between the brain and the bloodstream that carefully modulates what substances, including drugs, cross into the brain.

BULIMIA. An illness characterized by episodic binge eating, sometimes followed by self-induced vomiting.

CANNABINOID RECEPTOR. A receptor in the brain that binds naturally occurring substances called cannabinoids and also marijuana. Blocking it may be a treatment for obesity.

COGNITIVE SYMPTOMS. Problems with memory, attention, and speed of mental processes that are always seen in dementia (like Alzheimer's disease) and in subtler forms may be the core problems of schizophrenia.

CYCLIC ANTIDEPRESSANTS. The class of antidepressants that includes Anafranil, Tofranil, Norpramin, Aventyl, Pamelor, Pertofrane, Elavil, Sinequan, Vivactil, Surmontil, and Ludiomil. They are used mainly to treat major depression. They are infrequently prescribed today.

DELUSION. A false belief that no amount of reality, facts, or hard evidence will shake. This is a psychotic symptom.

DOPAMINE. A chemical neurotransmitter in the brain. Most of the antipsychotic drugs block the binding of dopamine to its receptors.

DYSTHYMIA. Chronic low-grade depression.

ELECTROCONVULSIVE THERAPY (ECT). A treatment for major depression in which the patient is given a small current of electric shock, inducing a seizure. It is called bilateral ECT if electrodes for the shock are placed on both temples of the head and unilateral ECT if the electrodes are placed on only one temple.

EUTHYMIC. Normal mood.

EXTRAPYRAMIDAL SYMPTOMS (EPS). Neurological symptoms caused by antipsychotic medications that include muscle spasms (dystonia), Parkinsonian symptoms (tremor, mucles rigidity), restlessness (akathisia), and decreased movement and facial expression (akinesia). All of the old antipsychotic drugs (e.g., Haldol, Stelazine, Thorazine, and Mellaril) can cause this; among the newer atypical antipsychotic drugs, EPS is much less common. It sometimes occurs with higher doses of Risperdal or Zyprexa, less often with Geodon and Abilify, almost never with Seroquel, and never with clozapine.

GAMMA-AMINOBUTYRIC ACID (GABA). A neurotransmitter that generally reduces brain activity. Benzodiazepine antianxiety drugs and many sleeping pills increase the effects of GABA in the brain.

GENERALIZED ANXIETY DISORDER (GAD). An anxiety disorder in which the patient feels continuously anxious for no apparent reason for at least six months.

GLAUCOMA. A condition involving increased pressure in the eyes. There are two types, chronic wide-angle and acute narrow-angle glaucoma. Patients with acute narrow-angle glaucoma should not take psychiatric drugs with anticholinergic effects.

GLUTAMATE. A very abundant neurotransmitter in the brain that is critical for memory and other cognitive functions. Too much of it can kill brain cells, as happens during strokes. Too little may cause memory problems.

HALF-LIFE. A measure of how long a drug remains in the body after it is taken. Some drugs are broken down and eliminated very quickly by the body and therefore are said to have a short half-life. Some drugs remain in the body for days or even weeks after they are taken and therefore have a long half-life.

HALLUCINATION. Hearing, seeing, or feeling things that are not really there. A psychotic symptom. Auditory hallucinations are common to patients with schizophrenia. Visual hallucinations sometimes occur in patients with Alzheimer's disease or in people who take amphetamines or cocaine.

HIPPOCAMPUS. A region in the brain critical for memory and mood regulation. It is one of only two places in the adult brain known to be capable of making brand-new neurons.

HYPERTENSIVE CRISIS. A sudden and severe increase in blood pressure produced when a person on a monoamine oxidase inhibitor antidepressant eats or drinks something on the restricted list.

HYPNOTIC DRUGS. Sleeping pills.

HYPOMANIA. A relatively mild "high" that may come on spontaneously in patients with a form of bipolar disorder or may be produced by taking antidepressants. When hypomanic, the patient is unusually energetic and talkative, may be irritable, and is overly optimistic, often with bad judgment.

HYPOTHALAMUS. The part of the brain that controls many important vegetative functions, including appetite and sleep. Some abnormalities in the functioning of the hypothalamus may occur in psychiatric illness, especially depression.

HYPOTHYROIDISM. A condition in which the thyroid gland is underactive.

INSOMNIA. Inability to fall asleep (initial insomnia) or stay asleep (middle insomnia), or waking up too early in the morning (terminal insomnia or early-morning awakening).

LIBIDO. Sex drive.

MAGNETIC RESONANCE IMAGING. (MRI). A brain-imaging technique that creates detailed pictures of brain structures. Important variants are functional MRI (fMRI), which shows the activity of different parts of the brain during different types of mental activity; and magnetic resonance spectroscopy (MRS), which measures the concentration of various brain chemicals including some neurotransmitters. None of these use radiation.

MAJOR DEPRESSION. A form of depression in which the patient cannot be cheered up, even temporarily. Often associated with loss of appetite and concentration, as well as insomnia. Responds to antidepressants and electroconvulsive therapy.

MANIA. A serious psychiatric condition in which the patient is "high." This usually occurs as part of bipolar disorder but can be caused by drugs. The patient with mania is extremely energetic, hyperactive, and talkative. He or she has an increased sex drive and very little need for sleep, and becomes grandiose. In very severe forms, the patient talks so fast and the mind races so rapidly that nothing he or she says makes much sense. The patient may hear voices (auditory hallucinations) or develop delusions.

MONOAMINE OXIDASE. An enzyme in the brain that breaks down neurotransmitters.

MONOAMINE OXIDASE INHIBITORS (MAOIs). Antidepressant/antianxiety drugs that interfere with the brain enzyme monoamine oxidase. They are used to treat depression and anxiety disorders that do not respond to other medications.

MOOD STABILIZERS. Medications used in the treatment of bipolar disorder for long-term maintenance that prevent the occurrence both of new lows (periods of depression) and new highs (periods of mania or hypomania).

NEGATIVE SYMPTOMS. A cluster of symptoms observed in some patients with schizophrenia that includes loss of motivation, apathy, and loss of emotion. Although controversy exists, it is said that negative symptoms do not respond to traditional antipsychotic drugs as well as other symptoms of schizophrenia such as hallucinations and delusions. Negative symptoms appear to respond to the new atypical antipsychotic drugs.

NEUROLEPTIC. A term sometimes used for antipsychotic drugs.

NEUROLEPTIC MALIGNANT SYNDROME (NMS). A medical emergency sometimes caused by antipsychotic medications (more often with the older drugs), characterized by muscle rigidity, fever, disorientation, and abnormalities on laboratory tests. The medication must be stopped and the patient is usually hospitalized for treatment.

NEURON. A type of brain cell. The other three main types of brain cells are oligodendrocytes (which make the myelin coating for axons), astroglia cells (which nourish neurons and help form the blood-brain barrier), and microglial cells (which are part of the brain's immune system).

NEUROTRANSMITTER. A chemical in the brain that crosses the space (synapse) between one brain cell and the next to enable communication between cells. Examples of neurotransmitters are acetylcholine, glutamate, GABA, noradrenaline (also called norepinephrine), serotonin, and dopamine. Psychiatric drugs often affect the levels of neurotransmitters.

NIGHT TERRORS (PAVOR NOCTURNUS). A sleep disorder in which the person, usually a child, wakes from stage 4 (deep) sleep in a state of terror with rapid breathing and heart rate. By definition, night terrors do not involve nightmares and the patient never remembers dreaming.

NORADRENALINE. A neurotransmitter that may be involved in depression and anxiety disorders. Many antidepressant drugs affect the level of noradrenaline in the brain. Also called norepinephrine.

OBSESSIVE-COMPULSIVE DISORDER (OCD). An anxiety disorder in which the patient suffers from the need to complete seemingly meaningless rituals, like hand washing, over and over again, or must incessantly entertain meaningless and anxiety-provoking thoughts.

ORTHOSTATIC HYPOTENSION. A drop in blood pressure resulting in dizziness or faintness produced after suddenly sitting up or standing up. Many psychiatric drugs cause orthostatic hypotension. It can be a serious side effect in elderly patients.

PANIC DISORDER. An anxiety disorder characterized by sudden unexpected anxiety attacks that are recurrent. Patients with panic disorder also develop worries about having panic attacks, called anticipatory anxiety, and may avoid situations in which they fear they will not be able to get help quickly in case of a panic attack, a situation called agoraphobia.

PARANOIA. A feeling or state in which someone believes others are trying to harm him or her when this is absolutely untrue. Some patients with schizoprehnia suffer from paranoid delusions: They persistently believe there are plots against them, and nothing can convince them otherwise. It can also develop in patients with psychotic depression, the manic phase of bipolar disorder, Alzheimer's disease, and drug abuse. Uneasiness with or mistrust of other people is not the same as paranoia.

PLACEBO. An inactive sugar pill used in research to test the effectiveness of new drugs. In a drug trial involving a psychiatric medication, a new medication must be shown to work better than the placebo to prove it is truly effective and satisfy FDA requirements. The use of placebo is considered unethical by some and is not permitted by some medical schools and teaching hospitals.

POSITIVE SYMPTOMS. Psychotic symptoms of hallucinations, delusions, thought disorder, and disorganized behavior seen in patients with schizophrenia.

POSITRON EMISSION TOMOGRAPHY (PET) SCAN. A brain-imaging technique that allows visualization of the activity of different parts of the brain at rest and during mental activity and also allows visualization of receptors for neurotransmitters. It uses radiation.

POST-TRAUMATIC STRESS DISORDER (PTSD). The cluster of symptoms that begin at least one month after experiencing or witnessing a life-threatening event.

PSYCHOPHARMACOLOGY. The branch of medicine that specializes in medications to treat psychiatric illnesses. Practitioners are called psychopharmacologists and usually are medical doctors with special training in psychiatry and psychopharmacology. There is no official or special certification for psychopharmacology and therefore anyone can theoretically call himself or herself a psychopharmacologist.

PSYCHOSIS. A severe psychiatric abnormality often defined as involving a break with reality and comprising hallucinations, delusions, thought disorder, and markedly bizarre behavior. It can occur as part of many psychiatric illnesses or may be caused by some drugs.

RAPID CYCLING. A form of bipolar disorder in which the patient experiences four or more episodes per year of mania or depression. It is said to be less responsive than regular bipolar illness to lithium and more responsive to Depakote.

REM (RAPID EYE MOVEMENTS). The stage of sleep in which almost all dreaming occurs. During this stage the eyes dart rapidly back and forth.

SCHIZOAFFECTIVE. A diagnosis for patients who combine features of schizophrenia and abnormal mood, either depression or mania.

SEROTONIN. A neurotransmitter that may be involved in depression and anxiety disorders. Many antidepressant drugs affect the level of serotonin in the brain. Atypical antipsychotic drugs also affect serotonin receptors.

SEROTONIN NOREPINEPHRINE REUPTAKE INHIBITORS (SNRIs). Medications used to treat depression, anxiety disorders, and pain that affect both serotonin and norepinephrine. Examples are the cyclic antidepressants Tofranil, Elavil, and Anafranil, which are infrequently used to treat depression, and the newer drugs Effexor XR and Cymbalta.

SEROTONIN REUPTAKE INHIBITORS (SSRIs). A group of antidepressant/antianxiety drugs whose main action is to affect serotonin. The group includes Prozac, Luvox, Paxil (also called Pexeva), Zoloft, Celexa, and Lexapro. They are also called SSRIs (selective serotonin reuptake inhibitors) because their *only* action is to affect serotonin.

SIDE EFFECTS. Unwanted physical and emotional changes caused by drugs that have nothing to do with their ability to treat an illness. Also called adverse effects.

SOCIAL PHOBIA. An anxiety disorder in which the patient has anxiety symptoms only in social situations, such as giving a presentation in front of a group, talking to people at a party, and answering a question in class. If many such situations are involved, the condition is called generalized social phobia. Also called social anxiety disorder.

SPECIFIC PHOBIA. An anxiety disorder in which a patient, for no good reason, fears and avoids specific objects to the point that it interferes with his or her ability to function normally. Examples are phobias of small animals, heights, and close spaces.

SYNAPSE. In the brain, the space between nerve cells. Neurotransmitters go across the synapse to convey electrical information from one neuron to another.

TAPERING. The process of slowly decreasing the dose of medication over several days or weeks until the medication is completely discontinued. This is done to reduce or avoid withdrawal symptoms.

TARDIVE DYSKINESIA (TD). A serious side effect of the traditional antipsychotic medications (and possibly the antidepressant Asendin) characterized by abnormal and involuntary movements. It usually does not occur until the patient has taken the drug many months and usually years, but elderly people can develop it more quickly. It usually goes away if the medication is stopped immediately, but not always. The Abnormal Involuntary Movements Scale (AIMS) is a physical examination that picks up early signs of tardive dyskinesia. The first symptoms usually involve movements of the face, mouth, and tongue. It is much less likely to occur with the newer "atypical" antipsychotic drugs and never occurs with clozapine, which is a treatment for tardive dyskinesia.

TEMPORAL LOBE EPILEPSY. A form of epilepsy involving the temporal lobe of the brain. During seizures the patient engages in some usually purposeless activity like banging on things, twirling around, or stomping his or her foot. As with all seizures, the behavior is involuntary. Anticonvulsant medication is given to control this. Also called psychomotor epilepsy and partial complex seizure disorder.

WITHDRAWAL SYMPTOMS. New symptoms that arise because a drug is discontinued. These almost always go away within two weeks of drug discontinuation. Tapering a drug rather than abruptly discontinuing it reduces and sometimes even eliminates withdrawal symptoms. Withdrawal symptoms are sometimes a reason that patients are reluctant to stop drugs like the benzodiazepine antianxiety drugs (e.g., Xanax, Klonopin). It occurs with many antidepressants (e.g., Zoloft, Celexa, Effexor XR, Paxil, and Cymbalta) and is a cause of drug abuse (alcohol, cocaine, opiates, cigarettes).

Suggestions for Further Reading

Agras, W. Stewart. *Panic: Facing Fears, Phobias, and Anxiety.* San Francisco: W. H. Freeman, 1985.

Amada, Gerald. *A Guide to Psychotherapy.* New York: Ballantine, 1983.

Amador, Xavier. *I Am Not Sick, I Don't Need Help! How to Help Someone with Mental Illness Accept Treatment,* 2d ed. Peconic, NY: Vida Press, 2007.

————. *When Someone You Love Is Depressed.* New York: Free Press, 1996.

Andreasen, Nancy. *The Broken Brain: The Biological Revolution in Psychiatry.* New York: Harper, 1984.

Antony, Martin M., and Richard P. Swinson. *The Shyness and Social Anxiety Workbook: Proven Techniques for Overcoming Your Fears.* Oakland, CA: New Harbinger, 2000.

Barlow, David H., and Jerome A. Cerny. *Psychological Treatment of Panic.* New York: Guilford Press, 1988.

Barondes, Samuel H. *Molecules and Mental Illness.* New York: Scientific American Library, 1993.

Berger, Diane, and Lisa Berger. *We Heard the Angels of Madness: A Family Guide to Coping with Manic Depression.* New York: William Morrow, 1991.

Bruno, Frank J. *The Family Mental Health Encyclopedia.* New York: John Wiley, 1989.

Burns, David D. *Feeling Good: The New Mood Therapy.* New York: New American Library, 1981.

Campbell, Robert J. *Psychiatric Dictionary,* 6th ed. New York: Oxford University Press, 1989.

Carroll, David L. *When Your Loved One Has Alzheimer's: A Caregiver's Guide.* New York: Harper, 1989.

Castle, Lana R., and Peter C. Whybrow. *Bipolar Disorder Demystified: Mastering the Tightrope of Manic Depression.* New York: Marlowe & Co., 2003.

Charney, Dennis S., and Charles B. Nemeroff. *The Peace of Mind Prescription: An Authoritative Guide to Finding the Most Effective Treatment for Anxiety and Depression.* Boston: Houghton Mifflin, 2004.

Diagnostic and Statistical Manual of Mental Disorders, 4th ed., rev. *(DSMIV-TR).* Washington, DC: American Psychiatric Press, 1994.

Duke, Patty. *Call Me Anna.* New York: Bantam, 1987.

Ehret, Charles F., and Lynne Waller Scanlon. *Overcoming Jet Lag.* New York: Berkley Books, 1983.

Falloon, Ian R.H., Jeffrey L. Boyd, and Christine W. McGill. *Family Care of Schizophrenia.* New York: Guilford Press, 1984.

Fawcett, Jan, Bernard Golden, and Nancy Rosenfeld. *New Hope for People with Bipolar Disorder: Your Friendly, Authoritative Guide to the Latest in Traditional and Complementary Solutions.* New York: Three Rivers Press, 2007.

Fieve, Ronald. *Moodswings.* New York: Bantam, 1982.

Fisher, Richard B. *A Dictionary of Mental Health.* Chicago: Academy, 1983.

Foa, Edna B., and Reid Wilson. *Stop Obsessing! How to Overcome Your Obsessions and Compulsions,* rev. ed. New York: Bantam, 2001.

Golant, Mitch, and Susan K. Golant. *What to Do When Someone You Love Is Depressed: A Practical, Compassionate, and Helpful Guide,* 2d ed. New York: Holt, 2007.

Gold, Mark. *The Good News About Depression.* New York: Bantam, 1988.

Goodwin, Donald W. *Anxiety.* New York: Oxford University Press, 1986.

Gorman, Jack M. *The Essential Guide to Mental Health: The Most Comprehensive Guide to the New Psychiatry for Popular Family Use.* New York: St. Martin's Press, 1998.

Graedon, Joe. *The People's Pharmacy.* New York: St. Martin's Press, 1985.

Green, Michael Foster. *Schizophrenia Revealed: From Neurons to Social Interactions.* New York: W. W. Norton, 2001.

Greist, John H., and James W. Jefferson. *Depression and Its Treatment.* Washington, DC: American Psychiatric Press, 1984.

Greist, John H., James W. Jefferson, and Isaac Marks. *Anxiety and Its Treatment.* Washington, DC: American Psychiatric Press, 1986.

Hallowell, Edward M., and John J. Ratey. *Delivered from Distraction: Getting the Most Out of Life with Attention Deficit Disorder.* New York: Ballantine, 2005.

———. *Driven to Distraction: Recognizing and Coping with Attention Deficit Disorder from Childhood Through Adulthood.* New York: Simon & Schuster, 1995.

Heimberg, Richard G., Michael R. Liebowitz, Debra A. Hope, and Franklin R. Schneier. *Social Phobia: Diagnosis, Assessment, and Treatment.* New York: Guilford Press, 1995.

Hobson, J. Allan. *The Dreaming Brain.* New York: Basic Books, 1988.

Hofmann, Stefan G., and Patricia Marten DiBartolo. *From Social Anxiety to Social Phobia: Multiple Perspectives.* Boston: Allyn & Bacon, 2000.

Jamison, Kay Redfield. *Touched with Fire: Manic-Depressive Illness and the Artistic Temperament.* New York: Free Press, 1996.

————. *An Unquiet Mind.* New York: Knopf, 1995.

Kass, Frederic I., John M. Oldham, and Herbert Pardes, eds. *The Columbia University College of Physicians and Surgeons Complete Guide to Mental Health.* New York: Henry Holt, 1992.

Katcher, Brian S. *Prescription Drugs.* New York: Avon, 1988.

Keefe, Richard S. E., and Phillip D. Harvey. *Understanding Schizophrenia.* New York: Free Press, 1994.

Kernodle, William O. *Panic Disorder,* 2d ed. Richmond, VA: William Byrd Press, 1993.

Ketcham, Katherine, and William F. Asbury. *Beyond the Influence: Understanding and Defeating Alcoholism.* New York: Bantam, 2000.

Klein, Donald F., Rachel Gittelman, Frederic Quitkin, and Arthur Rifkin. *Diagnosis and Drug Treatment of Psychiatric Disorders: Adults and Children,* 2d ed. Baltimore: Williams and Wilkins, 1980.

Klein, Donald F., and Paul H. Wender. *Do You Have a Depressive Illness?* New York: New American Library, 1988.

————. *Mind, Mood, and Medicine.* New York: New American Library, 1982.

Kline, Nathan S. *From Sad to Glad.* New York: Ballantine, 1981.

Knauth, Percy. A *Season in Hell.* New York: Harper, 1975.

Kocsis, James H., and Daniel N. Klein, eds. *Diagnosis and Treatment of Chronic Depression.* New York: Guilford Press, 1995.

Kovel, Joel. *A Complete Guide to Therapy.* New York: Pantheon, 1976.

Kramer, Peter D. *Against Depression.* New York: Viking, 2005.

————. *Listening to Prozac.* New York: Penguin, 1995.

Liebowitz, Michael. *The Chemistry of Love.* Boston: Little, Brown, 1983.

Lithium and Manic Depression: A Guide. Madison, WI: Lithium Information Center, 1982.

Luria, S. E. *A Slot Machine, A Broken Test Tube.* New York: Harper, 1984.

Marks, Isaac M. *Living with Fear.* New York: McGraw-Hill, 1980.

Morrison, James R. *Your Brother's Keeper: A Guide for Families Confronting Psychiatric Illness.* Chicago: Nelson-Hall, 1981.

Nathan, Peter E., and Jack M. Gorman, eds. *A Guide to Treatments That Work,* 3rd ed. New York: Oxford University Press, 2007.

Nathan, Peter E., Jack M. Gorman, and Neil J. Salkind. *Treating Mental Disorders: A Guide to What Works.* New York: Oxford University Press, 1999.

Papolos, Demitri F., and Janice Papolos. *Overcoming Depression.* New York: Harper, 1987.

Piersall, Jim, and Al Hirshberg. *Fear Strikes Out: The Jim Piersall Story.* Boston: Little, Brown, 1955.

Rapee, Ronald M. *Overcoming Shyness and Social Phobia: A Step-by-Step Guide.* Northvale, NJ: Jason Aronson, 1998.

Rapoport, Judith L. *The Boy Who Couldn't Stop Washing.* New York: Dutton, 1989.

Rosenthal, Norman E. *Winter Blues.* New York: Guilford Press, 1993.

Ross, Jerilyn. *Triumph Over Fear: A Book of Help and Hope for People with Anxiety, Panic Attacks, and Phobias.* New York: Bantam, 1994.

Rush, John. *Beating Depression.* New York: Facts on File, 1986.

Schou, Mogens. *Lithium Treatment of Manic Depressive Illness: A Practical Guide,* 5th ed. New York: Karger, 1993.

Sheehan, David. *The Anxiety Disease.* New York: Bantam, 1986.

Sheffield Anne. *How You Can Survive When They're Depressed: Living and Coping with Depression Fallout.* New York: Harmony, 1998.

Silverman, Harold M. *The Pill Book: Guide to Safe Drug Use.* New York: Bantam, 1989.

Solomon, Andrew. *The Noonday Demon: An Atlas of Depression.* New York: Scribner, 2001.

Steketee, Gail, and Teresa A. Pigott. *Obsessive Compulsive Disorder: The Latest Assessment and Treatment Strategies.* Kansas City, MO: Compact Clinicals, 2006.

Styron, William. *Darkness Visible: A Memoir of Madness.* New York: Vintage, 1992.

Torey, E. Fuller. *Surviving Schizophrenia: A Manual for Families, Consumers, and Providers,* 4th ed. New York: Harper, 2001.

Walsh, Maryellen. *Schizophrenia: Straight Talk for Families and Friends.* New York: William Morrow, 1985.

Wilson, R. Reid. *Don't Panic: Taking Control of Anxiety Attacks,* rev. ed. New York: Harper, 1996.

Index

Page numbers in boldface indicate extended discussion of a subject. A page number followed by ± indicates a table.